Risk and Resilience in Military and Veteran Families

Series Editor

Shelley MacDermid Wadsworth
Department of Human Development and Family Studies,
Military Family Research Institute,
Purdue University,
West Lafayette, IN, USA

More information about this series at http://www.springer.com/series/11919

Linda Hughes-Kirchubel
Shelley MacDermid Wadsworth
David S. Riggs

Editors

A Battle Plan for Supporting Military Families

Lessons for the Leaders of Tomorrow

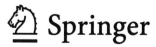 Springer

Editors
Linda Hughes-Kirchubel
Department of Human Development
and Family Studies
Military Family Research Institute
College of Health and Human Sciences
Purdue University
West Lafayette, IN, USA

Shelley MacDermid Wadsworth
Department of Human Development
and Family Studies
Military Family Research Institute
College of Health and Human Sciences
Purdue University
West Lafayette, IN, USA

David S. Riggs
Department of Medical and Clinical
Psychology
Uniformed Services University
of the Health Sciences
Bethesda, MD, USA

Risk and Resilience in Military and Veteran Families
ISBN 978-3-319-68983-8 (hardcover)   ISBN 978-3-319-68984-5 (eBook)
ISBN 978-3-319-99377-5 (softcover)
https://doi.org/10.1007/978-3-319-68984-5

Library of Congress Control Number: 2017960217

Printed on acid-free paper

This Springer imprint is published by Springer Nature
The registered company is Springer International Publishing AG
The registered company address is: Gewerbestrasse 11, 6330 Cham, Switzerland

To all who serve

Acknowledgements

We are grateful for the work of all those who contributed to this volume, including the participants and speakers who attended the conference, who in turn were greatly supported by MFRI staff. We also wish to acknowledge the assistance of an excellent panel of reviewers, whose time and expertise elevated the work of the authors:

Nathan D. Ainspan, Ph.D. Researcher, Author, and Writer on Veterans Transitions and Research Psychologist with the Transition to Veterans Program Office, Department of Defense

Patricia Montes Barron, B.S.N., M.S., Director of Family Readiness, Association of the United States Army

Adrian Blow, Ph.D., Associate Professor and Program Director, Couple and Family Therapy Program, Department of Human Development and Family Studies

Aggie Byers, Director of Military Spouse Employment Programs, Office of the Secretary of Defense, Military Community and Family Support Services (Retired)

Elspeth Cameron Ritchie, M.D., M.P.H., Chief of Mental Health, Community Based Outpatient Clinics, Washington DC VA

René A. Campos, CDR, U.S. Navy (Ret.), M.B.A., Director of Government Relations for Veterans-Wounded, Ill and Injured Health Care, Military Officers Association of America

Mary Carstensen, M.H.A., Master of Science National Resource Strategy, Director, National Veterans Intermediary, Bob Woodruff Foundation

Kathy Cox, Senior Manager—Walmart Giving

Jason Dempsey, Ph.D., Senior Advisor for Military and Veterans, School of Professional Studies, Columbia University

David DiRamio, Ph.D., Professor, Educational FLT Department, Auburn University

MAJ Scott A. Edwards, Ph.D., Chief Psychologist, Office of the State Surgeon, Indiana National Guard

Christopher Ford, M.S., M.A., CEO, National Association of Veteran-Serving Organizations

Ellen Galinsky, M.S., President and Co-Founder, Families and Work Institute; Chief Science Officer and Executive Director, Mind in the Making, Bezos Family Foundation

Vivian W. Greentree, Ph.D., Senior Vice President, Head of Global Corporate Citizenship, First Data Corporation

Catharine Grimes, M.B.A., Director, Bristol-Myers Squibb Foundation

Margaret C. Harrell, Ph.D., Director of Programs and Partnerships, Bob Woodruff Foundation

Stacy Ann Hawkins, Ph.D., Behavioral Research Scientist, Research Facilitation Laboratory, Northrop Grumman

Stacie Hitt, Ph.D., Assistant Head of Outreach and Assessment, College of Nursing, Purdue University

Johnson, C. Michael, M.A. Chief of Staff, University of Houston

Robert Koffman, M.D., M.P.H., Captain, MC, USN (retired), Red Cross Volunteer (Psychiatry), National Intrepid Center of Excellence, WRNMMC, Bethesda, MD

Rachel Lipsey, M.A., Military Legislative Assistant, Office of Senator Joe Donnelly, United States Senate

Andrew S. London, Ph.D., Associate Dean and Professor of Sociology, Maxwell School of Citizenship and Public Affairs, Syracuse University

Mallory Lucier-Greer, Ph.D., Associate Professor, Department of Human Development and Family Studies, Auburn University

Valerie Maholmes, Ph.D., Chief, Pediatric Trauma and Critical Illness Branch, Eunice Kennedy Shriver National Institute of Child Health and Human Development, National Institutes of Health

Jay A. Mancini, Ph.D., Professor Emeritus of Human Development at Virginia Tech, and Adjunct Professor of Human Development and Family Science at the University of Georgia

Gail H. McGinn, former (retired) Deputy Under Secretary of Defense (Plans), Office of the Under Secretary of Defense for Personnel and Readiness, Department of Defense

Sebastian Negrusa, Ph.D., Econ, Associate Director, National Security and Emergency Preparedness Division, The Lewin Group

Joyce Wessel Raezer, M.A., Executive Director, National Military Family Association

Eve E. Reider, Ph.D., Health Scientist Administrator, National Center for Complementary and Integrative Health, National Institutes of Health

Kathy Roth-Douquet, CEO, Blue Star Families

Trooper Sanders, M.Sc., founder, WiseWhisper

Elisabeth M. Stafford, M.D., F.A.A.P., F.S.A.H.M., Colonel (Retired) U.S. Army Medical Corps

Colonel David W. Sutherland, U.S. Army (Ret.)

Jay Teachman, Ph.D., Professor of Sociology, Western Washington University

BG(Ret.) Marianne Watson, Masters of Science National Security Strategy—National Defense University, working for Center for America, a nonprofit organization

Raymond Weeks, B.A., Vice President of Development at US Military Endurance Sports

Rosemary Freitas Williams, former Deputy Assistant Secretary of Defense—Military Community and Family Policy; former Assistant Secretary—Public and Intergovernmental Affairs

Dorinda Williams, Ph.D., LCSW-C, Director of Military Family Projects, ZERO TO THREE

Doug Wilson, former Assistant Secretary of Defense for Public Affairs and Co-Founder, Vets' Community Connections

Contents

Contributors

William Baas Comcast Corporation, Philadelphia, PA, USA

Keisha M. Bailey Department of Human Development and Family Studies, Military Family Research Institute, College of Health and Human Sciences, Purdue University, West Lafayette, IN, USA

Leah Barber American Red Cross, Washington, DC, USA

Jillian Bourque Department of Defense, US Army, The Pentagon, Washington, DC, USA

Rory M. Brosius ScoutComms, Inc., Fredericksburg, VA, USA

William T. Cahill Georgetown University Law Center, Washington, DC, USA

Bob Cartwright Intelligent Compensation, LLC, Pflugerville, TX, USA

Carl A. Castro University of Southern California, Suzanne Dworak-Peck School of Social Work, Los Angeles, CA, USA

Nida Corry Abt Associates, Durham, NC, USA

Stephen J. Cozza Center for the Study of Traumatic Stress, Department of Psychiatry, Uniformed Services University of the Health Sciences, Bethesda, MD, USA

Sherrill A. Curtis Curtis Consulting Group, LLC, East Rutherford, NJ, USA

Ellen R. DeVoe School of Social Work, Boston University, Boston, MA, USA

Eric M. Flake Developmental Pediatrics, Madigan Army Medical Center, Tacoma, WA, USA

Christopher Forsythe Department of Defense, US Army, The Pentagon, Washington, DC, USA

Abigail H. Gewirtz Department of Family Social Science & Institute of Child Development, & Institute for Translational Research in Children's Mental Health, University of Minnesota, St Paul, MN, USA

Brian Gilman Department of Defense, US Marine Corps, The Pentagon, Washington, DC, USA

Lisa A. Gorman Michigan Public Health Institute, Okemos, MI, USA

Michael L. Gravens Military Child Education Coalition, Harker Heights, TX, USA

Vivian Greentree First Data, Washington, DC, USA

Linda Hughes-Kirchubel Department of Human Development and Family Studies, Military Family Research Institute, College of Health and Human Sciences, Purdue University, West Lafayette, IN, USA

Jennifer L. Hurwitz Research and Policy Department, Blue Star Families, Encinitas, CA, USA

Christian Johnson Department of Defense, US Army, The Pentagon, Washington, DC, USA

Elizabeth Cline Johnson University of Houston, Sugar Land, TX, USA

Robin Johnson Department of Defense, US Army, The Pentagon, Washington, DC, USA

Sean Jones Department of Defense, US Air Force, The Pentagon, Washington, DC, USA

Karen G. Jowers Sightline Media Group, Vienna, VA, USA

Michelle R. Kees Military Support Programs and Networks, Department of Psychiatry, University of Michigan, Ann Arbor, MI, USA

Mary M. Keller Military Child Education Coalition, Harker Heights, TX, USA

Patricia N. Kime Arlington , VA, USA

Meredith Kleykamp Department of Sociology, University of Maryland, College Park, MD, USA

Leanne K. Knobloch Department of Communication, University of Illinois, Urbana, IL, USA

Koby Langley American Red Cross, Washington, DC, USA

Michael Lawson Department of Defense, US Army, The Pentagon, Washington, DC, USA

Richard M. Lerner Institute for Applied Research in Youth Development, Tufts University, Medford, MA, USA

Patricia E. Lester Nathanson Family Resilience Center, University of California Los Angeles, Los Angeles, CA, USA

Mary Lowe Mayhugh J1 Programs, National Guard Bureau, Arlington, VA, USA

Lesley McBain National Association of College and University Business Officers (NACUBO), Washington, DC, USA

Joyce Wessel Raezer National Military Family Association, Alexandria, VA, USA

David S. Riggs Department of Medical and Clinical Psychology, Uniformed Services University of the Health Sciences, Bethesda, MD, USA

Morgan T. Sammons National Register of Health Services Psychologists, Washington, DC, USA

Jason Schmidt Department of Defense, US Air Force, The Pentagon, Washington, DC, USA

Cristin Orr Shiffer Research and Policy Department, Blue Star Families, Encinitas, CA, USA

Kathryn McMurtry Snead Military and Veterans Partnerships, American Association of State Colleges and Universities, Washington, DC, USA

Hisako Sonethavilay Research and Policy Department, Blue Star Families, Encinitas, CA, USA

Kathrine S. Sullivan University of Southern California, Suzanne Dworak-Peck School of Social Work, Los Angeles, CA, USA

Terri Tanielian RAND Corporation, Arlington, VA, USA

Barbara Thompson Manassas, VA, USA

Thomas E. Trail RAND Corporation, Arlington, VA, USA

Jason T. Vail American Bar Association, Chicago, IL, USA

Shelley MacDermid Wadsworth Department of Human Development and Family Studies, Military Family Research Institute, College of Health and Human Sciences, Purdue University, West Lafayette, IN, USA

Anthony A. Wickham J1 Programs, National Guard Bureau, Arlington, VA, USA

About the Authors

Will Baas is a vice president of talent at Comcast where he heads all talent acquisition and talent management functions for Comcast's Northeast Division, which includes 23,000 employees supporting 8.1 million customers across five regions. Will's prior Comcast leadership positions include heading university relations, executive search, and diversity recruiting. Previously he held HR leadership positions for the Vanguard Group. Will began his career as an officer in the U.S. Navy; he currently is serving as a U.S. Navy Reservist holding the rank of Captain with over 26 years of total active and reserve service in the field of cryptologic warfare. He holds an undergraduate degree from the University of Pennsylvania and a master's degree in human resources from George Washington University.

Keisha Bailey is pursuing a Ph.D. in Human Development and Family Studies from Purdue University examining the intricacies of parent-child relationship—specifically, how adult guardians and adolescents navigate changes to family responsibilities brought on by developmental milestones like school transitions and family-level stressors like parental military deployment. Through her work with the Military Family Research Institute and as a 2017 Policy Intern for the Center for Families, Keisha engages with a broad spectrum of individuals including research participants and legislators to promote rigorous evidence-based approaches to improving the lives of families through policy and programming.

Leah Barber is a Senior Associate with Policy and Program Development for the American Red Cross, Service to the Armed Forces (SAF) where she develops and creates organization-wide guidance, policy, and programming. Leah co-created and manages the SAF Integration into the Home Fire Campaign as well as Cutout Clara, a new Red Cross social media program. She previously served in various positions in Germany, Oklahoma, South Korea, and Colorado and as an AmeriCorps member, specializing in emergency and social services. During this time, she responded to two national disasters: wildfires in California and flooding in Indiana. Leah received her undergraduate degree from Randolph-Macon Woman's College in Lynchburg, Virginia, and her M.P.A. from Upper Iowa University.

Major Jillian R. Bourque served as a Joint Chiefs of Staff Intern in the Chairman's Office of Reintegration, Policy Initiatives and Plans. Major Bourque was commissioned into the Ordnance Corps from the U.S. Military Academy at West Point, New York, in 2007. She has served in conventional and special operations units providing logistics support to the warfighter, including command of a support maintenance company. Her operational experience includes a combat deployment to Iraq and Afghanistan in support of Operations Iraqi Freedom and Enduring Freedom. Major Bourque holds a B.S. from the U.S. Military Academy and an M.S. from Georgetown University.

Rory M. Brosius is a Vice President at ScoutComms where she provides advisement to a variety of military and veteran serving clients on communications, advocacy, and philanthropic strategy. Rory previously served as a White House policy adviser to Michelle Obama and Jill Biden where she was the Deputy Director of Joining Forces, an initiative to engage all sectors of society to support service members, veterans, and their families. Rory has also worked in various capacities for both the Marine Corps and the Army. A military spouse and a social worker, Rory holds a bachelor's degree from Clemson University and a Master of Social Work from the University of Southern California. She is the recipient of a Presidential Volunteer Service Award, the Army Achievement Medal for Civilian Service, and a Marine Corps Certificate of Commendation.

Bill Cahill has spent the last decade working as in-house counsel in the health care services industry. Prior to working in the private sector, Bill served over 10 years (1997–2007) with the U.S. Senate Committee on Veterans' Affairs, including time as Health Policy Counsel and Chief Counsel to the Committee. He advised the Chair and Members of the Committee on Presidential nominations, committee procedure, and legislation affecting the health care services and benefits provided to military veterans and their dependents. Bill resides in Severna Park, M.D., with his wife, Courtney, and two sons, Liam and Brennan.

Bob Cartwright (SPHR/SHRM-SCP) is President and CEO of Intelligent Compensation, LLC, a client centric compensation, performance, and HR management consulting firm located in the Greater Austin, Texas area. Bob has 30+ years' experience consulting with for-profit and not-for-profit organizations across the country. Bob speaks throughout the United States and is quoted as a business/compensation expert in various media outlets around the country. He has also authored and coauthored articles on business topics and veteran employment issues. His professional affiliations include State Council Member Texas SHRM; Board Officer/Treasurer Texas Association of Business and Chambers of Commerce; and National Volunteer Leader for SHRM on Veteran Employment and Military Family Integration issues.

Carl A. Castro is currently Associate Professor and Director of the Center for Innovation and Research on Veterans and Military Families in the School of Social

Work at the University of Southern California. He retired from the Army after serving for 33 years, where he obtained the rank of colonel. Dr. Castro received his Ph.D. from the University of Colorado in 1989. He began his military career as an infantryman in 1981 and has completed two tours in Iraq, as well as serving on peacekeeping missions to Saudi Arabia, Bosnia, and Kosovo. He is currently Chair of a NATO research group on Military Veteran Transitions, a Fulbright Scholar, and member of several Department of Defense advisory boards. He has authored over 200 scientific articles and reports on numerous military topics. His current research efforts focus on assessing the effects of combat and operations tempo (OPTEMPO) on soldier, family, and unit readiness, and evaluating the process of service members' transition from military to civilian life.

Nida Corry, Ph.D. is a licensed Clinical Psychologist and Senior Associate at Abt Associates. Her work has focused on the design and implementation of epidemiological research and evaluation of national policies. She is currently the Project Director of the Department of Defense Millennium Cohort Study Family Assessment Component and has published widely in trauma recovery and has recent articles in the *American Journal of Epidemiology*, *JAMA Psychiatry*, and *International Journal of Methods in Psychiatric Research*. Dr. Corry completed her Ph.D. in Clinical Psychology from Purdue University, her clinical internship at Duke University Medical Center, and a postdoctoral fellowship at the Johns Hopkins University School of Medicine.

Stephen J. Cozza, M.D. (COL, U.S. Army, Retired) is a graduate of the U.S. Military Academy at West Point and Professor of Psychiatry at the Uniformed Services University of the Health Sciences (USUHS). He serves as the Director, Child and Family Program, Center for the Study of Traumatic Stress, USUHS. Dr. Cozza is principal investigator on studies examining the characteristics of child neglect in military communities, the impact of parental combat injury on children and families, the effectiveness of a family-based intervention with combat injured families, as well as the impact of U.S. military service death on surviving family members.

Sherrill A. Curtis is an author, coach, speaker, trainer, business consultant, and recognized expert in, and advocate for, career transitioning veterans. She spearheaded national award winning, grant and survey programs including "Mission Career Success"; "Serving Women Who Served"; and "Recruiting Veterans with Disabilities: Perceptions in the Workplace" (Cornell/SHRM 2011). Sherrill's research and publications include "10 Steps to Becoming a Military-Ready Employer" (SHRM 2012). She co-founded and co-chairs the Annual Stand Down in Morristown. Her practice exclusively serves socially conscious, business and individual clients who offer products, services, and skills that improve the quality of life for others.

Ellen R. DeVoe is an Associate Professor and Director of the Ph.D. Program at the Boston University School of Social Work (BUSSW). Her scholarship has focused on sexual abuse, the impact of domestic and community violence on children and families, and intervention research. Dr. DeVoe's work has been supported by the National Institute of Mental Health, Centers for Disease Control, Robert Wood Johnson Foundation, and the Department of Defense. During the last decade, she has directed the Strong Families Strong Forces project designed to support military and veteran families who have served in the post-September 11th era.

Eric M. Flake, M.D. is the program director of the only Department of Defense (DoD) Developmental Behavioral Pediatrics Fellowship at Joint Base Lewis McChord, Tacoma, Washington, and the medical director of the only DoD Autism Center JBLM CARES. He attended the military medical school (USUHS) graduating in 2001. Dr. Flake is board certified both in Pediatrics and Developmental and Behavioral Pediatrics. Dr. Flake has published numerous articles and presentations regarding the psychosocial effects of deployment on children. Dr. Flake is an Associate Professor at the Uniform Services University and Clinical Assistant Professor at the University of Washington. He currently serves on the Executive Council for the Uniformed Services Section of the American Academy of Pediatrics (AAP) and member of the science advisory board for the Military Child Education Coalition.

Chris Forsythe served in the Office of the Chairman, Joint Chiefs of Staff as the Director-South/Community Integration for the Chairman's Office of Reintegration. He holds a B.A. from the University of North Carolina-Chapel Hill and four master's degrees. He commanded the 82nd Financial Management Company (82nd FMCo) at Ft. Bragg, which successfully deployed in support of OIF for over 14 months. Upon relinquishing command, Colonel Forsythe served as the G8/Resource Management Officer for the U.S. Army John F. Kennedy Special Warfare Center and School (Airborne). He then commanded the Columbia Recruiting Battalion and was responsible for the mission of recruiting qualified applicants to serve in both the Regular Army and Army Reserves.

Brian Gilman served as Director, National Organizations and Interagency Collaboration, Chairman's Office of Reintegration in the Office of the Chairman of the Joint Chiefs of Staff. A career intelligence and reconnaissance officer, he has served in Infantry and Reconnaissance units and has commanded at the platoon, company, and battalion levels. His operational experience includes deployments with Marine Expeditionary Units to the Western Pacific and Southwest Asia. His combat deployments include two tours in Iraq as well as two tours in Helmand Province, Afghanistan. Colonel Gilman holds a B.S. in Environmental Engineering from Montana Tech, an M.A. from the Naval War College, and Master of Strategic Studies from the U.S. Army War College.

Lisa A. Gorman is a Senior Research Scientist at the Michigan Public Health Institute (MPHI). Dr. Gorman works collaboratively with families, public health, universities, policy makers, and other community partners on innovative solutions to improve health outcomes and quality of life for families who face chronic health conditions. She has been PI or co-investigator on several studies involving National Guard service members and families including *Risk, Resiliency and Coping in National Guard Families* funded by the Office of the Assistant Secretary of Defense for Health Affairs. Prior to joining MPHI, she was a contractor for the Michigan National Guard Family Program office. She is also a licensed marriage and family therapist in private practice.

Michael L. Gravens retired from the U.S. Army in 2006 after 35 years of military service. He entered the business world as the senior business development director for a Central Texas information technology company that specializes in defense logistics technology with global contract responsibilities. He has had a long association with the Military Child Education Coalition (MCEC) and joined the team in 2011 as the Communications Director. In this role, he is responsible for the strategic communications of the organization in all arenas to include national, state, and local media, defense and federal agencies, as well as Coalition partnerships with other nonprofit organizations.

Vivian Greentree, Ph.D. is a Senior Vice President and Head of Global Corporate Citizenship at First Data Corporation, where she oversees the strategy and implementation of First Data's philanthropic, diversity and inclusion, social responsibility, responsible sourcing, and sustainability efforts. Before assuming this role, Vivian joined First Data as the Head of Military and Veteran Affairs in February 2014. In that role Vivian created First Data Salutes, a company-wide military engagement strategy to provide the military community with access to career opportunities and best-in-class education resources, while offering premier business solutions to veteran-owned businesses. In recognition of the program's successes under Vivian's leadership, in 2017 First Data was ranked #1 on *Military Times'* Best for Vets: Employers. Vivian is a veteran, having served in the Navy as a Supply Corps officer. She is married to a Naval Officer and they have two little boys, ages 10 and 13.

Linda Hughes-Kirchubel is the director of external relations at the Military Family Research Institute (MFRI) at Purdue University, where she creates strategies and tactics that advance MFRI's strategic mission. She previously worked as a journalist for newspapers in California and Indiana and won national recognition for her work. Hughes-Kirchubel is pursuing her Ph.D. at Purdue's Brian Lamb School of Communication and researches stigma, resilience, and disenfranchised grief in marginalized communities. A military family member, she is married to a retired U.S. Army lieutenant colonel with 28 years of service, and mother to an Air Force staff sergeant.

Jennifer L. Hurwitz is a Research and Policy Analyst at Blue Star Families. An Air Force spouse for the past 19 years, she has volunteered and worked in a variety of roles that help to support military families. Military spouse underemployment is an issue that she has experienced firsthand due to the ten military moves she, her husband, and daughter have made. After years of reinventing herself at each duty station—working as a speech-language pathologist, teacher, university professor, and researcher—she finally discovered Blue Star Families, an organization that fully understands these challenges. Jennifer has a master's degree in Communication Disorders and Sciences from Eastern Illinois University and a doctorate in Educational Leadership from the University of Nevada, Las Vegas.

Beth Johnson is the executive director of public relations and community partnerships for the University of Houston at Sugar Land. In this role, she serves to establish and strengthen relationships with community stakeholders, prospective donors, local officials, and the private sector. Prior to her time with UH, Johnson held positions in communications, public relations, and external affairs with the Military Family Research Institute at Purdue University, the Office of Development and Alumni Affairs at George Mason University, Salsa Labs, Inc., and the Marine Corps Marathon. Johnson is proud to come from a military family where her father served in the Coast Guard, her brother in the Army, and her husband in the Marine Corps.

Christian Johnson served as Regional Director-North in the Chairman's Office of Reintegration under the Office of the Chairman of the Joint Chiefs of Staff. He began his career as an Infantry Officer and transitioned to the Adjutant General Corps where he served in various headquarters-level human resource assignments to include family programs, veteran employment, and national recruitment marketing. His combat deployment experience was one tour in 2007 at Bagram Air Base, Afghanistan, as a liaison officer with the 82nd Airborne Division. Lieutenant Colonel Johnson holds a B.A. from Liberty University and a master's degree from the National Graduate School.

Robin Johnson served as the Regional Director-West for the Chairman's Office of Reintegration. In this capacity, she was responsible for coordinating community-based methodology to assist veterans and military families to effectively reintegrate into civilian communities. After enlisting in the Ohio National Guard, she earned her commission as a Quartermaster Officer through the Ohio State University ROTC in 1999. Her 16 years on active duty include combat deployments in support of Operations Enduring Freedom and Iraqi Freedom. Previously, she served as the Special Assistant to General Martin E. Dempsey, the 18th Chairman of the Joint Chiefs of Staff. She has an M.B.A. from Webster University.

Sean Jones served as Strategy Chief for the Chairman's Office of Reintegration, Joint Chiefs of Staff. He executed the Chairman's initiative for supporting the successful reintegration of veterans and their families. He led strategic planning, coordination, and collaboration with other agencies. His staff assignments include tours at Joint Task Force-Bravo, Air Combat Command, International Security Assistance Force Joint Command, the Air Staff, and the Joint Staff. He has deployed in support of Operations Allied Force, Southern Watch, and Enduring Freedom. He commanded the 6th Force Support Squadron, MacDill AFB, FL. He is a graduate of Wake Forest University, the Air Command and Staff College, and the School of Advanced Air and Space Studies.

Karen G. Jowers has covered family issues for *Military Times—Army Times, Navy Times, Air Force Times*, and *Marine Corps Times*—for 28 years. A senior reporter, her beat includes numerous quality of life topics and issues such as deployments; moves; personal finance; spouse employment; child care and education; housing; military stores; and morale, welfare, and recreation. Before *Military Times*, she reported for other newspapers covering a wide variety of military and civilian beats, in Virginia, Florida, Georgia, and Guam. She has received several awards in her career, including the National Military Family Association's award for support to military families. She has a bachelor's degree in English from Appalachian State University.

Michelle R. Kees is a Clinical Psychologist and Associate Professor at Military Support Programs and Networks (M-SPAN) in the Department of Psychiatry at the University of Michigan. Dr. Kees' expertise centers on risk and resilience in female veterans, military spouses, caregivers, and families; peer programs supporting access to services for veterans; and large-scale dissemination of evidence-based programs. She is the Principal Investigator for HomeFront Strong, a state-wide resiliency intervention for military and veteran spouses/partners, and also for PAVE (Peer Advisors for Veteran Education), a nationwide peer program for student veterans returning to college on the Post 9-11 GI Bill.

Mary M. Keller President and CEO of the Military Child Education Coalition (MCEC), was one of the founders of the organization in 1998, which was created in response to the educational needs of military-connected children and youth. As an area superintendent, school administrator, and K-12 as well as higher education professional for over 21 years, she was uniquely positioned to witness the challenges military families faced in times of transition due to moves, deployment, or separation. She earned her doctorate from Texas Tech University and holds several professional certifications, including superintendency, mid-management supervision, and teacher education as well as a mediation certification from the Texas Bar Association.

Patricia N. Kime is a journalist and author whose work has appeared in more than two dozen publications, including the *Washington Post, USA Today, Defense News, Military Times*, and *Kaiser Health News*. She has covered military and veterans health care since 2011, reporting on combat-related illness and injuries and Defense and Veterans Affairs health policy. As a military spouse, Kime volunteered with several military family support organizations and held key leadership positions within them. She holds a bachelor's degree in international relations from the University of Virginia.

Meredith Kleykamp is an associate professor of Sociology and the director of the Center for Research on Military Organization at the University of Maryland. She received a Ph.D. in sociology from Princeton University. Her research centers on the consequences of military service for later life outcomes and the transition from military service to civilian life. Her research has been funded by the National Science Foundation and the Army Research Institute and has been published in a variety of outlets including the *American Sociological Review*, *American Journal of Sociology*, *Social Problems*, *Social Science Research*, and others. She previously taught at the University of Kansas and U.S. Military Academy.

Leanne K. Knobloch is a professor in the Department of Communication at the University of Illinois. Her research addresses how people communicate during times of transition within close relationships, with a particular focus on how military families navigate the deployment cycle. Her scholarship has been honored by the Gerald R. Miller Award for Early Career Achievement from the International Association for Relationship Research, the Golden Anniversary Monograph Award from the National Communication Association, and the University Scholar Award from the University of Illinois. She is a member of the Science Advisory Board of the Military Child Education Coalition.

Koby Langley serves as a Senior Vice President at the American Red Cross, overseeing worldwide care and support services for our military and veteran families on more than 118 Military Installations, and 100 VA Hospitals and Clinics worldwide. He previously served as the Director of Wounded Warrior, Veteran and Military Family Engagement at the White House and as a member of the Department of Defense Senior Executive Service where he worked as Acting Deputy Assistant Secretary and Senior Advisor for the Office of Wounded Warrior Care and Transition Policy. Langley has also worked as a Special Assistant to the Secretary of the Department of Veteran Affairs. He is a two-tour combat veteran and Bronze Star recipient for meritorious service.

Michael Lawson served as a Special Assistant to the Chairman of the Joint Chiefs of Staff and Director, Chairman's Office of Reintegration. A career combat arms officer, he has served in field artillery units spanning the globe and has commanded at the company, battalion, and brigade levels. Colonel Lawson's operational experience includes numerous assignments to the Republic of Korea. His combat deployments include tours in support of Operations Desert Storm, Desert Shield, and Iraqi Freedom. Colonel Lawson holds a B.A. from Stockton State College, and M.S. degrees from George Washington University, and the School of Advanced Military Studies (SAMS), and Strategic Studies from the Advanced Strategic Leadership Studies Program at SAMS.

Richard M. Lerner is the Bergstrom Chair in Applied Developmental Science and the Director of the Institute for Applied Research in Youth Development at Tufts University. A 1971 Ph.D. in developmental psychology from the City University of

New York, Lerner has more than 700 scholarly publications, including more than 80 authored or edited books. He was the 2013 recipient of the American Psychological Associations (APA) Urie Bronfenbrenner Award for Lifetime Contribution to Developmental Psychology in the Service of Science and Society and the 2014 recipient of the APA Gold Medal for Life Achievement in the Application of Psychology.

Patricia E. Lester is the Nathanson Family Professor of Psychiatry, Director of the Division of Population Behavioral Health, Director of the Nathanson Family Resilience Center, and Co-Director of the UCLA CARES (Child Anxiety Resilience Education and Support) Center. A board certified child and adolescent psychiatrist, her research and clinical work have been dedicated to development, evaluation, and implementation of family-centered prevention and treatment for families facing impact of military deployments, traumatic events, and parental illness.

Mary Lowe Mayhugh served in the Army for nearly 37 years. She has worked closely with Senior Leaders in the Department of Defense, Veterans Administration, and the White House, leading studies and shaping policy to improve programs for Military Service members and their families. She has served in multiple countries, including Kosovo, Iraq, Kuwait, and Afghanistan. She holds an M.B.A. from Touro University of California and a Master's in Science from National Defense University. She currently works for MITRE Corporation as a Principal in the Center for Connected Government and resides in Washington, DC, with her husband Kevin.

Lesley McBain, Ph.D. is an Assistant Director, Research and Policy Analysis at the National Association of College and University Business Officers (NACUBO) in Washington, DC. She has previously worked in various research-, survey-, and policy-related roles at the U.S. Department of Education, the Cooperative Institutional Research Program (CIRP) within the Higher Education Research Institute at UCLA; the American Association of State Colleges and Universities (AASCU)/Servicemembers Opportunity Colleges (SOC); and the College Board. She earned a Ph.D. from UCLA, with a dissertation focusing on veterans education policy, the civil-military gap, and national higher education associations. She also holds an M.A. from UCLA and an M.S. from Drexel University.

Joyce Wessel Raezer became Executive Director of the National Military Family Association in 2007 after serving in Government Relations since 1995. She guides the Association's initiatives that serve the families of the seven Uniformed Services. Joyce has represented military families before Congress and government agencies. She serves on the Strategic Board for the DoD Millennium Cohort Program. In 2004, she authored a chapter on "Transforming Support to Military Families and Communities" in *Filling the Ranks: Transforming the U.S. Military Personnel System.* An Army spouse, Joyce earned a B.A. from Gettysburg College and an M.A. in History from the University of Virginia.

David S. Riggs, Ph.D. is Professor and Chair, Department of Medical and Clinical Psychology (MPS) at the Uniformed Services University of the Health Sciences. He also serves as the Executive Director of the Center for Deployment Psychology (CDP). At MPS, he leads a program to train psychology students to deliver outstanding patient care and contribute to clinically relevant science in psychology. At CDP, he oversees the development and delivery of training for behavioral health professionals, preparing them to care for warriors and their families. Dr. Riggs has held clinical research positions at the University of Pennsylvania and Boston Veterans Administration Medical Center. His work concentrates on trauma, violence, anxiety, and the impact of PTSD and other anxiety disorders on families.

Morgan T. Sammons, Ph.D. ABPP, is the Executive Officer of the National Register of Health Service Psychologists. He has a long history of leadership and advocacy in the profession, including many years' experience working with the National Register. He has served as Systemwide Dean of the California School of Professional Psychology and is a retired U.S. Navy Captain. Dr. Sammons is a diplomate of the American Board of Professional Psychology (Clinical) and a Fellow of the American Psychological Association. He contributes regularly to professional literature and presents widely on issues pertaining to clinical practice and the advancement of psychology.

Jason Schmidt served as the Deputy Director for the Chairman's Office of Reintegration on the Joint Chiefs of Staff, where he worked to ensure the successful reintegration of veterans and military families by facilitating inter-service and inter-agency coordination, fostering community solutions through effective public-private partnerships, and the furthering of civilian-military understanding. He has deployed in support of contingency operations in Southwest Asia and Iraq. His previous Pentagon assignments include duty at the Air Force Senior Executive Service Management Office. He is a graduated Air Force Fellow and served as Commander of the 51st Force Support Squadron at Osan Air Force Base, Republic of Korea.

Cristin Orr Shiffer is Senior Advisor for Policy and Survey at Blue Star Families, a nonpartisan, nonprofit military family organization with over 100,000 members. A subject matter expert on military spouse employment and the relationship between military families and national security, Ms. Shiffer leads Blue Star Families' annual Military Family Lifestyle Survey. Ms. Shiffer's graduate studies and subsequent research focus on the impact of military families on the organizational and institutional goals of the U.S. Department of Defense. Prior to joining Blue Star Families Ms. Shiffer held positions with a leading foreign policy research institute and as a Congressional staff member. She is married to an active duty Navy pilot.

Kathryn McMurtry Snead (Kathy) is Vice President for Military and Veterans Partnerships for the American Association of State Colleges and Universities (AASCU) and Director of Servicemembers Opportunity Colleges (SOC), a Department of Defense (DoD) funded contract managed by the Defense Activity for

Non-Traditional Education Support (DANTES) and sponsored by AASCU. Snead serves on the Secretary of Veterans Affair's Advisory Committee on Education where she has been appointed Committee Chair, 2014 through 2016. Snead joined the Nonprofit Leadership Alliance Advisory Board in 2016. Kathy earned a bachelor's degree from Wake Forest University, a master's degree from the University of Georgia, and her doctorate from Syracuse University.

Hisako Sonethavilay is the Research and Policy Manager at Blue Star Families (BSF) where she aides the Senior Advisor in advancing BSF's key legislative/policy work and research initiatives including the annual Military Family Lifestyle Survey. Hisako's interest in the field stems from her own experiences and challenges as a Marine Corps spouse and her background in family-focused community social work, research, and advocacy. Hisako holds a Master of Social Work degree from George Mason University and an active License in Social Work (LSW) from the state of Virginia. Hisako and her family are currently stationed at Camp Pendleton, CA.

Kathrine S. Sullivan is a Ph.D. candidate at the University of Southern California Suzanne Dworak-Peck School of Social Work. Kate has an M.S.W. from the University of North Carolina and a B.A. from Williams College. Kate's research interests include risk and resilience in military and veteran families and predictors of adverse and resilient outcomes among military- and veteran-connected youth. Her dissertation, funded by a Ruth L. Kirschstein National Research Service Award from the National Institute of Child Health and Human Development, focuses on health and mental health outcomes associated with profiles of risk and resilience among U.S. Army spouses and children.

Terri Tanielian, M.A. is a senior behavioral scientist at the RAND Corporation and leading national expert in military and veteran health policy. She led RAND's study Invisible Wounds of War: Psychological and Cognitive Injuries, Their Consequences, and Services to Assist Recovery as well as Hidden Heroes: America's Military Caregivers, and has conducted several needs assessments of issues facing veterans and their families. She led the Deployment Life Study, a study of military families across the deployment cycle, and a study examining community-based models for expanding mental health care for veterans and their families. Tanielian has an M.A. in psychology from the American University.

Barbara Thompson is the former director of the Office of Military Family Readiness Policy, where Ms. Thompson was responsible for programs and policies that promote military families' well-being, readiness, and quality of life. In this capacity, she had oversight for child development and youth programs, serving 700,000 children daily at more than 300 locations worldwide. Ms. Thompson had purview over military family readiness programs, including spouse well-being and career advancement, military family lifecycle and transition support, and community capacity building to support geographically dispersed military members and their families. She also had oversight of the Family Advocacy Program and Exceptional Family Member Program.

Thomas E. Trail, Ph.D. is an associate behavioral scientist at the RAND Corporation. His research focuses on interpersonal relationships, including between spouses, friends, and group members, with a particular focus on how stress affects relationship processes and health outcomes. Recent research includes investigating the relationship between risk and resilience factors among military couples, an evaluation of education programs for military spouses, the potential impact of integrating women into combat roles on unit cohesion, and investigating the health and well-being of unpaid military caregivers. He received his Ph.D. in social psychology from Princeton University and his M.S. in applied/experimental psychology from Virginia Tech.

Jason T. Vail is a Senior Attorney in the American Bar Association Division for Legal Services and serves as Chief Counsel to the Standing Committee on Legal Assistance for Military Personnel, working to enhance the scope and availability of civil legal services for military personnel and their families. Initiatives include creation of ABA Home Front, an online legal resource; ABA Military Pro Bono Project, a first-of-its-kind national pro bono program for active duty military; and ABA Veterans' Claims Assistance Network, a pro bono project assisting veterans with disability claims. Jason received his J.D. cum laude from Gonzaga University School of Law.

Shelley MacDermid Wadsworth, Ph.D., M.B.A. is a professor in Purdue University's Department of Human Development and Family Studies and directs both the Military Family Research Institute and Center for Families. Her research focuses on relationships between work conditions and family life, with a military family emphasis. MacDermid Wadsworth is a fellow of the National Council on Family Relations and a recipient of the Work Life Legacy Award. She served as the civilian co-chair of the Department of Defense Task Force on Mental Health, and on the Returning Veterans Committee of the Institute of Medicine and the Psychological Health External Advisory Committee to the Defense Health Board.

Anthony A. Wickham graduated from West Point and is completing a successful 30-year military career, including one tour to Iraq. He became the Chief of J1 Programs, where he has oversight of family, Yellow Ribbon reintegration, transition assistance, employment, and suicide prevention programs for the National Guard. He earned an M.B.A. from Boise State University and holds a Master of Strategic Studies degree from the U.S. Army War College. He is married and has three sons, the oldest of whom serves in the U.S. Navy.

Chapter 1
Introduction to a Battle Plan for Supporting Military Families

Linda Hughes-Kirchubel and Shelley MacDermid Wadsworth

Since September 11, 2001, all branches of our federal government, as well as state and local governments, corporations, advocacy groups, philanthropies, researchers, and many others have taken action to support military families during and following their service. Often, these efforts were mutually supportive, but sometimes they competed or conflicted with each other. While many efforts were successful, others failed to achieve their potential or were misdirected. A nation eager to support military and veteran families sometimes fell short, even with the noblest intentions and goals.

In an effort to address this, the Military Family Research Institute at Purdue University called together experts representing many sectors to present, discuss, and reflect in order to construct the contingency plan for families for the next big conflict. The goal was to define the messages and action items for future professionals about the steps they should take and the strategies they should use to determine their courses of action. The focus of the gathering was not on specific programs or policies that should be created or enacted, but rather the processes that should be used and the issues that would need to be considered when trying to make good choices. The event was called the Battle Plan for Supporting Families Symposium, and this book is the product of that symposium.

The 2-day symposium included presentations organized into four sessions: federal government; education, industries, and associations; states and communities; and knowledge generation and dissemination. Following each group of presentations, working groups discussed forward-focused questions prepared in advance. Working group leaders recorded notes, and moderators led brief report-out sessions. Following each session, table notes were posted for all participants to review and

L. Hughes-Kirchubel, M.A (✉) • S.M. Wadsworth, M.B.A., Ph.D.
Department of Human Development and Family Studies, Military Family Research Institute, College of Health and Human Sciences, Purdue University, West Lafayette, IN, USA
e-mail: lhughesk@purdue.edu

© Springer International Publishing AG 2018
L. Hughes-Kirchubel et al. (eds.), *A Battle Plan for Supporting Military Families*, Risk and Resilience in Military and Veteran Families, https://doi.org/10.1007/978-3-319-68984-5_1

endorse three responses as most important. Each day ended with the reflection of an expert discussant, beginning on the first day with Admiral Michael Mullen, formerly the 17th Chairman of the Joint Chiefs of Staff, and Mrs. Deborah Mullen; and on the second day with Faith McIntyre, director general of the policy and research division of Veterans Affairs Canada.

Many of the chapters in this volume were written by symposium presenters and participants with the goal of digging deeply into the programs, policies, and practices mobilized in response to the Global War on Terror. We asked authors to reflect carefully and with a critical eye and to envision themselves guiding the next generation of leaders who find themselves encountering a nation at war. We asked them to consider questions like: What key needs did you face? For which needs were you well or poorly prepared? What were good ideas were tried and worked—and what didn't work? What didn't get tried that should have been? Which gaps never got addressed? And how did we make ourselves better in durable ways? Finally, we asked authors for recommendations: What should the next generation of leaders do first, or find out first?

The chapters that follow are not simply extended versions of symposium presentations, but have been crafted in collaboration with expert colleagues across multiple domains. Each has been reviewed and revised with beneficial guidance by outside experts. In this chapter we provide a brief summary of each of the succeeding chapters, situated within the structure of the symposium, providing a brief explanation of the session where it first appeared, and the questions and endorsements that informed it.

1.1   Part I: Federal Government

The first section of this volume focused on the federal government. Panelists included Nicole Malachowski, at the time the executive director of the Joining Forces campaign; Barbara Thompson, at the time the director of the Department of Defense (DoD) Office of Family Readiness Policy; Susan Sullivan, the deputy assistant secretary for data governance and analytics for the Department of Veterans Affairs (VA); William Cahill, formerly Chief Counsel to the Senate Committee on Veterans Affairs; and Joyce Raezer, executive director of the National Military Family Association (NMFA).

Discussion questions for this session were:

- How do we get ahead of the early flood of new resources, staying focused on the things that will help the most families the most vs. efforts that may "feel good" or offer high PR value?
- How do we make sure we're considering all the factors in a new conflict that are likely to affect families—possibly in ways we've not seen before?

After discussion, dozens of top takeaways emerged from the discussion, but following a series of endorsement activities, the most popular recommendations were to develop mechanisms for vetting existing and emerging military and veteran family resources; to prioritize research, metrics, and data; and to create mechanisms for more centralized or better coordinated resource management. In response to the second question, participants overwhelmingly favored the use of "table top, realistic simulations of circumstances and possible solutions" as a way to consider all the factors in a new conflict that are likely to affect families.

Chapter 2 focuses on the White House's Joining Forces campaign. In this chapter, Rory Brosius documents how First Lady Michelle Obama and Dr. Jill Biden, wife of then-Vice President Joe Biden, launched a nationwide effort aimed at improving supports for service members, veterans, and their families through the production of activities aimed at three pillars: employment, education, and wellness (The Obama White House Archives, 2017).

This was not the beginning of efforts to support military and veteran families during the Global War on Terror, of course; those began at the same moment the OIF/OEF conflicts began—or even before, given substantial prior efforts to ensure that families were ready for everything military service would ask of them. Many Department of Defense (DoD) family support programs were launched or expanded during the Bush administration, and President and Mrs. Bush's advocacy continues through their work at the George W. Bush Institute. In June 2017, the Bush Institute hosted Stand To, a national veterans and military family convening, where Mrs. Bush delivered remarks saying:

> Our military is the strength of our nation, our service members are the strength of our military, and our caregivers are the strength of our veterans and wounded warriors.
>
> Military families are American families. They have the same priorities – to create a nurturing home, to take care of their loved ones, to find a strong education for their children, and to be financially secure. And they do so with more difficulties and more obstacles. As you work to improve veterans' transition, I ask that you also consider how you too can support the hidden heroes – the spouses, fathers, mothers, children, and loved ones who serve our country too. Their devotion to our men and women in uniform, and their commitment to their marriage, their family, and to our country is an inspiration to us all.

The Joining Forces campaign took military family support efforts to a new level in the Obama administration. Although the offices of the First and Second lady had little in the way of formal authority or budget, they used the "bully pulpit" of their positions—in collaboration with the President—to convene leaders, exert influence over federal agencies, raise the visibility of military and veteran families, and propel new collaborations between government and nongovernmental organizations. In each of the three pillar areas, significant initiatives were undertaken, many with impressive results. In this chapter, Ms. Brosius reflects on the specific strategies used by Joining Forces, and how future leaders could best benefit from the resulting lessons. Chapter 3 considers the DoD's response to post-9/11 deployments, the subsequent outcomes, and lessons for the future. DoD's mission includes ensuring that families are ready to surmount any challenges presented by military service. Armed with this knowledge, DoD leaders are responsible for establishing programs and policies to support military family members. Lead author Barbara Thompson uses her experience as a leader in the Pentagon to reflect about the sudden shock of the

9/11 bombings, the unexpected challenges presented when large numbers of reserve component service members from all over the country deployed, and the persistent lag between policies and constantly changing family circumstances. As a result, the meaning of "family readiness" also has evolved, with implications for the activities that should be undertaken during periods of relative calm, as well as those needed in the urgent atmosphere of the launch of a conflict.

In Chap. 4, the National Guard Bureau's Anthony Wickham and Mary Lowe Mayhugh offer a thoughtful look at how the war on terror changed the way services are provided to National Guard and other geographically dispersed military families. During the war, National Guard families experienced more than 700,000 deployments. Wickham and Mayhugh examine the organizational response to their needs, as well as the implications for the future role of the National Guard in supporting families, identifying lessons to be learned from rapidly developing and implementing a large array of programs and partnerships.

In Chap. 5, former staff members of the Office of the Chairman of the Joint Chiefs reflect about initiatives aimed at veterans. Their broad familiarity with efforts throughout the country gives them an excellent vantage point from which to comment. They analyze recent trends and offer recommendations about how best to institutionalize the momentum achieved in recent years, highlighting innovative examples of transition and reintegration supports that have been created by veteran serving organizations, nonprofits, and community service providers. They express optimism that an inflection point is approaching where sustainable momentum for supporting veterans' transitions has been achieved—a view not shared by every chapter author. The recommendations in this chapter focus heavily on supporting, promoting, facilitating, and institutionalizing collaborations between military and other organizations.

In Chap. 6, Cahill details the challenges of navigating Congress while responding to the urgent needs of wounded service members and military-affiliated families during wartime. As Cahill notes, Congress has historically operated with the assumption that the VA would provide care and services to wounded service members and their families. In practice, there were significant and troubling complexities of whether, when, and how families could receive assistance from VA or DoD, and considerable variation across branches of service and other factors. The chapter includes several recommendations aimed at minimizing disconnects between DoD and VA and maximizing Congressional response.

NMFA's Joyce Raezer contributes the final chapter of this section, which delves into the story of military family advocacy after 9/11. Raezer explains that advocacy is "about anticipating consequences, engaging and listening to the grassroots, doing one's homework to understand options, and building networks of partners to help further one's cause." She includes examples of actions resulting in both success and frustration, in hopes both will be instructive to the next generation of military family advocates. She also offers helpful observations about the role of established organizations and how they may best collaborate with the new organizations that will inevitably emerge in times of war.

1.2 Part II: Industries, Associations, and Education

The second session of the symposium focused on industries, associations, and education. Panelist included: Will Baas, vice president of talent acquisition at Comcast; Jason Vail, senior attorney in the American Bar Association's Division for Legal Services and chief counsel to the Standing Committee on Legal Assistance for Military Personnel; Kathy Snead, vice president for Military and Veterans Partnership for the American Association of State Colleges and Universities (AASCU); and Morgan Sammons, executive officer of the National Register of Health Service Psychologists.

Participants discussed the following questions:

- How can we quickly get at the real issues, when our most common first pressures often come from highly imperfect sources: the loudest voices, sensational media stories, opportunists, or briefings that are chopped dozens of times before reaching leaders?
- How do we fully exploit synergies across programs and sectors?

Answers to the first question focused heavily on the importance of data, as participants endorsed ideas that stressed the need for creating opportunities for strong research, and actively disseminating it through ongoing communications with key decision makers, leaders, journalists, and the general public. Participants endorsed the creation of a "brain trust" of research experts, as well as training leaders to consult evidence as they work to make decisions and policies.

In response to the second question, participants stressed the need for increased communication opportunities across sectors. For example, participants suggested that leaders use the Substance Abuse and Mental Health Services Administration (SAMHSA)'s Policy Academies as a model for interagency strategic plans that meet families' needs. Participants also urged the adaptation of a collective impact model.

Chapter 8 focuses on corporate programs aimed at supporting military members, veterans, and their families. Sherrill Curtis, Vivian Greentree, Will Baas, and Bob Cartright chronicle how the role of employers has evolved over more than a decade of war, from "doing the right thing" to hiring and supporting military-connected employees as a competitive business strategy. They identify disconnects in family needs and employer strategies caused by rapidly shifting patterns of deployment and transition as the conflicts in the Middle East evolved. They also share detailed insights about the ways that military culture does not fully prepare service members for corporate cultures, offering helpful suggestions for employers and military leaders to consider so that future transitions can be smoothed.

Chapter 9 focuses on educating America's "next great generation" and was written by Kathy Snead and Lesley McBain. The authors discuss three key issues that surfaced during the initial phases of Operation Iraqi Freedom (OIF) and Operation Enduring Freedom (OEF): institutional policies allowing service members and family members access to, withdrawal from, and readmission into educational environments without educational or financial repercussions; financial support mechanisms and strategies to fill initial education benefit funding gaps; and transition programs and supports for military service as well as civilian support communities for veterans whose terms of enlistment were satisfied. They recognize "disconnects" between institutional policies and the diversity among today's college students—including military-connected students—and offer recommendations for prompt, well-tuned actions in the future.

Chapter 10 focuses on behavioral healthcare in the "long war." Morgan Sammons and David Riggs examine behavioral health responses to the psychological injuries military members experienced during wartime deployments, especially those related to the blast injuries that were so prevalent in Iraq and Afghanistan. With advances in battlefield medicine and trauma medicine increasing survival rates to more than 90%, TBI and PTSD became the "signature injuries" of the conflict, and experts continue to work to lessen their impact. In this chapter, the authors discuss six broad areas of improvement that US leaders should pursue in response to the lessons of the long war. A particularly thorny problem is the "perverse" system of incentives embedded in existing disability systems.

In Chap. 11, Vail details the unique role of professional associations in assisting military families, illustrating how such organization can engage large membership groups in work that benefits military-connected families, from the expertise necessary to conduct studies of needs and how to meet them, to performing direct services for military families. He uses the ABA as a case study, specifically its Standing Committee on Legal Assistance for Military Personnel, which has played an active role in the effort to ensure access to justice for military families in need of civil legal services. The committee has developed several innovative programs that are responsive to these needs, and can provide a helpful model for other professional associations seeking to serve military-connected families. The ABA also provides generally applicable guidance and lessons learned that can be of assistance to other professional associations in the area of military family assistance. Of particular interest in this chapter are the mechanisms that allowed the ABA to quickly respond after operations began in Afghanistan.

1.3 Part III: States and Communities

Panelists for this session included Kathryn Power, regional administrator for SAMHSA; Koby Langley, senior vice president for the American Red Cross Services to the Armed Forces; Mary Carstensen, senior consultant to the Bob Woodruff Foundation on Military, Veterans and Wounded Warriors; and Mary

Keller, president, CEO, and one of the founders of the Military Child Education Coalition (MCEC). Following the presentations, the audience was asked to discuss:

- How do we spur innovation, supporting entrepreneurial thinking but also aggressively pushing for program refinement?
- We know resources will eventually dwindle, how do we begin working now to find maximum cost efficiencies?

With respect to the first question, participants endorsed listening to grassroots voices as a way to spur innovation, support entrepreneurial thinking, and aggressively push for program refinement, pointing out that a movement to help caregivers began with a chorus of caregivers who needed help. Creative individuals amplified these voices and spurred innovation. With regard to the second question, participants urged future leaders not to gut family support programs because "family readiness equals service member retention." Participants also recommended a cross-agency succession committee to protect and transfer institutional knowledge.

In Chap. 12, Michael L. Gravens and Mary M. Keller examine the nonprofit sector, which has played a vital role in filling gaps and meeting otherwise unfulfilled needs of military and veteran families. The past 17 years have seen tremendous growth in organizations focused on providing support in wellness, healthcare, employment, housing, and education. The chapter argues that it is imperative for there to be collaborative efforts between the public and private sector—including nonprofits—to be mutually supportive of military members, veterans, and their families. They call on nonprofits to be innovative in their thinking, strategic in their planning, and efficient and relevant in their operations.

Chapter 13 focuses on community mobilization. Koby Langley and Leah Barber reflect upon the mobilization of community service providers, and the ways in which they found that sector unprepared for the challenges of the post-9/11 world. The rush to fill service gaps created so many programs and resources that the amount of information was overwhelming for the very people that the organizations sought to help. Rather than too few available services, the problem became how best to determine ways to connect the right service to the right person at the right time. This chapter discusses ways for community organizations to be better prepared for future conflicts, emphasizing that the needs of families and veterans will continue to increase as the effects of more than a decade at war continue to be felt.

Chapter 14, by Linda Hughes-Kirchubel and Elizabeth Cline Johnson, describes post-9/11 philanthropic efforts that emerged in support of service members, veterans, and their families. Drawing on the expertise of philanthropic leaders, the authors detail military and veteran families' needs, analyze the philanthropic response, and offer examples of both successful efforts and efforts that failed to achieve their full potential. After discussing gaps that remain, the chapter concludes with recommendations for future philanthropic leaders to consider, including overlaying military cultural competence on existing philanthropic services, programs, and initiatives; working to develop true public/private partnerships with the DoD, the VA, and other organizations that serve military and veteran families; and prioritizing the use of data, evidence-informed practices, and needs assessments to drive deeper understandings of the military and veteran space.

Since January 2010, the America Joins Forces with Military Families Retreat, commonly referred to "White Oak" because it was first held at the White Oak plantation, has provided a recurring forum for cross-sector, multi-organization discussions to highlight new thinking, build networks, and update frameworks to best serve America's military and veteran families. These meetings are the focus of Chap. 15, written by Jennifer Hurwitz, Cristin Orr Schiffer, and Hisako Sonethavilay. The chapter provides an historical overview of the retreats and describes why such cross-sector discussions are critical to successful support of service members, veterans, and their families. Systematic data gathered about the retreats reveal common themes, lessons learned, and resulting achievements. Recommendations focus on methods for effectively engaging public, private, and nonprofit actors, ensuring military families are understood as a central and necessary component of future force planning, and continuing efforts to bridge the civilian-military divide in local communities.

1.4   Part IV: Knowledge Generation and Dissemination

Panelists for this session were Dr. Stephen J. Cozza, professor of psychiatry and associate director of the Uniformed Services University's Center for the Study of Traumatic Stress; Meredith Kleykamp, associate professor of sociology and the director of the Center for Research on Military Organization at the University of Maryland; Terri Tanielian, senior behavioral scientist at the RAND Corporation; and Carl Castro, assistant professor and director of research for the University of Southern California's Center for Innovation and Research on Veterans and Military Families. Following the presentations, the audience discussed the following questions:

- How do we ensure we are leveraging the most current advances in science/technology (e.g., neurology/resiliency, medical, family research, communication)?
- What other stakeholders are most crucial to meaningful impact of any successful knowledge generation response?

Group discussions and a subsequent endorsement activity generated consensus about several priorities. First, participants were eager for there to be a designated government organization as a primary "home" for funding and championing military family research, in contrast to the current fragmented landscape. They also encouraged the creation of a "brain trust" of research advisors who could promote collaborations and prepare strategic agendas for research. Participants emphasized the importance to future leaders of ensuring that research is communicated and disseminated to policy makers and funders in an understandable and digestible way, and the importance of policy makers using evidence in their decision-making. With regard to "what other stakeholders are most crucial to meaningful impact," participants gave top priority to media, federal data holders, and private funders.

In Chap. 16, Cozza and co-authors discuss academic research, with specific attention to primary data collection. They note that the ability of clinicians, policy makers, community service providers, commanders, and researchers to meet the needs of military children has been limited by outdated research, inappropriate comparison groups, uneven systems of care, and a lack of evidence-based practices to guide intervention. However, strategic partnerships emerged as academics, practitioners, and military leaders united in a common mission to support military children and families. The authors identify challenges to gathering high quality data from families and outline best practices for future scholarship. Lessons learned include the importance of understanding and respecting military family culture, building trust, fostering lasting community relationships, building collaborative multidisciplinary academic research teams, and sustaining a program of scientific research about military families.

Meredith Kleykamp discusses other challenges of serving military families through research in Chap. 17, presenting an overview of the academic sector and the cultural demands that shape the kinds of research scholars produce. Because good research depends on having high quality data and access to study populations, the utility of academic research is constrained when access to both is limited. Given the enormous amounts of administrative data maintained by government sources—all compiled with taxpayer funds—some of these constraints on access should be avoidable. A dilemma for academics is the need to balance responsibilities to their own institutions and professions while also using their skills to address immediate community needs. Kleykamp offers several recommendations for ensuring that a community of researchers will be available and can be mobilized when needed for future conflicts.

In Chap. 18, Terri Tanielian, Thomas E. Trail, and Nida Corry note that while policy institutes have long been designing and conducting large-scale studies to inform evidence-based decision-making on behalf of military families, significant knowledge gaps remain. They identify multiple factors that have hampered the prompt collection of high quality data throughout the current conflict. They provide several recommendations to address these problems, including crafting a strategic research agenda on military families, streamlining and modernizing regulatory processes, and providing greater access to data and findings. Beginning to implement these recommendations now will help to ensure that necessary knowledge and research infrastructures will be in place and ready before the next major conflict occurs.

In Chap. 19, Carl Castro and Kathrine Sullivan argue that new, larger, and more robust empirical studies of military families must be undertaken to address significant knowledge gaps. They argue that lack of funding for military family research is at least partly due to lack of clarity of military family researchers' goals and insufficient attention in research designs to benefitting military families. The authors explain how military research priorities are established and key features of proposals that are fundable by the DoD. They also recommend that DoD personnel appreciate the importance of family research and ensure it is included in the strategic research plan. The authors describe some of the challenges of research about military families and provide a set of recommendations to senior DoD leaders to ensure that military family research remains a high priority.

The final chapter of this section, and the volume, focuses on journalism. Authors Karen Jowers and Patricia Kime describe the tensions of covering military family issues in times of war, when revealing important news can compete with respecting national security and protecting families from further trauma. These challenges are intensified in a world with social media, where completely unfounded claims can be seen by millions of followers before professional journalists can produce confirmed and properly sourced reports—the pressure to "break news" is unrelenting and stressful. Journalists experience ethical dilemmas about which images to report so as to accurately report but not violate family privacy, about whether or how to ensure that service providers they write about are credible, and about reporting the news in a way that will seize readers' attention about family challenges, but also accurately reflect family strengths. Finally, it is important to remember that journalists have served in dangerous circumstances and sometimes sacrificed their lives. Jowers and Kime close with guiding questions that newsrooms can use to develop policies in advance so that regrettable errors will not be made in the haste to cover breaking war news.

The preparation of the chapters in this book has been a labor of both love and challenge for many of the authors. Reflecting about accomplishments over the past 17 years of armed conflict is inevitably accompanied by recognition of missed opportunities, false starts, and problems not fully addressed. Readers will learn the "inside story" about many sectors of the military and veteran community, finding thoughtful insights on which to draw, each accompanied by a fervent wish that military-connected families will be supported even better the next time there are large deployments—and that veterans and their families who have already served will be effectively supported today and in the years to come. Across the chapters, readers will find multiple common themes, but also creative sector-specific suggestions. Information from the broad range of sectors represented in the volume makes it clear that effective support for military and veteran families requires participation, cooperation, and collaboration far beyond DoD, VA, or even the federal government.

This book is intended to serve as a battle plan for future leaders with the responsibility of supporting military and veteran families during war. We hope that the assembled wisdom from today's community of leaders presented here will serve future leaders—and more importantly, military and veteran families—well.

Acknowledgments This work was supported in part by a grant from Lilly Endowment Inc.

Part I
Federal Government

Chapter 2
Joining Forces: Lessons Learned

Rory M. Brosius

2.1 Introduction

On the campaign trail in 2008, spouse of Senator Barack Obama, Michelle Obama participated in a series of roundtable discussions with working mothers across the country. These sensing sessions were designed to identify the needs and challenges of working families across the USA. For Mrs. Obama, this was one of the first times she had heard the voice of military families. Roundtable participants candidly shared the challenges of military life: managing major household moves every 2–3 years, running households during multiple deployments and heightened operational environments, and encountering barriers to meaningful employment. This was a particularly challenging time for military families who were living through the surge of 20,000 additional troops in Iraq as well as extended deployments for ground troops. When the time came to determine platforms and initiatives, Mrs. Obama, along with Dr. Jill Biden, spouse of then Senator Joe Biden, chose to work collaboratively to support veterans, service members, and their families.

By the time the Obama Administration began, there had been significant work in the realm of veterans, service members, and their families as the nation had been at war consistently for 7 years in Iraq and Afghanistan. Despite that, it could be opined that we were not significantly prepared for what a war of this duration would mean for military families. Amongst the issues which military families shared with Dr. Biden and Mrs. Obama were details of 7–18 month deployments with insufficient dwell time between them in which to recover, growing mental health issues amongst returning service members and family members, and insufficient economic opportunity and job security for military spouses.

R.M. Brosius, M.S.W (✉)
ScoutComms, Inc., Fredericksburg, VA, USA
e-mail: rbrosius@scoutcommsusa.com

© Springer International Publishing AG 2018
L. Hughes-Kirchubel et al. (eds.), *A Battle Plan for Supporting Military Families*, Risk and Resilience in Military and Veteran Families,
https://doi.org/10.1007/978-3-319-68984-5_2

While it was not always abundantly clear what all of the distinct needs of these individuals were, an emerging "sea of goodwill" seemed to indicate that the civilian community wanted to step up to support these families. A white paper published by the Warrior and Family support division in Office of the Chairman of the Joint Chiefs of Staff noted that "[t]oday, unlike any generation in history, citizens across the country are supportive in word and deed of the American Active Duty, Reserve, and National Guard Solider, Sailor, Airman, Marine and Coast Guardsman" (Copeland & Sutherland, 2011). There also existed an early sense in the military and veteran support organization community that a force to streamline these efforts and lift the issues with a sense of purpose and unity would be necessary.

If government support of military families was to be a priority, it was imperative that the tone be set from the highest level. Family readiness issues, while not always at the forefront of defense conversations, needed to be held up by the Commander in Chief as a necessary part of the conversation regarding American presence in warfighting efforts. From a national security perspective, a Pentagon report showed that the majority of new military recruits in 2012–2013 had one or more close family members who had served in the military (Defense Human Resources Activity, 2014). If the country desired to maintain an "all-volunteer force," one could postulate that care for families should be at the forefront of defense conversations so that the experience of these potential recruits is largely positive, and not one of exceptional hardship or lackluster support.

As Commander in Chief, President Obama made such care and support for military families a key national security priority. In May 2010, he commissioned Presidential Study Directive 9 (PSD-9) which directed National Security Staff to examine the needs of military families and all federal government departments to examine what could be done to support the military and veteran community (Office of the President of the United States, 2011, p. 1). Every cabinet secretary was tasked with examining his or her agency's support of military families, and creating a commitment, unique to that agency, to accelerate efforts to bolster support. By January 2011, PSD-9 was released jointly by the President, First Lady, and Dr. Jill Biden. A press release issued by the White House indicated that the result of the report,

"… will be a unified Federal Government approach to help ensure:

- The U.S. military recruits and retains America's best, allowing it to maintain the high standards which have become a hallmark of our armed forces.
- Service members can maintain both strong families and a high state of readiness;
- Family members can live fulfilling lives while supporting their service member(s); and
- The American people better understand and appreciate the experience, strength, and commitment of those who serve and sacrifice on their behalf.

This document provides the Federal Government's response to that challenge by identifying four strategic priorities that address the primary challenges facing our military families.

1. Enhance the well-being and psychological health of the military family.
2. Ensure excellence in military children's education and their development.
3. Develop career and educational opportunities for military spouses.
4. Increase child care availability and quality for the Armed Forces" (The White House, 2011).

Two years into the administration, and four months following the release of PSD-9, the Office of the First Lady of the United States and the Office of Dr. Jill Biden launched Joining Forces. The initiative called on all Americans to rally around service members, veterans, and their families and support them through wellness, education, and employment opportunities. Joining Forces was designed to work hand in hand with the public and private sectors to ensure that service members, veterans, and their families have the tools they need to succeed throughout their lives. With no congressional authority or budget, the initiative sought to mobilize and centralize public and private efforts to support the military connected and to offer an agenda of needs. The First Lady and Dr. Biden sought to mobilize communities to support service members, veterans, and their families by encouraging citizens to "do what you do best."

Strategically, it was important to identify discrete issue areas in which private, public, and nonprofit partners could commit to and rally around action. The national security and policy council staffs, experts in the field, and multiple stakeholder engagements informed the areas of most pressing need. These issues and areas of concentration roughly mirrored the findings of PSD-9, and three pillars were established for Joining Forces as employment, education, and wellness. For the Administration, amongst a gamut of concerns, record high unemployment numbers amongst the youngest veterans, difficulty in gaining academic credit for military children due to their mobile lifestyle, accessibility of child care, and mental health support were urgent policy issues that would require a high level of focus and coordination across sectors and the federal government.

In addition to these discrete pillars, Joining Forces was also at its heart a public awareness campaign. Comments from senior military leaders and research released around the time of the Joining forces launch revealed a disconnect between the civilian community and the military community. During a statement to cadets at the US Military Academy at West Point, Chairman of the Joint Chiefs Admiral Mike Mullen stated, "I fear they do not know us, I fear they do not comprehend the full weight of the burden we carry or the price we pay when we return from battle" (Mullen, 2011). Coming from the senior most military leader in our country, this statement was concerning. Data gathered and released appeared to lend further credence to this view. The report, *The Military-Civilian Gap: War and Sacrifice in the Post-9/11 Era*, noted "…more than nine-in-ten [civilians] express pride in the troops and three-quarters say they thanked someone in the military. But a 45% plurality say neither of the post-9/11 wars has been worth the cost and only a quarter say they are following the news of the wars closely. And half of the public say the wars have made little difference in their lives" (Pew Research Center, 2011, p. 8). While most civilians were aware of the ongoing conflicts in Iraq and Afghanistan and were supportive of the military community, there did seem to be a lack of understanding of the nuance of military service and lifestyle; thus, translating that support into concrete action to address some of the obstacles faced by the veteran and military community was challenging.

Joining Forces' creation was a response to both specific policy needs and the concept of the civilian-military divide. And while this initiative was started at time of great international conflict, a volatile national security environment, and heightened operational tempo for service members, many of the issues that the initiative dealt with were not necessarily outcomes of wartime, but outcomes of the challenges facing military families during war AND peace. From uncertain work schedules, to routine duty station changes, to stress and trauma, the military community faced and continues to face a myriad of issues outside of and apart from deployments to combat areas of operation. Obviously, when a nation is at war, there is heighted attention paid to the armed forces, but what happens when we are in a state of protracted global military operations—not technically at war, but not technically at peace? The personnel and readiness policies of today's military—those that dictate the rhythm and frequency of duty station changes, recruitment, and retention—lag behind massive changes in society, and often still focus on nuclear, single earner, military families who reside on military posts.

What was sought by Joining Forces was a national call to action and a plan to address both the wartime and military lifestyle obstacles facing modern military families therefore easing some of the challenges and increasing the readiness of our military fighting force. Through structured work and collaboration in education, employment, and wellness, Joining Forces attempted to heighten connectivity between resources, identify and fill programmatic and policy gaps, and increase coordination amongst players in the private and public sectors.

2.2 Employment

From the outset of Joining Forces, the veteran unemployment rate drove rapid, targeted and multi-sector work to get out-of-work veterans back into the workforce. External factors such as the great recession had had a significant impact on unemployment across the population of America, but it seemed particularly troubling that young service members could return from multiple combat deployments, transition from the military, and find themselves in dire economic straits without a job prospect in sight. Additionally, White House staff learned what the military community had known all along, that military spouses were consistently un- or underemployed and those in skilled professions faced daunting amounts of bureaucratic red tape that slowed or even stopped their career growth. Joining Forces staff, along with colleagues across White House policy councils, the Department of Veterans Affairs (VA), the Department of Defense (DOD), and the Department of Labor (DOL) found themselves in the thick of these issues nearly immediately. These entities quickly scoped the issue, identified growth industries, and developed a strategy for engagement of the private sector job creators.

The First Lady and Dr. Biden set a priority to engage with service members, veterans, and their families on a regular basis as well as engaging with those in the public, private, and nonprofit sectors who were committed to supporting the military-connected community. Dedicated staff were detailed from the Department of Defense or hired to direct the day-to-day work of Joining Forces. Staff cultivated regular opportunities for Mrs. Obama and Dr. Biden to engage with stakeholders through open and closed events. Having the megaphone of high-visibility political figures meant that CEOs could be convened, goals set, and hiring commitments established. They were, in a sense, the "closers," brought in to ask business leaders to open their doors and create opportunities for veterans and military spouses. The presence of Mrs. Obama and Dr. Biden and their personal gravitas increased the likelihood that opportunities would be pursued with speed and efficiency and that requests for assistance were heard and action plans set in place. The convening power of the Executive Branch, which hosted meetings of groups like the Business Roundtable, presented opportunities to educate employers regarding veteran and military spouse employments. In addition to garnering commitments from trade associations, Fortune 500 companies, and specific employment sectors, Joining Forces was also able to amplify existing veteran hiring efforts such as those spearheaded by the Chamber of Commerce Foundation and the JPMorgan Chase 100,000 Jobs Coalition.

Early on in Joining Forces efforts, the strategy was quite basic: asking employers to hire veterans and military spouses. While these efforts were strong—over 1.5 million were hired in the span of 5 years, especially as the economy improved—there was a realization that more advanced issues also would need to be addressed. CEOs and businesses originally answered the call to hire veterans and military spouses based on the need and patriotism. It quickly became apparent, however, that there was a strengths-based argument to be made in support of businesses hiring these individuals. Joining Forces moved, along with many of those who worked in veteran and military spouse hiring to make the "business case" for hiring, highlighting attributes such as team-leadership, timeliness, and mission-orientation as being nearly innate in the veteran and military spouse communities. A friendly sense of competition and unlikely alliances between normally competitive businesses formed, allowing for sharing of best practices and building of coalitions in specific industries such as industrial construction, defense contracting, science and technology, and private equity. Eventually, leaders like Blackstone, Disney, and others forged relationships in data and process sharing that allowed them to learn from one another about veteran and military spouse recruitment, hiring, and retention.

On the user side of the equation, Joining Forces sought to amplify best-in-class resources and tools for veterans and military families, especially those designed to translate military service or the military spouse experience (volunteerism, unpaid work experiences, etc.) into terms that private employers would understand. Championing federal programs like the Department of Defense's Military Spouse Employment Partnership (MSEP) and private sector employment focused programs like the United States Chamber of Commerce's Hiring our Heroes, the First Lady and Dr. Biden sought to spread the word about high-quality, underutilized programming.

Concurrently to hiring commitment efforts, there was a vast push in the whole of federal government to work together to create a more streamlined transition process for veterans, and increased efforts by the Department of Defense and the Department of Labor to support military spouses. Legislation like the *VOW Act of 2011* dictated a review and substantial improvements in service member transition preparation and further improved the Transition Assistance Program (TAP). Changes to the transition process dictated that all service members complete a mandatory, multiday transition workshop that focused on resume preparation, job searches, and benefits awareness. These transition workshops were also opened to the participation of military spouses who recognized their role and importance in a successful military family to veteran family transition. Service-specific initiatives like the Army's Soldier for Life and the Marine Corps' Marine for Life programs also had a heavy early focus on employment and the creation of "alumni" programs, networking opportunities, and post-military career preparedness.

The First Lady and Dr. Biden also issued a call to states to address licensing and credentialing barriers that impacted veterans and military spouses in skilled careers ranging from commercial truck drivers to nurses. The fact that a service member was not able to take an industry credential out of their military service and apply it to a civilian career, or that a military spouse would have to pay-for and take licensing exams across multiple states in a span of just a few years was troubling. During the National Governor's Association meeting in 2012, the First Lady and Dr. Biden called on governors from all 50 states to take either executive or legislative actions to streamline licensing and credentialing to help spouses and veterans overcome tedious, expensive, and sometimes needless bureaucratic red tape. While the call to action was one very important step in this process, work could not have progressed without the support and constant strategic engagement spearheaded by the Department of Defense State Liaison Office (DSLO). Having a full-time staff devoted to issues that were controlled and largely dictated by state entities was imperative to the success of this effort. The DSLO was also a key player in other state-by-state issues tackled by Joining Forces, such as the Military Child Education Compact, which will be discussed later in this chapter. Significant improvements were made in licensing and credentialing, with all 50 states eventually taking some level of executive or legislative action to streamline licensing and credentialing, although each state approached this differently and with different careers and vocations in mind.

Despite all of the progress made in the veteran and military spouse employment space, at the time of publication, still much remains to be done. Military spouses still experience unacceptable rates of un- and underemployment. A study commissioned by the U.S. Chamber of Commerce Foundation found that while military spouse unemployment had fallen from 23% in 2015 to 16% in 2017, it also found that underemployment continued to be an issue for this population (Public Opinion Strategies and the U.S. Chamber of Commerce Foundation, 2017, p. 7). Licensing and credentialing remains a focus of the Department of Defense and the creation of advocacy groups like the Military Spouse Juris Doctorate Network (MSJDN), a network of military spouse attorneys advocating for licensing accommodations across the country, continue to work for specific improvements for various job fields. It is also important to recognize that employment, particularly military spouse employment, is not just a war-related issue. The challenges and obstacles faced by veterans and military spouses are largely not caused by deployments or battles but rather an outgrowth of the military lifestyle. By modernizing personnel policies on the government side and developing more virtual/mobile career opportunities on the employer side, there is hope that veterans and military spouses will continue to see sustainable improvements in their employment circumstances.

2.3 Education

As an educator, Dr. Jill Biden was a passionate advocate for the needs of students across a variety of spectrums. In addition to championing Administration efforts on Community Colleges, Dr. Biden led Joining Forces efforts in the educational space. As in employment, there were both veteran/service member and military family member aspects to education, and Joining Forces chose to focus efforts on both the unique needs of military-connected students and veteran/military family utilization of the Post-9/11 GI Bill.

Through their earliest convening with experts in the space, White House officials were told about the daunting educational situation of military children, who, on average, move three times more than their civilian counterparts (Military Child Identifier, n.d.). Constant military relocations, which sometimes dictated that children attended schools in multiple states or countries over the course of just one academic year, meant that parents consistently faced challenges like ensuring that their children received credit for previous academic work, that they were medically qualified to attend school (i.e., had received the vaccinations required by a new system), and were eligible to play sports or participate in extra-curricular activities. Spouses of the country's most senior military leaders, as well as organizations like the Military Child Education Coalition, a nonprofit organization committed to programming to improve the educational and career opportunities of military-connected youth, persistently trumpeted the need for improvements for these students, particularly in smoothing inconsistent educational policies that hindered the academic progress of military kids. As in employment, state-by-state advocacy was needed both to educate leaders and to change educational policies that created unfair or unnecessary barriers to academic completion for military children. Alongside the DoD, the Military Interstate Children's Compact Coalition (MIC3), and the Military Child Education Coalition, the First Lady and Dr. Biden advocated for states to sign on to the interstate compact as it addressed the key areas of enrollment, placement, attendance, eligibility, and graduation. By the end of Joining Forces in 2017, all 50 states had signed on to the compact, though implementation of the compact and knowledge of its content varied considerably across states and school districts. Going forward, participation by many states in the compact will "sunset," making it imperative for advocacy organizations as well as federal government partners to continue to focus on state engagement if support is to continue.

In keeping with the types of commitments seen across Joining Forces, the National Math and Science Initiative (NMSI) also expanded programmatic offerings for military children to offer more transferable, universally recognized Advanced Placement (AP) STEM courses. In collaboration with the Department of Defense, NMSI identified school systems with large military populations and provided training for teachers to increase the quality of education received by military kids. During the 5-year commitment made in 2011, NMSI eventually placed programs in 200 schools and reached more than 60,000 military-connected youth. As most military children face geographic moves every few years, this programming allowed them to take courses that would be recognized by other secondary schools as well as colleges and universities, and introduced them to academically rigorous programming regardless of where their family was stationed around the globe. After a year in the program, students enrolled in NMSI programming "show an 85% increase in qualifying AP math and science exam scores, 11 times the national average" (NMSI, n.d.).

Joining Forces also sought to advance military cultural competency amongst educators who encountered military-connected youth in their classrooms. Dr. Biden worked with American Association for Colleges of Teacher Education (AACTE) and the Military Child Education Coalition to promote "Operation Educate the Educators," which sought to raise awareness of the needs of military-connected youth and helped to prepare teachers to lead in the classroom. With an original commitment of more than 100 colleges and universities, the program grew and impacted the next generations of teachers who will enter the classroom with a heightened awareness and responsiveness to the social, emotional, and academic needs of military-connected children.

While deployments, injuries, and the impact of war are certainly evident in our military child population, as with military spouse employment, military child education obstacles are often simply a function of the highly mobile military lifestyle. As military families increasingly choose to live off-base and the Department of Defense Education Activity (DoDEA) closes its schools in the United States, continued advocacy and attention must be paid to ensuring that military children who are educated in civilian communities have the support and structure needed to thrive developmentally. Assuming that core personnel policies will continue to dictate duty station changes every few years, programs like the Interstate Compact, NMSI, and Operation Educate the Educators have the potential to provide great value to military children, if continued and implemented properly and consistently. In the future, we must ensure the "care and feeding" of programs and initiatives designed to minimize the impacts of geographic moves of the academic progress of military youth. If at the resolution of the current conflict, programs for military-connected youth and military families more broadly, lapse, it will be challenging for future leaders to rebuild these partnerships and programs in a timely manner when a future conflict increases the urgency of the need for them.

Regarding veteran employment and transition, Dr. Biden was particularly supportive of programs and initiatives designed to ease the transition of service me7mbers into higher education using 2009s improved Post-9/11 GI Bill. Championed by many Veterans Service Organizations (VSOs), the Post-9/11 GI Bill expanded education benefits for transitioning service members and qualifying family members, providing: tuition, allowances for housing similar to those received by active duty service members, allowances for books and supplies, and access to "Yellow Ribbon" funds that would supplement funding to cover costs at schools with higher tuition rates. While the newly updated GI Bill was a popular modernization of a valued program, it suffered some growing pains in terms of confusion regarding new benefits, delayed payments to veterans, and transferability issues.

While Joining Forces held no congressional or policy authority, Dr. Biden and the First Lady were able to spur the development of resources designed to ease burdens for military and veteran families. In the case of the Post-9/11 GI Bill, Dr. Biden helped to launch the U.S. Department of Veterans Affairs GI Bill Comparison tool, a website that could inform the educational choices of GI Bill recipients by disclosing tuition and fees, housing allowances, loan default rates, and graduation rates for colleges and universities. Eventually, a companion "complaint system" was also launched, again to help inform student veteran consumers about issues that could impact their choice of school.

To be sure, economic opportunity is often nested within educational opportunities, and in the military and veteran communities this is no different. Going forward, there will be tough choices about what programming to support given budgetary constraints, changing mission sets, competing priorities, and compassion fatigue. At the time of publication, the United States has been at war for 16 years, and there are ongoing discussions about proposed changes to the GI Bill to ensure the benefit will continue to be available to future generations of service members to the broadest audience possible. From a recruitment perspective, if educational opportunity continues to be a driver for prospective American service members, the GI Bill will need to be solvent for future generations.

2.4 Wellness

In some ways, the wellness pillar of Joining Forces was the most broadly defined of the initiative's efforts. Actions were undertaken to support holistic wellness of military and veteran families, with particular focus on caregivers of wounded warriors; mental health of service members, veterans, and their families; homelessness; and military cultural competency for healthcare providers. As with the other pillars of Joining Forces, great care was taken to leverage the work of partners across a variety of sectors to optimize support to the military-connected community while also acting as quickly and efficiently as possible.

A 2008 RAND report titled *Invisible Wounds of War* designated Post-Traumatic Stress Disorder (PTSD) and Traumatic Brain Injury (TBI) as the signature wounds of Iraq and Afghanistan (Tanielian & Jaycox, 2008, p. 3). Service members also suffered from traumatic physical injuries inflicted by Improvised Explosive Devices (IEDs), and those wounded faced years or decades of recovery. Very early in the Obama Administration it was recognized that in the realm of both mental and physical health, community providers, and sometimes even providers in DOD and VA facilities, needed more knowledge about the signature wounds of the wars, and sometimes lacked knowledge about the military lifestyle that could impact the health of their patients. The early strategy used for the wellness pillar of Joining Forces was similar to that of early efforts in the employment pillar, focusing on mobilizing existing communities in unified efforts for an attainable, yet ambitious goal.

In 2011 and 2012, Joining Forces worked to build a coalition of healthcare providers committed to building awareness of the signature wounds and military cultural competency in current and future providers. Organizations like the American Nursing Association, the Association of American Medical Colleges, the American Association of Colleges of Nursing, the National Association of Social Workers, and the American Psychological Association made commitments to support the health and well-being of troops and their families through opportunities for current providers to gain knowledge through the use of apps and the continuing education credits, development of curricula for students, and the production of promotional collateral. This strategy encouraged a variety of providers to become involved in the support of service members and their families.

The Association of American Medical Colleges' (AAMC) signature commitment to Joining Forces was the organization of "Joining Forces Wellness Week," an effort to organize a variety of health organizations to educate both current and future providers about issues in the military/veteran health and wellness space. Over the course of 5 years, and with the support of the Center for Deployment Psychology (CDP) at the Uniformed University of the Health Sciences, what began as a small on-site training effort during the week of AAMC's annual conference became a multi-organizational virtual and on-site training opportunity for a variety of health professionals. Utilizing the expertise of CDP in online education, Joining Forces Wellness Week produced five, 1-h trainings offered daily during the week of Veterans Day for free continuing education credits (CEUs). The provision of free CEUs added an aspect of incentive to providers who were willing to take the time to enroll and participate in these trainings.

For those who suffered wounds, either visible or invisible, their family members were often providing the day-to-day care necessary during and after recovery. For some, "recovery" will last a lifetime and the need for care may increase. During discussions with stakeholders and military families early on in Joining Forces, it was clear that caregivers of the wounded would require support of their own. Both Mrs. Obama and Dr. Biden, along with their husbands, visited facilities like Walter Reed, Brooke Army Medical Center, and Landstuhl to meet with those who had been wounded and their families. During one of Mrs. Obama's visits to Ft. Belvoir in 2013, she sat down for a discussion with caregivers of patients at the Intrepid Spirit Center, which focused on brain injuries. It was during that roundtable that Mrs. Obama heard unvarnished and candid stories about the struggles of caregivers. Issues emerged during that conversation, including social isolation, depression, employment struggles, and their own health problems. As former First Lady

Rosalynn Carter and former Senator Elizabeth Dole had both engaged in this issue, the visit to Ft. Belvoir and the work that followed seemed to open the aperture for collaboration with other high-profile individuals.

Nearly 6 months after the visit to Ft. Belvoir, joined by former First Lady Rosalynn Carter and former Senator Elizabeth Dole, Mrs. Obama and Dr. Biden announced a series of government and private sector commitments to support the needs of America's military and veteran caregivers. A RAND report entitled *Hidden Heroes* was commissioned by the Elizabeth Dole Foundation and was issued around the time of the event. The report identified discrete areas for improvement such as future financial and legal planning, caregiver friendly environments, and the health and well-being of caregivers (Ramchand et al., 2014). In addition to commitments from partners like TAPS, MOAA, and Easter Seals, the federal government made commitments to provide in-person and virtual peer-to-peer support groups. Individual organizations like the Elizabeth Dole Foundation and the Rosalynn Carter Institute for Caregiving were integral to the success and continuation of this work. Even as Joining Forces came to an end in January 2017, these groups have continued to drive forward the research blueprints and programmatic improvements for caregivers of veterans and wounded warriors.

In the initial stages of planning how Joining Forces, Dr. Biden and Mrs. Obama would engage in a specific effort for mental health awareness, there was an understanding that a discussion of military mental health must also include discussions about mental health more broadly. While both Mrs. Obama and Dr. Biden felt passionate about addressing the pressing need to shine a light on the mental health of service members, veterans, and families, they also felt a broader discussion addressing the mental health of Americans could assist in the lowering of barriers for military-connected individuals. It seemed that while the military community faced barriers to open discussion of mental health: fear of command intervention, concern that one would be labelled as weak or unfit for duty, or simple shame, the same types of concerns, shame, and embarrassment existed in the civilian community around this topic. The announcement of "The Campaign to Change Direction," a collective impact public awareness campaign organized and led by the nonprofit organization Give an Hour, was launched in March 2014 to address the culture change needed to increase both the awareness of mental health issues and the conversations that were necessary to encourage people to speak up, speak out, and get help for mental health issues. The First Lady and Dr. Biden lent their voices to the campaign and participated in both video and print public service announcements and appeared at Change Direction events encouraging people and organizations to commit to learning the "5 Signs" and starting conversations about mental health.

The identification of the "signature wounds" focuses efforts to address highly publicized negative health outcomes, such as high suicide rates and drug and alcohol abuse. That being said, the laser focus on these two types of injuries may have made efforts slightly myopic. In retrospect, and for future knowledge, cultural competency and knowledge of particular diagnoses were not the only areas in which improvement was needed to improve wellness outcomes for military-connected individuals. In the future, availability of and access to quality care, understanding barriers that can keep military and veteran connected individuals out of healthcare, and implementation of existing, along with rapid development of new, evidence-based treatment protocols in mental health are likely to also be key pieces to this puzzle.

As was previously mentioned, Joining Forces wellness efforts were more holistic than simply physical and mental health. Nested within the Administration's overall goals in homelessness were efforts specifically focused on veteran homelessness, which was identified as an area in which Joining Forces support and ability to unite public and private partners would be helpful. In 2010, President Obama pledged to end veteran homelessness by 2015; and, in 2014, the First Lady challenged Mayors, City Managers, and other state and local officials to concentrate efforts to make the goal a reality. Working with the US Interagency Council on Homelessness (USICH), Community Solutions, and the National Coalition for Homeless Veterans, Federal Agencies responsible for homelessness efforts, private sector stakeholders, and internal White House staff in the office of Intergovernmental Affairs, the Joining Forces team worked to draw attention to the issue and encourage the coordination needed to drive down veteran homelessness. Although the goal to end veteran homelessness by 2015 was not met, significant progress was made. By the end of the Obama Administration, veteran homelessness rates were cut by more than half, and 35 communities including two states had effectively ended veteran homelessness.

With limited resources and staffing, Joining Forces was clearly not able to address all issues relating to the wellness and health of military and veteran families. As in education and employment, wellness issues selected were in response to stressors and conditions related to both the military lifestyle and the ongoing war. Lessons learned in several of the wellness areas of interest, specifically mental health and veteran homelessness, also had the potential to scale out of the military space and address broader societal issues.

2.5 Conclusion and Recommendations

From the beginning of Joining Forces it was understood that government alone would not be able to provide sufficient, impactful, and effective support to service members, veterans, and their families. A call to action to all varieties of organizations and individuals, and the convening power of the White House, allowed an office with nearly no budget and no congressional authority to positively impact the lives of military-connected individuals and their families. Achievements in veteran and military spouse hiring, ending veteran homelessness in multiple communities, and bringing together a coalition of the willing to support caregivers of wounded, ill, or injured service members were a testament to not only the Joining Forces effort, but the efforts of so many committed partners. The bully pulpit of the office and the visibility of the First and Second ladies drew attention to hard work that was already in progress when Joining Forces began in 2011 and has continued beyond the end of the Obama Administration in 2017. Having very high visibility "champions" for service members, veterans, and their families allowed more mainstream attention to be paid to an issue, which was not always understood with much nuance in the civilian community.

For future understanding, there was no need to "recreate the wheel," when Joining Forces began. The expertise of senior leaders and advisors both within and external to the White House who oversaw the conceptualization and implementation of Joining Forces sought to use the bully pulpit to add value to existing efforts, rather than as an opportunity to create redundant programming. The ability of senior leaders to quickly scope the issue, survey key stakeholders and experts, and examine policy implications is imperative to the success of any future efforts in this arena. These leaders also tried to collaborate, learn from, and build upon the successes of those that were already doing work to support service members, veterans, and their families. Key to the success of future work will be a keen and systematic approach to building an understanding of the "geography," complexity, strengths and weaknesses of the network of potential partners. Work from inside the government is only as strong as the collaborative and sustainable relationships we build with partners.

Mrs. Obama and Dr. Biden used national news and pop culture vehicles to address issues integral to the well-being of the military and veteran community. In some ways, especially when it came to discussing the knowledge gap between the civilian military-connected populations, they sought to bring the issues "into the living rooms" of Americans, to promote a better understanding of not only the challenges but also the strengths of service members, veterans, and their families. Cover stories on magazines like *Glamour* and *Redbook* as well as television appearances on programs like *Late Night with David Letterman*, *Sesame Street*, and *NCIS* offered different and creative vehicles in which to reach the American people about the issues facing service members, veterans, and their families. High-visibility trips to bases and the invitation of service members, veterans, and their families to White House events also allowed the First Lady and Dr. Biden to use the interest of the public to bring attention to the issues Joining Forces sought to address.

Successes of the initiative were also made possibly by an administration that made the support of veterans, service members, and their families a high priority. Service members, veterans, and their families were nested as a community of interest within a broad range of Administration domestic policy priorities including healthcare, education, and economic opportunity.

While we are still engaged in the Global War on Terror, many lessons have been learned by the veteran and military support community over the past 16 years. The terror attacks of September 11, 2001 thrust a peacetime military into more than a decade of protracted war. The negative outcomes for both warfighters and families required that those working in support spaces move quickly; and, while the collection of data and empirically based interventions are ultimately essential to success, during this war, the need to act quickly to support families and individuals often overtook the ability to surmount regulatory hurdles, collect data, assess outcomes, and adapt or develop evidence-based practices. As we look to future conflicts, several areas of concentration could have the potential to more effectively support service members, veterans, and their families.

Public–private partnerships, and the invitation of corporate, nonprofit, research, and educational organizations to planning discussion are key in building strong, agile relationships and programming which support service members, veterans, and their families. While there were a broad variety of responses to the war effort itself, some positive and some negative, most Americans did seem supportive of individual service members, veterans, and their families. Engaging the "coalition of the willing" about where and how they could support the military/veteran community was helpful in coalescing around purposeful goals while also creating a feedback loop and opportunities for improvement and collaboration. Bringing together willing corporate partners and allowing an opportunity for the exchange of information with best-in-class support organizations often gave way to unique partnerships that paved the way for advancements.

Ensuring that structures built within agencies to support service members, veterans, and their families during this conflict remain resourced through the next conflict is integral to the ability of the government to respond in the event of the next conflict. While budget constraints and policy focuses will invariably shift from administration to administration, the resourcing of these offices is essential to our national security. Understanding that a full-staff may not be possible during peacetime, it is imperative that the government maintains a baseline of support, so as not to "start from zero" in the event of the next conflict. Each global conflict is different, but the knowledge that there will be commonalities in stressors impacting service members, veterans, and their families can help to focus efforts to support them during peacetime. Maintaining a staffing presence, however minimal, will also reduce activation time in the event of the next conflict. Having a proverbial "voice at the table" for issues of the military-connected community is an important way to be sure that the issues of these communities continue to be heard and acted upon regardless of peace or war.

Without appropriate data, leaders during the GWOT phase were hindered in how quickly they could act with certainty. There was pressure to act and relieve the stresses of these families, but not always a strong *scientific* evidence base to inform action. While some data could be scaled or cross-walked from the general population (i.e., general health information, nontraditional learner information), there were problems and issues that we grappled with that did not translate directly to existing evidence bases. Collecting data and requiring that programs track outcomes with regard to service members, veterans, and their families will help to identify trends, opportunities for external and internal support, and emerging needs.

Ultimately, hindsight is 20–20, and the opportunities and challenges faced by service members, veterans, and their families will depend largely on the geopolitical landscapes of the future. There is hope that we will learn from one of the longest periods of warfare in history to ensure that service members, veterans, and their families will operate from a strategic advantage rather than disadvantage.

Acknowledgments The author and the editors wish to express appreciation to Colonel Nicole Malachowski, United States Air Force and Executive Director of Joining Forces from June 2015 to May 2016, who presented about Joining Forces at the "Battle plan" symposium.

References

Copeland J., & Sutherland D. (2011). *Sea of goodwill: Matching the donor to the need* [White paper]. Retrieved March 1, 2017, from First in Families of North Carolina: http://www.fifnc. org/programs/Sea_of_Goodwill.pdf.

Defense Human Resources Activity. (2014). *New recruit survey wave 1 findings* [PowerPoint slides]. Retrieved March 1, 2017, from https://timedotcom.files.wordpress.com/2016/03/new_ recruit_wave1_briefing_final_7-23-2013.pptx.

Military Child Identifier. (n.d.). Retrieved from http://www.militarychild.org/student-identifier.

Military Family Mission. (n.d.) Retrieved from https://www.nms.org/Our-Approach/Military-Mission.aspx.

Mullen, M. (2011). *Commencement address*. Speech presented at United States Military Academy at West Point Commencement in West Point, New York. Retrieved March 1, 2017, from http://wppcco.us/11_Graduation.html.

Office of the President of the United States. (2011). *Strengthening our military families: Meeting America's commitment. (Presidential Study Directive 9)*. Retrieved March 1, 2017, from Military OneSource: https://www.dol.gov/dol/milfamilies/strengthening_our_military_families.pdf.

Pew Research Center. (2011). *The Military-Civilian gap: War and sacrifice in the Post 9/11 era*. Retrieved March 1, 2017, from Pew Research Center: http://www.pewsocialtrends.org/files/2011/10/veterans-report.pdf.

Public Opinion Strategies and the U.S. Chamber of Commerce Foundation. (2017). *Military spouses in the workplace: Understanding the impacts of military spouse unemployment on military recruitment, retention and readiness*. Retrieved June 15, 2017, from Hiring Our Heroes: https://www.uschamberfoundation.org/sites/default/files/Military%20Spouses%20in%20the%20Workplace.pdf.

Ramchand, R., Tanielian, T., Fisher, M. P., Vaughan, C. A., Trail, T. E., Epley, C., et al. (2014). *Hidden heroes: America's military caregivers*. Santa Monica, CA: RAND.

Tanielian, T. L., & Jaycox, L. (Eds.). (2008). *Invisible wounds of war: Psychological and cognitive injuries, their consequences, and services to assist recovery* (Vol. 720). Rand Corporation. Retrieved from http://books.google.com/books?hl=en&lr=&id=DHfiWi2AcdAC&oi=fnd&pg =PP1&dq=Tanielian+Invisible+Wounds+of+War+Psychological+and+Cognitive+Injuries,+T heir+Consequences,+and+Services+to+Assist+Recovery&ots=QGc6R8Q64g&sig=g6OH4H ZswOvNapFVez9EtIlohQA.

The White House. (2011). *Presidential initiative supports military families* [Press release]. Retrieved from https://obamawhitehouse.archives.gov/the-press-office/2011/01/24/presidential-initiative-supports-military-families.

Chapter 3
Lessons Learned Inside the Pentagon

Barbara Thompson and Keisha M. Bailey

3.1 Background

Within DoD, the Office of the Deputy Assistant Secretary of Defense for Military Community and Family Policy (MC&FP) reports to the Assistant Secretary of Defense for Manpower and Reserve Affairs (M&RA) under the auspices of the Under Secretary of Defense for Personnel and Readiness (P&R). The Under Secretary is the principal advisor to the Secretary of Defense on all matters relating to military and civilian personnel policies, such as end strength, recruitment goals and standards, pay and bonuses, delivery of medical entitlements, readiness of the Force, and the well-being of military families.[1] MC&FP is directly responsible for the DoD's Quality of Life (QoL) policies, programs, and services on military installations worldwide, sites serving reserve component members and their families, and the virtual delivery of such services and programs.

The military services, comprising the Army, United States Marine Corps, Navy, and Air Force, execute, i.e., operationalize, the vast majority of these family support programs available to their particular Service families as well as sister Service military families who are assigned to a particular installation. Regardless of Service or Component, family support programs as required by policy must be delivered to

---

[1] There are four other major functions that support military family readiness that are included in the P&R portfolio, i.e., medical benefits, financial readiness, commissaries, and military children's education that will not be addressed in this chapter.

B. Thompson, M.S. (✉)
Manassas, VA, USA
e-mail: barbarathompson02017@gmail.com

K.M. Bailey, B.A.
Department of Human Development and Family Studies, Military Family Research Institute, College of Health and Human Sciences, Purdue University, West Lafayette, IN, USA
e-mail: baile167@purdue.edu

© Springer International Publishing AG 2018

L. Hughes-Kirchubel et al. (eds.), *A Battle Plan for Supporting Military Families*, Risk and Resilience in Military and Veteran Families, https://doi.org/10.1007/978-3-319-68984-5_3

military families who are in need. MC&FP is also responsible for analyzing demographic and programmatic data addressing the general development and functioning of military families across the DoD. Principle objectives adhered to by MC&FP include ensuring military families are knowledgeable about the challenges they may face; equipped with the skills to function in the face of such challenges; are aware of the resources available to them to manage such challenges; and know how to access those resources when needed. One of the directorates that supports the mission of MC&FP is the Office of Military Family Readiness Policy (OMFRP). This directorate, originally named the Office of Family Policy, was established by the Military Family Act of 1986 which for the first time, codified family policy as a function of the Office of the Secretary of Defense and mandated professional personnel be designated to provide policy and oversight for family support programs. The National Defense Authorization Act of 2010 also established the Office of Community Support for Military Families with Special Needs. Over the last 30 years, the responsibilities and functions of OMFRP have evolved to meet the ever-changing needs of military families. Today, there are five multidisciplinary teams of subject matter experts who address child and youth programs, prevention of domestic violence and child abuse and neglect, family readiness and well-being which includes spouse education and career opportunities, support for families with special needs, and the Military Family Readiness Council. The teams within OMFRP develop DoD policies, provide oversight for programs that fall under the guidance of these policies, leverage resources to enhance the overall readiness and well-being of military families, provide recommendations and guidance to senior leadership, and support multiple components of the Military Family Readiness System (MFRS). The MFRS is defined as the network of agencies, programs, services, and individuals that collaborate to address the unique challenges associated with military service.[2] Military families, regardless of activation status or location, must be able to access information and services to support their successful navigation of the military lifestyle. In a perfect web of family support, the DoD, the military services, and local community agencies work together to connect the military family to the right resource at the right time, meeting the imminent need and gaining trust for future interventions.

3.2   History

Unexpected life-altering events took place on September 11, 2001 in the United States. In Washington DC, the DoD mobilized to provide immediate care and assistance for the families affected by the terrorist attack that occurred at the Pentagon. Similar assistance was initiated in New York City for the victims of the World Trade Center—without consultation between cities. DoD staff from MC&FP and staff from military family support programs located in the National Capital Region followed protocols learned

---

[2] See Department of Defense(DoD). (2012). DoD Instruction 1342.22 Military Family Readiness (published on July 03, 2012). Available at www.dtic.mil/whs/directives/corres/pdf/134222p.pdf

from previous emergency family assistance events; however, they also had to quickly adjust and adapt to meet the unique challenges of this particular disaster. Most responses to emergency assistance do not start out as a reaction to a large-scale terrorist attack nor are they geared to be sustained for such a protracted period of time. This effort required an immediate response from many entities to meet the needs of families reeling from the unanticipated, brutal loss of their loved ones. Neither the response nor the needs ended a month later when the Pentagon Family Assistance Center (PFAC) closed. There are many lessons learned and protocols to follow that have been documented in the PFAC after action report (Office of the Secretary of Defense, 2003). The scope of the effort expanded to the larger military community due to the start of large-scale deployments in support of Operation Enduring Freedom. Previous experience and subject matter expertise were sufficient to meet the needs identified during a short-term conflict, but no one imagined the length of this conflict. In hindsight, milestones and events mark shifts in how resources were delivered to meet the evolving needs of military families.

There was no playbook for this prolonged conflict and the impact it would have on military families, especially those who were geographically isolated from military installation support. This resulted in an ongoing assessment and reassessment of the needs and gaps in services and populations served as the operation grew and intensified. The lessons learned from the acute response to 9/11 and outlining the long-term assistance required to address the strain of multiple, long-term deployments will better inform future leaders across all disciplines and organizations as they move forward to offer assistance. What has been learned can be applied to family assistance facing any community-level catastrophic events, whether it is a natural disaster, mass shooting, terrorist attack, or industrial accident. No one can anticipate the what, where, and when of how the next tragedy will challenge providers of family support in both the military and civilian communities. Nevertheless, we can and must be prepared to address the evolving human needs of both military and civilian families that manifest when a family is undergoing stress.

3.3   Response: MC&FP Led

Before the wars in Iraq and Afghanistan, family support had become a standard service provided on military installations around the world where military family members had resided since the early seventies, but gaps in services and resources became readily apparent in the wake of multiple, lengthy, dangerous deployments. Under normal circumstances, MC&FP's primary role is to develop policies based on research, trend analysis, and law. When post-9/11 conflicts occurred, leadership recognized the importance of developing and operationalizing immediate courses of action that would augment what the military services were doing to support military families. Support services such as financial counseling, relocation guidance, spouse employment support, information and referral, deployment assistance, exceptional family member services, life skills education, and emergency family assistance had been delivered through specialists at military family support centers.

Knowing that military family support centers were available during limited hours and that a family "emergency" could happen at any time, MC&FP decided a virtual, more robust family support program needed to be offered 24/7/365 to augment what the staff at the military family support centers were providing. In addition, MC&FP leadership recognized that military life challenges had been exacerbated as a result of these extended separations under life-threatening conditions. Two initiatives were developed simultaneously to address these needs. MC&FP implemented Military OneSource and the Military Family Life Counselor program as the bedrock of what could be done from the Office of the Secretary of Defense. Over time as more needs emerged, additional services were added to both programs and they were modified to meet the demand. This section will amplify what took place with regard to these support programs over time.

With the wars, the landscape of family support evolved to meet the needs of family members who were geographically dispersed from the military family support system and to meet the needs of a younger generation who showed a preference for support that was user-friendly, technologically advanced, and immediately accessible. Today, the DoD response includes support that goes beyond the traditional face-to-face service delivered at military family support centers. Because 70% of military families live off of the installation and because the reserve component is largely remote from installations, family support is now also delivered by phone, or online through chat rooms, video chat, webinars, and self-paced interactive tools. Two initiatives were developed with these capabilities in mind:

3.3.1 Military OneSource (MOS)

Military OneSource (http://www.militaryonesource.mil; 1-800-342-9647) is uniquely positioned among all other family support services in that it offers 24/7/365 access to master's degree consultants who are trained in providing support services to military families. An extension of existing installation services, MOS provides free, convenient access to confidential support in person, online, or phone to provide information and referral to a wide array of services and resources, such as nonmedical counseling, financial counseling, tax preparation, specialty consultations for adoption, elder care, special needs, spouse career counseling, relocation assistance, transition assistance, and health and wellness coaching, the Sesame Workshop materials, articles, books, special needs kits, podcasts, and webinars.

3.3.2 Joint Family Support Assistance Program (JFSAP)

The Joint Family Support Assistance Program was initially mandated by the National Defense Authorization Act (NDAA) of 2007 to address the needs of geographically dispersed service members and their families. Congress leverages funding levels and provisions in the annual NDAA to impact service members and their families by directing the Secretary of Defense to follow through on their recommendations for studies, pilots, change in policies, etc. In the case of JFSAP, subject matter experts from MC&FP met with a select group of State Family Program directors and staff from the National Guard Bureau to identify the needs and what could be done to mitigate these challenges. This program was designed to provide high-quality, mobile support teams and assistance in 50 states and four territories to augment existing family support programs. It is important to note that ongoing analyses must be done throughout the life of a program to determine if the program/resource developed to meet a gap in family support is working as planned, is still needed, or does it require a new approach to better serve military families. This was done with JFSAP and modifications were made to the design and delivery of direct support with more reliance on surge support for nonmedical and financial counseling to increase the numbers of service members and families being served and better aligned to where they lived. Also, JFSAP's mission to develop a community support network evolved into a separate effort, Community Capacity Building, to maximize the efforts of both DoD and non-DoD helping professionals to support military members and their families regardless of their activation status or residence. Community agencies play a key role in supporting military members and their families. In order to enhance the relationships among DoD and civilian helping professionals, a self-directed training is offered on Military OneSource's My TrainingHub (https://myhub.militaryone-source.mil/MOS/f?p=SIS:2:0:). Families and communities must be aware of what the DoD can and cannot do, as a means of developing and maintaining the most effective and available resources to support service members in the face of current and uncertain future threat environments. For example, the DoD does not provide direct financial assistance to families who may need extra support during unforeseen crises. The Military Aid Societies and nonprofit agencies do provide monetary or resource support to meet the financial needs of military families.

Because many military members served and are serving in combat situations, they are at risk of serious injury and death. Many have returned with invisible injuries, such as traumatic brain injuries (TBI) and post-traumatic stress (PTS). More have returned with muscular-skeletal injuries and amputations. These life-altering injuries not only affect the service member, but also every member of his or her family. MC&FP took action in 2005 to provide direct support to service members and their families at the behest of Deputy Secretary Wolfowitz while the military services were developing their response to the growing needs of wounded, ill, and injured (WII) service members.

3.3.3 Military Severely Injured Center

A call center was set up to address the immediate needs of severely WII service members. Representatives from the Military Services, TSA, Red Cross, Military OneSource, Health Affairs, and the Department of Veterans Affairs (VA) manned the center to find answers to the issues at hand, from looking into promotion status, to finding nonprofit support to overcome financial challenges, to smoothing travel security screenings for WII service members. Family members called to the bedside of their loved ones were also in need of support. MC&FP recognized that families needed guidance as they awaited a diagnosis or worked to adapt to long-term care plans. Counselor advocates were deployed to major military treatment facilities (MTFs) and the four Veterans Affairs (VA) Polytrauma Centers to provide direct assistance to the families. Because WII service members were transitioning from Walter Reed and Bethesda to VA Polytrauma Centers in Tampa, Richmond, Palo Alto, and Minneapolis for catastrophic, multiple injuries such as amputations and TBIs or spinal paralysis and PTS, MC&FP knew the families needed support in this unchartered territory. In addition, the staff at the VA Polytrauma Centers were inexperienced dealing with young service members, young families, and young children in their hospitals. These professionals assumed a case management role intent on getting families the resources and support they needed so that families could concentrate on recovery and reintegration. The center was in operation for 2 years until senior leadership made the decision to discontinue its mission because the military services had implemented their support for WII service members and their families. Military OneSource continues to provide specialty consultation for WII service members and their families to resolve issues that they are facing.

The high level of stress experienced by military families due to conflict since 2001 resulted in a review of the adequacy of the Department's counseling services to meet the increased need of support. However, the stigma associated with seeking psychological healthcare and these resources were deeply rooted in the military culture.[3] MC&FP realized that resources were needed to address stress-related work-life challenges in the early stages to prevent exacerbation of the stress which could trigger a higher level of intervention. The following two programs were launched and continue to this day.

3.3.4 Military Family Life Counselors (MFLCs)

This program was designed to use licensed clinicians to deliver face-to-face, confidential, nonmedical counseling focused on problem-solving for military families coping with normal reactions to the stressful challenges of deployments, separations, and reintegration. MFLCs possess a master's degree or PhD in a mental health field and are licensed or certified to practice independently. Services are delivered on military installations and at reserve component events. This service augments the nonmedical counseling Military OneSource provides virtually as well as face-to-face in the local community in the United States. This program evolved to provide

---

[3] The Virginia Polytechnic Institute and State University conducted the Military Family Needs Assessment from September 2009 through April 2010. The study found that service members were worried about potential negative consequences and stigma to use those resources. Final report is available at http://download.militaryonesource.mil/12038/Project%20Documents/MilitaryHOMEFRONT/Reports/MFNA_2010_Report.pdf

face-to-face financial counseling. To better serve families with children, Child and Youth Behavioral Military Family Life Counselors (CYB-MFLCs), who are licensed clinicians with child and youth training and experience, are embedded in military child development programs, youth centers, Department of Defense Education Activity (DODEA) schools, and public schools that serve military children. Their work helps staff and parents respond to behavioral challenges, as well as helping children with coping skills. The three MFLC counseling specialties (non-medical counseling to cope with life challenges, financial counseling and education, and child and youth prevention counseling for children, staff, and parents) are delivered normally on 30, 45, 60, 90 day rotations and on 180, and 360 days under special circumstances. The MFLC program provides a response to an individual, couple, or family whose needs for counseling do not meet the level of severity to require a clinical intervention. MFLCs do not keep traditional counseling records, and the confidentiality helps to address the stigma associated with seeking counseling that exists in the military. The ease of access and the confidential component promote a culture that encourages delivery and receipt of counseling, and helps to eliminate barriers to seek counseling support. The program provides an entry point to a continuum of counseling support that includes prevention, early intervention, and referrals to treatment when needed, to enhance coping and build resilience.

3.4 Response: MC&FP Supported Activities

3.4.1 Project Families OverComing under Stress (FOCUS)

Project FOCUS provides resilience training to military children and their parents who have experienced deployment. In guided sessions and group workshops, the program teaches practical skills in a natural setting, such as the Family Support Center to meet the challenges of deployment and reintegration, to enhance communication and solve problems effectively, and to successfully set goals together to create a shared family story. Published results of program effectiveness show improvements in communication, affective responsiveness and involvement, role clarity, and problem-solving—all characteristics linked to the core family resilient processes, as well as reductions in parent and child distress and improvements to their adaptive functioning overall.

3.4.2 Respite Care

A growing body of research demonstrates that parental deployments impact children's and families' day-to-day functioning as a result of separation, reconfigurations of the family system, routines, and household responsibilities, financial strains, ambiguous loss and fear for a loved one's safety (Flake, Davis, Johnson & Middleton,

2009; Huebner, Mancini, Wilcox, Grass & Grass, 2007; Riggs and Riggs, 2011). The management of stressors faced by the stay-at-home parent or caregiver directly impacts the well-being of the military child. Losing half of the family support system when the fathers and/or mothers deploy can negatively affect the coping skills of the stay-at-home parent/guardian when challenged with all of the day-to-day family responsibilities. This is particularly difficult if the child also has special health or educational needs. Due to the length of the military parent's absence, it became critical to provide respite care so the stay-at-home parent/guardian would have a break from these responsibilities and opportunities for self-care. In support of the war effort, military child development centers and youth centers offered extended hours of care, to include some nights and weekends, in order to support mission readiness schedules and to provide much needed respite care to families. Up to 16 hours/month of respite child care was offered as well as up to 40 hours/month of respite care for families with a member who had special needs. Respite care was offered through the child development system or through contractual arrangements with the National Association of Resource and Referral Agencies. Additional resources were provided through Overseas Contingency Operations (OCO) funding so the cost would not be shouldered by the family.

3.4.3   New Parent Support Program

This is a DoD-sponsored program facilitated through the Family Advocacy Program to support expectant parents and those with children birth through age 3. Nurses and social workers conduct voluntary home visits to help new parents better understand the needs of their babies and toddlers, how to best meet their needs, and what to expect on a child's developmental journey. For young families away from their extended families, this program helps to ensure a healthy start for the very youngest military children.

Throughout the post-9/11 conflicts, many groups of government and civilian entities prioritized and strategized how to best understand the difficulties faced by military families, how to mitigate these difficulties, and how to strengthen family systems. Over the course of post-9/11 conflicts, there were many large scale as well as smaller scale strategic planning efforts. This section will highlight a few of these initiatives:

3.5   MC&FP Strategic Planning Events:

- Guard and Reserve Task Force Meeting (May 19–20, 2009): This two-day meeting brought together representatives from MC&FP, the active duty family support, and the Guard and Reserve communities to focus on the realities and needs of the reserve component community.

- Joint National DoD Family Readiness Conference (Sep 1–3, 2009): This world-wide forum was organized to share innovative resources and information on practice guidelines and tools to improve military family readiness for internal and external DoD helping professionals. Presentations and computer labs provided innovative information in the following categories:

  - Long-term effects of deployment on children and families
  - Family Support
  - Personal Finance
  - Education
  - Healthcare and mental health access
  - Spouse Employment

- National Leadership Summit on Military Families (Nov 9–10, 2009): This summit was one of the steps taken in an ongoing effort to transform military family support and readiness programs to eventually lead to more effective coordination and implementation. Summit participants included more than 200 senior military family policy makers, family program leaders and their staff, military family researchers, and military family members. The focus was on strengthening the well-being and resiliency of military families during an era of protracted conflict with the goal of transforming family support and readiness programs in ways that enhance their effectiveness, efficiency, and overall impact. The identified top five issues and challenges were:

  - Challenges of the deployment cycle
  - Psychological health of military families
  - Access to services and consistency of support
  - Communication challenges
  - Frequent relocation

  The following goals and scope of family support and readiness were identified:

  - Evaluate support program to learn which models are effective and built on success
  - Communicate critical information to military family members
  - Establish collaborative partnerships
  - Address psychological health needs of military families
  - Develop and implement programs that support military children and youth

  The Summit's participants voted to prioritize recommendations for DoD family support programs:

  - Create a coordinated, strategic map of all existing programs to identify redundancies and opportunities for consolidation. Develop metrics of success and evaluate all programs to determine which ones are working.
  - Design and implement a strategic communications plan.
  - Review the Department's focus on behavioral health services to ensure access, availability, and education to encourage early identification, and to reduce stigma associated with mental health treatment.

Finally, the participants put forward the following priorities:

– Categorize and evaluate programs to enhance effectiveness, consistency, and
  return on investment.
– Develop and implement a strategic communications strategy that reaches
  families with what they need to know, and connects them with those who have
  the capacity and resources to provide support.
– Strengthen the Department's ability to provide for the psychological well-
  being of military personnel and their families (with a particular focus on the
  health of children in these families).

3.6   Community-Led Strategic Planning Events

• Blue Star Families White Oak Retreats (February 2010–2016): Five retreats have
  been held since 2010 to address the needs of military families across multiple
  sectors to include government, the nonprofits, and philanthropy. Representatives
  came together to identify priorities and facilitate solutions to support the veteran
  and military community. "White Oak" is recognized as a process by which positive transformation can be accomplished.
• National Military Family Association Summit—When Parents Deploy:
  Understanding the Experiences of Military Children and Spouses (May 12–13,
  2010): NMFA organized a Blue Ribbon Panel of experts and advocates from inside
  and outside the military community to develop a set of recommended actions. The
  results from in-depth interviews and discussions at the summit included innovative
  and pragmatic ideas that could be undertaken by government, communities, and
  individuals to make a positive difference in the lives of military families.
• Presidential Study Directive 9—Strengthening Our Military Families (Office of
  the President, 2011): President Obama made the care and support of military
  families as a top national security policy priority and called together subject matter experts from every cabinet of the federal government to review what resources
  could be leveraged to support military families, ways to identify new opportunities to augment what the DoD provides through a coordinated approach. This
  government-wide effort addressed:

  – The well-being and psychological health of the military family
  – Excellence in military children's education and their development
  – Career and educational opportunities for military spouses
  – Child care availability and quality for military families

• Joint National DoD Family Resilience Conference (Apr 27–29, 2011): This
  high-quality professional conference was co-sponsored by MC&FP and the
  USDA. This venue offered opportunities to connect, to acquire new tools and
  techniques, to build greater awareness to better focus on vulnerable and military
  family populations. Representatives from Cooperative Extension, universities,
  nonprofit agencies, military, and federal and local government were involved in
  the following communities of practice:

- Family Risk and Resilience
- Youth and Teens
- Family Support
- Parenting
- Community Capacity Building
- 4H
- Child Development

While these are some of the many initiatives undertaken by MC&FP or supported by MC&FP, there are many, many more that were put into place by MC&FP, the military services, and nonprofit organizations. The ongoing military conflicts during this period taught all involved that the urgency to implement and deliver was the driving force in a proactive response. However, we learned that by not using existing evidence informed programs or embedding an evaluation component into the delivery of new programs made it difficult to validate the effectiveness of the programs and services that were provided and to justify future funding. By fostering academic collaborations that can adequately inform results from evaluations and studies, leaders and policy makers will be able to better understand and implement the most effective, efficient and supportive programs, policies, and resources for military families. The last 15 years have seen the development of a very robust research program, as researchers investigated a wide variety of military service related influences. One of the most far-reaching and prolific initiatives undertaken by MC&FP for the larger P&R enterprise is the ongoing work with the Land-Grant Universities:

3.6.1 DoD-United States Department of Agriculture (USDA) Partnership

In November 2009, US Secretary of Agriculture Vilsack announced the formation of the USDA and DoD Extension-Military Partnership to focus on community capacity building in support of military families, workforce development, and strengthening family, child care, and youth development programs. In May 2010, the Under Secretary of Defense for Personnel and Readiness and USDA signed a Memorandum of Understanding to formally launch an interagency partnership. The mission of the partnership between DoD and the National Institute of Food and Agriculture (NIFA), Cooperative Extension, and the Land-Grant University (LGU) system is to advance the health, well-being, and quality of life for military service members, families, and their communities through coordination of research, education, and extension programs. This partnership made it possible for DoD to collaborate with USDA's LGU researchers in program evaluation and other subject areas and the Cooperative Extension Service in providing joint programs and resources for military families. This interagency effort also fulfilled the Government Accountability Office's recommendations to address future cross-cutting issues and challenges in military family support, particularly for those who are geographically dispersed. MC&FP commissioned Pennsylvania State University Clearinghouse for Military Family Readiness (http://militaryfamilies.psu.edu) to develop evaluation plans for family readiness programs that may need assistance in preparing for full-scope program evaluation as well as running programs through a continuum of evidence to help policy makers choose evidence informed resources to meet the needs of military families. MC&FP also engaged the University of Minnesota with Military REACH—Supporting Families with Research and Outreach (https://reachmilitaryfamilies.umn.edu) to identify and synthesize research and provide research briefs on military family issues to support policy makers making program decisions.

Future efforts to support military families need to address evaluation to assess potential outcomes and the partnership with the LGUs offers a prime vehicle to do this, as well as leveraging the LGUs to develop new resources, such as The Virtual Lab School (https://www.virtuallabschool.org), Early Childhood Curriculum, and a universal parenting program, Thrive.

3.7   Lessons Learned

The following suggestions are not to be dusted off and reviewed when a challenging event occurs that could potentially rock family stability. Unfortunately, those involved with military families were slow to react and build upon the realization of the impact military families have on mission success, and ultimately national security. Family support professionals, their leadership, and military leadership need to be immersed in the touchpoints of family functioning, adept at identifying gaps at every level of delivery, and willing to evaluate the relevance of the delivery system. It is in the DoD's best interest to embed what is known about protective factors for fully functioning family systems into the MFRS so that military families are ready and resilient to cope, overcome, and thrive as a family unit regardless of the challenge at hand. The following broad lessons learned and the needed courses of action to be undertaken to put that knowledge into practice are not listed in any priority or sequence—they are all important and critical to the success of meeting the needs of military families.

1. We must better understand the sociological differences of the generations of service members and their families who are to be served:

   - Identify family structures, i.e., nuclear family is no longer the norm; marriage is not seen as the "sacred" next step in relationships; LGTBQ families.
   - Identify how each generation prefers to communicate, i.e., how can we have access to updated contact information/email addresses for outreach; how can we engage in best communication practices, such as content strategies, user experience, and mobile access to ensure we are reaching our intended audience?

- Identify how each generation wants to receive information, i.e., how can we better rely on digital platforms where military families seek information; how can we identify the language they use; how can we better leverage nonprofit and military services' media platforms to amplify the messages?
- Identify how each generation wants to receive services, i.e., face-to-face, electronically, officially, through the MFRS, etc.
- Identify where they live, i.e., embedded in civilian communities; on installations; geographically isolated from organized support.
- Identify the entire family population—not just ID holders, i.e., parents, siblings, significant others, intimate partners.
  - Identify the legal impediments for providing support to non-ID holders.
  - Identify ways to provide support when not legally authorized.

2. Ensure the service members and family members are aware and understand what resources are available to support them.

- Identify what programs are currently available.
- Understand the efficacy of available programs.
- Determine which sector is responsible for program maintenance and coordinate a strategy for the program based on updated information about family needs
- Actively reach out to military families to share available resources and how to access.

3. With multiple efforts to improve the quality of life for military families it is critical to coordinate among different components, services, and others providing support to ensure efficiency and comprehensive services along the continuum of service—not just when an emergency family assistance event takes place.

- Conduct ongoing review of existing research.
- Conduct ongoing analysis of surveys that provide feedback from service members and spouses on their needs and gaps in services.
- Conduct focus groups to gather input from military families regarding the status of programs provided by the MFRS.
- Convene task forces concerned with particularly vulnerable groups to focus on realities and needs.
- Convene family support professionals to explore promising practices and share successes of existing partnerships and programs.
- Continue ongoing work with the LGUs and other research experts to support evaluation, analysis of research on military families; developing evidence informed resources to improve the delivery of family readiness system support, review and publication of promising practices on the Clearinghouse of Military Family readiness website.
- Armed with this information and analysis—make required changes—through statute, policy, delivery of services through the MFRS.

4. The military chain of command must be trained on the importance of family resilience and well-being and its impact on the mission. Too often, they are only focused on the mission to be executed and not fully immersed in the human capital toll.

   - This topic and the available resources to help every echelon of leadership support family resilience and well-being needs to be added to military leadership training curricula.
   - Include military family support requirements as one of the appendices in the military battle plan so efforts will not be sidelined.

5. When developing policy and operational guidelines for the DoD:

   - Identify the core needs to embed into policy.
     - What is needed during contingencies.
     - What is needed during peacetime.

   - There should be ongoing dialogue with the military services with regard to needs assessment, addressing gaps in services; standardization of programs and resources.
   - Ensure oversight that policies are followed, are practiced, and refined when needed.
   - Establish and maintain collaborative relationships, working groups, task forces, across disciplines—everyone must be fluid and responsive.
   - We must address the roles of OSD and the military services and determine the core missions which need a driving focus for delivery, e.g., PFAC and each party's role and responsibilities.

6. Establish a system of ongoing professional development for service providers both internal to DoD and those in local communities, across disciplines to ensure their proficiency and knowledge when working with military families.

   - Expand the Military Family Learning Network to other communities of practice. (https: militaryfamilies.extension.org)
   - Ensure professional development is offered virtually with CEUs.

7. Depending on the particular upheaval, there will be special populations who will need a more intense level of support:

   - Young adults who sustain catastrophic injuries, e.g., Military Severely Injured Center.
   - Special operators who are older and experience more dangerous deployments on a more recurring basis.
   - Families with young children and children with special needs, e.g., respite care.
   - Surviving family members.
   - Reserve component members and their families not near installation-based support, e.g., JFSAP.
   - Populations newly identified—how do we adapt and be flexible to meet their needs?

8. To overcome the lack of alacrity of the federal bureaucracy and for early identification of the gaps in services:

   - Develop sustained relationships with vetted nonprofit agencies so their ongoing work during peacetime can be ramped up and incorporated into the larger MFRS.
   - Expand internal efforts to build partnerships, remembering the centrality of family.

9. Government systems are constrained so the ability to react quickly to an unknown event can be hampered by the stove piped organizations within a federal agency as well as across the federal landscape. (For additional information, please review Chaps. 1 and 19 in current volume)

3.8 Recommendations

Defense departments and military academies around the world are renowned for their contingency planning; teaching strategy and tactical maneuvers to ensure a successful mission outcome; and analyzing military historical documents to build on experience and lessons learned to be prepared to overcome unforeseen challenges. Family support professionals need to apply these same principles to family support courses of action with a thorough review and analysis of the results from multiple summits, task forces, convenings, Reports to Congress, research, etc.—the battle plan next steps are all there, but not in any organized fashion. This wealth of information was not available when post-9/11 conflicts began and expanded. And, when an event that shakes family stability to its core is underway, there is no time to sift through a compendium of source documents to build on lessons learned or to revise policies. Action is needed to deliver resources and services that meet the needs of families undergoing tremendous stress. It is imperative to glean insights and counsel now since the U.S. Military continues operations in Iraq and Afghanistan—this conflict is not over. And, we must continue to review, modify, and enhance this knowledge base to be better prepared to enact a battle plan regardless of the challenges the next event brings to the family support community. What better way than to take the lessons learned outlined in this chapter and prioritize the courses of action listed to address what were the gaps when approaching the development of a Battle Plan?

In addition to the ongoing efforts to embed the courses of action outlined in the Lesson Learned section into practice, the following ideas are just gaining attention for further dissemination:

- Given what we are learning about Adverse Childhood Experiences (ACEs), the earlier we can identify service members who have had ACEs during their formative years, support can be provided to prevent additional trauma due to military stress to maintain their resilience and to protect their families. In addition, military children need to be screened for ACEs during their regular pediatric visits to ensure families are given the support in real time so that children can reach their full potential.

- Embed the Thrive parenting curriculum into the fabric of the MFRS—parents need the tools and knowledge to meet their children's developmental potential. It is particularly important to fully engage the service member in his or her role as a parent and not rely solely on the stay-at-home parent since children will fare better when parents are in sync with their parenting styles and goals for their children. Facilitators can be groomed across the MFRS—in pediatric clinics, New Parent Support staff, training and curriculum specialists at the child development center, staff at the family support centers, school personnel, and volunteers can all make a difference.
- Ensure all echelons of military leadership are trained on the impact military family members have on mission readiness; what resources are in leadership's "toolbox" to help service members meet the needs of their family members; their role in identifying gaps in services; what the MFRS is and who to contact for support; and how to manage expectations in times of unusual stress.
- Garner support from the current Congress and the White House, building off the success of Joining Forces and the PSD-9.
- Build on what we know that supports the development of strong family functioning/resilience into the programs offered in the MFRS so families are better prepared to meet the challenges of every day military life.

3.9 Reflection

Reflecting on what we will need to take into the future, we have a responsibility to our senior leaders to ensure they have the most accurate information and analyses from both OSD and the military services when making decisions regarding family support services, irrespective of who delivers subject services. Senior leaders need to question and listen to their subject matter experts and colleagues from both OSD and the military services before services are ramped up or curtailed. A primary example of failure to do so is the closure of the Military Severely Injured Center under the false assumption that the military services had "stepped up" their support for WII service members and their families. No analyses were done to assess the viability of four separate support programs. And, the need for an umbrella program, such as the Military Severely Injured Center, to catch those who may not be served through the delivery of their particular services' program, was ignored. We can no longer look at military family support in isolation—what we do impacts the larger military community. Since the military is becoming a smaller, leaner joint force, as directed in the 2012 Defense Strategic Guidance, all entities—the military services, OSD, the federal government, and community resources—must be in sync, collaborating, and not duplicating efforts.

Since 2001, there were many battles fought, not just in Iraq and Afghanistan, but within the Personnel and Readiness community and with the military services.

Without a doubt, stovepipes hurt the delivery of family support. Who is responsible for service member and family well-being—the particular Military Service or OSD or both? Who owns policy and who owns operations—OSD or the military services or both? Why are there differences in services and resources between the military services and between components? Many years of mistrust and role clarity had to be overcome because there was much to do and that will continue in the future. Keeping family well-being in the forefront of many competing priorities within the DoD will take a concerted, unified, multidisciplinary, and cross-sector approach to be successful. Hopefully, cooperation and collaboration among family support entities will continue to prosper within OSD, the military services, the federal government, and community agencies to become the standard modus operandi during peacetime which will offset the turbulence generated during times of conflict.

True leadership is not about receiving credit for what has been accomplished, but building coalitions and supporting relationships to efficiently and effectively meet the mission. Ultimately, it takes many dedicated individuals and systems to maintain ongoing communication and to synergize their efforts to connect the right resource to the right person at the right time.

3.10 Conclusion

After Operation Desert Storm—Frederick F.Y. Pang, Assistant Secretary of Defense for Force Management Policy, testified that, "The cycle of war, drawdown, mobilization and war repeated throughout this century has taught us that:

1. It is difficult to accurately foresee emerging threats to our national security.
2. Our military must always be ready to fight and win the next war, and therefore deter it.
3. Our people are our most important resource, and if we support them in peacetime as we have in wartime, they will perform with excellence and valor when called to protect our national interests" (Pang, 1995, p. 11).

Secretary Pang's insights are well worth remembering today as America considers its commitments to the military community in the wake of war since 2001 and helps prepare for the ramifications of the next violent conflict.

References

Flake, E. M., Davis, B. E., Johnson, P. L., & Middleton, L. S. (2009). The psychosocial effects of deployment on military children. *Journal of Developmental & Behavioral Pediatrics, 30*(4), 271–278.

Huebner, A. J., Mancini, J. A., Wilcox, R. M., Grass, S. R., & Grass, G. A. (2007). Parental deployment and youth in military families: Exploring uncertainty and ambiguous loss. *Family Relations, 56*(2), 112–122. https://doi.org/10.1111/j.1741-3729.2007.00445.x.

Office of the President. (2011). *Strengthening our military families: Meeting America's commitment.* Presidential Study Directive 9. Washington DC: Office of the President. Retrieved May 1, 2017, from http://www.militaryonesource.mil/footer?content_id=279111

Office of the Secretary of Defense. (2003). *Response to the Terrorist Attack on the Pentagon: Pentagon Family Assistance Center (PFAC) After Action Report.* Retrieved June 29, 2017, from militaryonesource.mil/12038/MOS/Reports/Crisis%20Report-new.indd.pdf

Pang, F. (1995). *Testimony to Senate Committee on Armed Services Subcommittee on Manpower and Personnel, March 16.* Retrieved from https://archive.org/stream/departmentofdefe061996unit#page/n5/mode/2up/search/The+cycle+of+war%2C+drawdown%2C+mobilization

Riggs, S. A., & Riggs, D. S. (2011). Risk and resilience in military families experiencing deployment: The role of the family attachment network. *Journal of Family Psychology, 25*(5), 675–687. https://doi.org/10.1037/a0025286.

Resources

The 1st, 2nd, and 3rd Quadrennial of Quality Life Reviews. Retrieved from http://www.militaryonesource.mil/footer?content_id=279112.

Military Family Readiness Reports to Congress. Retrieved from http://www.militaryonesource.mil/footer?content_id=279106.

Chapter 4
National Guard Service Member and Family Readiness After Action Review: Lessons Learned and a Way Forward

Anthony A. Wickham and Mary Lowe Mayhugh

4.1 Background

An era of persistent global conflict after 9/11 resulted in the nation's heavy reliance on the National Guard to meet National Security Requirements. Most policies and programs, however, were last updated in the 1980s, which created significant friction points in the effective execution of deploying and integrating units and overall levels of service member and family readiness in the Reserve Components. This necessitated massive changes and attention in how the services and the National Guard resourced and supported readiness programs for military families. In order to improve systems and access to programs, the National Guard, in conjunction with the Army and the Air Force, developed the Family Readiness Program to promote readiness, quality of life, and the resilience of military families. These programs specifically focused on education, wellness, communication, resource allocation, and community collaboration.

The National Guard Family Readiness Program is now central to providing services for service members and their families during mobilizations, deployments, and steady-state operations. The dispersion of National Guard armories across the country provides a national network to support community collaboration efforts and execution of service-based support programs and services.

Between 2001 and 2014, approximately 50,000 nonprofit organizations were established to respond to meet the demand for services stemming from the multiple deployments of service members (Carter & Kidder, 2015). Support came in many forms, including monetary donations, millions of volunteer hours, and physical donations of comfort items. Conversations at the national, state, and local levels focused on concerns about program effectiveness and return on investment. Each

A.A. Wickham (✉) • M.L. Mayhugh
J1 Programs, National Guard Bureau, Arlington, VA, USA
e-mail: anthony.a.wickham.civ@mail.mil

© Springer International Publishing AG 2018
L. Hughes-Kirchubel et al. (eds.), *A Battle Plan for Supporting Military Families*, Risk and Resilience in Military and Veteran Families, https://doi.org/10.1007/978-3-319-68984-5_4

state worked to develop a process to ensure enduring, quality programs were in place to respond to the need of service members, veterans and their families (SMVF).

The National Guard Bureau (NGB) recognized early on the importance of garnering the support of communities to serve all SMVF, especially the 1.3 million who are geographically dispersed (Brown et al., 2015). The National Guard strengthened existing local, state, and national collaboration efforts and developed these partnerships. They collaborated with other governmental agencies and nongovernmental organizations to establish new partnerships that respond to the needs of service members and their families. The National Guard brings an element of community involvement unique from other service or branch based on the Adjutant General's role as the head of the state Department of Military Affairs. The Guard is in every state and territory, including those states without an active duty installation (i.e., Iowa, Michigan, New Hampshire, Oregon, Vermont). NGB continually developed these platforms as a result of unmet needs as the Reserve Components transitioned from a strategic to an operational force. These platforms provide access points that have connections with other federal/DoD organizations, military services, state/local governments, and non-governmental organizations. Subsequently, a new initiative titled Joining Community Forces (JCF) was established to formalize grassroot collaboration efforts and establish them into cohesive geographically based support networks.

4.2   History and Key Events

4.2.1   Stretching Legacy Programs, 2001–2003

In 2001, the family program in each state consisted of one state family program director and one family readiness resource assistant. Volunteers augmented these offices. Families were expected to be resilient and find needed resources. Limited, unstructured support was provided by unit volunteer-based family support groups. Many of the unit-based family support groups, however, did not have the experience to deal with the challenges of deployments and quickly became overwhelmed with the caseload after 9/11.

Deployments in the National Guard skyrocketed from 13,829 personnel in Fiscal Year 2001 (FY01) to more than 46,400 in FY02, and further to more than 95,400 in FY03. Most units had not deployed overseas since the 90s during Operation Desert Storm. These large deployments created a significant amount of stress on peacetime response systems. Families were directly impacted and drove the need at the state and unit level for assistance to address physical and behavioral health, relationship, legal, financial, and many other support challenges.

The groundswell of support from local businesses, corporations, foundations, and individuals also created numerous challenges. Tracking federal, state, and local resources and support services tested the abilities of small staffs to keep information accurate and timely. New requirements evolved, requiring the National Guard to evaluate numerous offerings to ensure the goods and services were sustainable and meeting the needs of SMVFs. This created a need to develop manageable networks encompassing diverse groups, with different and at times opposing agendas.

The National Guard Bureau reassessed current response systems and, as a result, expanded existing programs and implemented several new initiatives focused more heavily on the Reserve Component and geographically dispersed Active Component Service members and families. These programs included Family assistance centers, airman and family readiness program managers, child and youth coordinators, family readiness program assistants, deployment cycle support coordinators, air wing integrators, expanded chaplains' offices, Strong Bonds (a marriage enrichment program usually implemented by Chaplains), transition assistance advisors, directors of psychological health, survivor outreach support coordinators, state resiliency coordinators, military funeral and honors officials, Yellow Ribbon Reintegration Program, Wounded Warrior Care services, and Employer/Employment Support. States also created Inter-Service Family Assistance Committees (ISFACs), which served to improve community collaboration and focus resources. As states identified gaps in resources or support, many created statewide councils, foundations, and programs to identify resources and organize support efforts.

4.2.2   Finding and Filling Gaps, 2004–2007

Deployments continued to increase; the National Guard deployed more than 95,800 personnel in FY04, over 111,500 in FY05 and deployments remained above 40,000 through FY07. Multiple deployments began to create additional unit challenges, including employment assistance for returning service members. The turbulence of deployments generated emerging challenges in the areas of employment and children struggling in school.

National Guard leaders and service members' relationships with employers strained due to unpredictable schedules and changes to deployment plans. Curtailments, deletions, and/or re-missioning further impacted training, strained resources (time, money), and increased unit level turbulence for military members, families, and employers. Families and employers planned well in advance to support deployments; however, many had to respond to last minute date changes. These changes left employers either having staffing gaps or personnel overages because of temporary hires.

Unemployment, especially among first term service members, typically 18- to 24-year-olds, was a shortfall that not previously experienced. This created an emerging trend of underemployment for service members and transitioning veterans. A substantial number of service members return from deployment better qualified, but often to jobs with comparatively much lower responsibilities and pay. Many states instituted employment programs such as South Carolina's Palmetto Employment to organize employment seminars and hiring events necessary to address increasing unemployment rates. Their efforts resulted in a reduction of service member unemployment nationally from 12.1% in 2011 to 9.0% in 2013 (Bureau of Labor Statistics, 2014).

States reported that local schools also struggled with issues raised by deployed service members' children. In response to numerous National Guard Children becoming "Suddenly Military" with the deployment of a parent, the National Guard teamed with the Military Child Education Coalition (MCEC) to conduct regional training sessions for school administrators, principals, and counselors. The training of local school administrations focused on how to properly deal with the challenges faced by children of deployed service members.

4.2.3   Covering New Challenges, 2008–2011

Surges in both Iraq and Afghanistan increased the number of unit deployments, subsequently reducing dwell time (time between deployments) to 2 years for many high demand units. National Guard mobilized 61,228 service members in FY08, 62,147 in FY09, 57,505 in FY10, and 45,269 in FY11. Abbreviated dwell time between these deployments degraded reintegration periods between deployments, especially for families. The surge period took a toll on service members, families, and employers due to perceived and real lack of predictability and insufficient time for reintegration, planning, and transition back into the community.

States identified a need to provide more in-depth behavioral health support and instituted an overall resiliency that included families. NGB partnered with the US Public Health Service and is assigned a colonel level, career Public Health Service Officer to implement a comprehensive national level program to address the mounting case load level. The officer executes a national contract to resource all the states and territories with a Psychological Health Adviser(s). During this time, National Guard behavioral health professionals served over 94,000 service members through group education and information venues and acted as Subject Matter Experts to State senior leaders and commanders, medical personnel, and Family Program staffs. They also provided more than 24,120 consultations to service members and families in need.

Service members and support networks were faced with new challenges because of the length of the conflict, resources needed for those with multiple deployments, and the necessity to build a resilient force. The National Guard formalized resiliency training both within units and for Family Program staff members.

4.2.4   Maintaining and Honing Outreach, 2012–2015

As overseas deployments and mobilizations decreased to about 21,200 in FY13, 15,032 in FY14 and then to about 8,300 in FY15, DoD identified requirement to sustain and in some instances expand family support programs. The 2014 Quadrennial Defense Review states, "America … will care for our men and women in uniform and their families - both during and after their service" (Office of the Secretary of

Defense, 2014, p. 48). Likewise, the Chairman of the Joint Chiefs of Staff (CJCS) Second Term Strategic Direction to the Joint Force "Keeping Faith with Our Military Families," stated: "We must keep faith with our military families. They must know that their sons, daughters, fathers, mothers, brothers, and sisters will be the best led, trained, equipped, and ready force in the world. They will never be sent into harm's way without the full preparedness and support of this Nation" (Warrior and Family Support Office, 2012, p. 4). Outcome-based metrics solidified those programs that were making positive impacts for geographically dispersed families.

Research identified further gaps in the Active Duty installation support network. A 2015 Rand study titled "Access to Behavioral Health for Geographically Remote Service members and Dependents in the U.S." used geospatial analysis to determine that there are over 1.3 million currently serving service members and families beyond a 30-minute travel time of an Active Duty Military Treatment Facility (Brown et al., 2015). Base Realignment and Closure Programs and reductions in availability of on post housing resulted in more service members and families residing off of Active Component installations. In 2015, OSD reported that 68% of service members resided off of installations (Office of the Deputy Under Secretary of Defense, Installations and Environment, 2017). This created challenges for service members and families accessing programs and services on the installation. Further, Army Command Policy, AR 600–20, states, "The NGB is the Army's lead agency for the establishment and execution of Family assistance for Total Army Families at all levels of contingency and mobilization" (Department of the Army, 2014, p. 51), further substantiating the need for new methods of community-based service delivery models, such as JCF.

The National Guard identified the need for a more integrated approach to support geographically dispersed families. Former National Guard Bureau Chief General Craig McKinley initiated the NGB Joining Community Forces (JCF) program in 2012 to meet outreach requirements outlined in Department of Defense (DoD) policies (Department of Defense 2012). NGB defines JCF as "a communication initiative focused on grassroots providing direct, tailored support to service members, veterans, and families." The overarching purpose of JCF is to encourage governmental, non-governmental, businesses and nonprofits to collaborate within each state to support veterans, service members, and their families. The goal is to create a "no wrong door" network of support at the state and community levels.

4.3 Responses and Strategies

4.3.1 National Guard Programs Supporting Families

As deployments continued and program gaps were identified, the National Guard implemented a series of support programs and community collaborative efforts to improve and maintain the readiness of geographically dispersed military families. These ranged from information and referral to reintegration support and covered the entire military life-cycle from assessment to funeral honors.

Family Assistance. The keystones of readiness support to families are the Army National Guard Family Assistance Center specialists, and the Air National Guard Airman and Family Readiness Program managers. These family readiness access points are located throughout each state. Their mission is to provide information, referral and follow-up to service members, their dependents, and veterans. Family Assistance Centers are located in armories throughout each state, and Air National Guard Airman and Family Readiness Program Offices are located at each Air National Guard Wing. This concept works well, because these offices were able to coordinate many existing resources in the states to provide assistance in the numerous areas that families needed during the deployment cycles.

The Family Readiness Support Assistant (FRSA) Program for the Army began in 2003 to address family readiness in times of mobilization and deployments. The stress of deployments on existing resources, coupled with fewer volunteers, drove the need for developing a FRSA services program. The FRSA's main role is to provide the Commander or Rear Detachment Commander (RDC), the Family Readiness Liaison (FRL), and Family Readiness Group (FRG) leader with administrative assistance in support of family readiness programs and activities. FRSAs also worked closely with the Family Assistance Centers to provide appropriate referrals for unit leaders and family members. In addition, Army National Guard (ARNG) FRSAs provide critical volunteer management and resilience training to ARNG family members and volunteers, such as Comprehensive Soldier & Family Fitness Resilience Training. In 2007, the FRSA Program was expanded to reach more Army Commands in all three components, Active, Army Reserve, and National Guard.

In 2005, the Army National Guard hired Child and Youth Program Coordinators to promote and sustain the quality of life and resilience of National Guard children by providing secure, timely, flexible, and high-quality support services and enrichment programs. Youth Programs also promote individual leader development, resulting in more resilient youth. By 2015, Child and Youth programs served 66,055 military children and youth. These numbers included children from all components and services, including Active Duty military and the Coast Guard.

Between 2008 and 2012, more than 1.4 million National Guard and Reserve service members and their families benefited from the deployment cycle information, resources, programs, services, and referrals offered by the Yellow Ribbon Reintegration Program. The Yellow Ribbon Program was instrumental with ensuring service members and their families were prepared and supported throughout deployments.

Relationship issues also became a major concern for returning service members. In 2004, the US Code was amended to allow command funding for "chaplain corps-led programs to assist members of the armed forces … in building and maintaining a strong family structure" (Title 10, ~1789). The Strong Bonds program seeks to strengthen relationships between married service members and their families and provides assistance for single service members. The Active Army completed the third year of a five-year longitudinal study evaluating the outcomes of the Strong Bonds training program. Preliminary outcomes show a 50% lower rate in divorce and an increase in marital satisfaction for participants. There were 250 Strong Bonds events conducted in FY15 serving 8,832 service and family members.

Veterans' issues began to surface for returning service members as they demobilized and sought to obtain medical assistance from the Department of Veterans Affairs (VA). As a result, Congress authorized additional funding to establish state Transition Assistance Advisors (TAA). These personnel help service members access employment, relocation, health care, behavioral health care, health and life insurance, financial assistance, career change, education and training, VA benefits, and disabled veteran benefits. In FY15 alone, the TAA Program resulted in 3915 Veteran Health Administration (VHA) enrollments, 14,720 VHA referrals, 16,112 Veteran Benefits Administration referrals, 7817 Veteran Center referrals, and over 28,000 referrals to other agencies.

As casualties increased, it became increasingly difficult to provide long-term support to the families of our fallen service members from installation-based locations. Consistency through the Casualty Assistance Officer (CAO) system was not only challenged by the amount of casualties, but also by the dispersion of survivors due to Reserve Component deployments. In 2005, the Army established Survivor Outreach Service (SoS) Coordinators throughout the nation to provide numerous services to families of the fallen. SoS Coordinators provided support to 43,000 surviving family members in FY15.

Public Law 106–65 requires that every eligible veteran receive a military funeral honors ceremony upon the family's request. In 2006, the Military Funeral and Honors program began providing the ceremonial paying of respect and the final demonstration of the country's gratitude to those who, in times of war and peace, have faithfully defended our nation. In FY14, the Army National Guard rendered services at 125,000 funerals for fallen comrades. Overall, in FY14 the Army National Guard supported 85% of the Department of the Army and 52% of DoD funeral honor requirements.

4.3.2   *Joining Community Forces (JCF)*

Joining Community Forces supports a "no wrong door," holistic approach to provide referral, resources, and programs to our SMVFs in their communities, leveraging the impact of community-based resources. JCF provides:

- An integrated outreach system which focuses on geographically dispersed SMVFs
- A nested platform to coordinate and communicate public and private sector initiatives that support readiness, wellness, and resiliency
- A cohesive community centric solution, allowing national, regional, state, and local entities to provide timely and effective support to SMVFs in the communities where they live

Many states found the best success with their JCF efforts when they leveraged the governor's office to establish legislation and state agency leads. Further analysis uncovered the need for a state coordinator. Program leads included but are not limited to the State National Guard Joint Force Headquarters, the state Veterans Affairs office and in some cases nonprofit organizations. Most legislation included service standards and outcome guidance. Many states created JCF Advisory Boards at both the state and community level. Board membership included state agencies, non-governmental, business and nonprofit organizations representing programs aimed at improving employment opportunities, education, and wellness.

Through the JCF initiative, the National Guard integrates a web of support for Reserve and Active Duty service members and their families who live outside the active duty installation catchment areas. JCF links service members, veterans, and their families to federal, state, and community-based resources through a framework of assistance centers in local communities and the National Guard Bureau website. The newly developed Service Provider Network provides a map of nearby assets that support our military families at: http://www.joiningcommunity-forces.org/spn.

4.3.3   Corporation for National Community Service (CNCS) and National Guard Bureau Partnership

At the national level, the Corporation for National Community Service (CNCS) established a partnership with the NGB providing Volunteers in Service to America (VISTAs) in support of the JCF collaboration efforts. CNCS provided enough VISTA personnel authorizations for each state to request VISTA support. These assets are still available by request and are no cost to the National Guard. The VISTA personnel and other volunteers (not directly assigned in any capacity to the military) can discuss veteran, service member, and family needs with nonprofit and other organizations.

States reported predominantly positive experiences with the VISTA program and were instrumental in the expansion of JCF and Land Grant programs. Some states used a third party such as the American Legion Auxiliary to assist with writing grant proposals needed to request VISTA personnel. The VISTA personnel (all college graduates) provided quality support and build local relationships needed to expand services provided by the State NG Family Program Offices. Some states experienced difficultly in funding the travel and emergency funding ($500) per VISTA. Many states used their 501(c)3 relationships to cover this refundable cost. As federal and state budgets decrease, the value of VISTA personnel increases, and they significantly benefit the states.

4.3.4   State-Established 501(c)3 Nonprofit Organizations

After 9/11, many corporations, businesses, communities, and individual donors reached out to governors' offices and the state National Guard Headquarters to see how they could support deployed service members. Offerings included monetary contributions, products and services and volunteer hours to support those in need. Subsequently, many states established nonprofit 501(c)3 organizations in order to receive direct support on behalf of their service members and families. Some states established new 501(c)3 organizations for the specific purpose of providing direct support to service members and their families while others partnered with existing nonprofit organizations to accomplish the same goal. Creating nonprofit entities (partnerships) within a state allowed interested parties to engage, thus eliminating any need for solicitation.

Many states did not establish a nonprofit 501(c)3 or partner directly with an existing organization. Some states struggled with relinquishing direct ownership and authority determining how their members would receive support. Many states addressed or mitigated this issue by including former service members on the nonprofit advisory board. Others decided their best option was to provide support solely through community engagement, collaboration, and partnerships in-lieu-of the establishment of a new nonprofit organization. Nonprofits can be established toward assisting the military in several areas such as youth and family programs to include scholarships and youth camps, patriotic projects that perpetuate the memory of our deceased veterans, emergency relief funds, and professional training classes.

4.3.5   Family Program Accreditation

There was also a need for family program standardization and delivery consistency regardless of state or location. Subsequently, the Office of Secretary Defense, Military Community and Family Policy, funded the State National Guard Family Program Offices across the 54 states, territories and the District of Columbia to achieve international accreditation standards by the Council on Accreditation. The three primary areas accredited were administration and management, service delivery/administration, and service standards to members. This accreditation process established international standards ensuring the same level of support no matter where a veteran, service member, or family member accessed the "system."

4.3.6   Collaboration

At the national level, "White Oak" meetings began in 2010 with the purpose of bringing together government agencies and national leaders to focus on cross-sector, multi-organizational solutions for military families and recent veterans. Other initiatives include but are not limited to SAMHSA Policy Academies, USDA's

4H programs, USDA's extension offices, Community Blue Print, VA's Veteran Economic Community Initiative (VECI), etc. Reductions in appropriations will place demand on government agencies to increase collaboration and partnerships and to identify efficiencies.

4.4 Evaluation and Results

4.4.1 Yellow Ribbon Reintegration

90-day Window Proved Too Long

Early in the deployment cycle, initial OSD guidance to the states was that service members should be allowed to readjust back to their families and communities without being contacted by their unit for the first 90 days. Lamentably, states found that service members challenged with reintegration problems were involved in some sort of crisis (foreclosures, loss of job, domestic violence, divorce) prior to the 90 day mark. With enough evidence, OSD changed the policy leading to changes in Yellow Ribbon guidance, notably to conduct the first reintegration event at the 45-day window after their return. This change enabled the chain of command to better identify service members who needed resources and get them assistance.

Yellow Ribbon Events for Service Members Who Have Had Multiple Deployments

Service members undergoing multiple deployments initially had to attend the entire Yellow Ribbon briefing cycle, including veteran benefits and other items as they returned from each deployment. Feedback from the service members led to changes in guidance. These service members attended an abbreviated event that provided them specific information which was more relevant to the issues they were facing with deployments.

4.4.2 Continued Need for Assets in the States

The Army National Guard G1 gathers monthly metric data from their Family Assistance Centers across the USA in support of an annual DoD report on the Family Readiness System. The data below highlights the volume by service branch that the Family Assistance Centers provided support of remote military members and their families, regardless of service.

In addition, geographically dispersed service members and families have found they can rely on National Guard Family Assistance Centers for information and

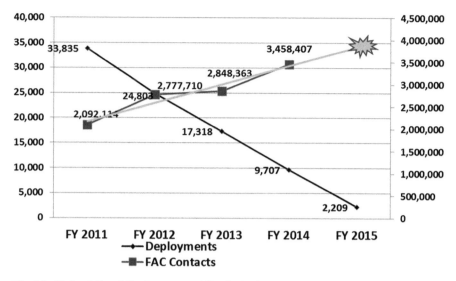

Fig. 4.1   National Guard Deployments and Family Assistance Center Contacts

Table 4.1   Army National Guard Family Assistance Center Quick Tracker Contacts

	FY11	FY12	FY13	FY14
Air Force	17,398	26,866	29,645	30,750
Army	2,056,864	2,720,348	2,768,119	3,372,680
Coast Guard	690	3209	3597	4983
Marine Corps	5841	15,217	23,656	20,776
Navy	11,035	12,017	20,450	29,162
Veterans	64,665	85,583	103,751	122,290
Total:	2,156,493	2,863,240	2,949,218	3,580,641

referral. Even as deployments continue to reduce, Family Assistance Center contacts continue to increase (see Fig. 4.1 and Table 4.1). These differences are attributed to families identifying Family Assistance Centers as effective entry points to local networks of support for a variety of needs.

4.5   Lessons Learned

4.5.1   Maintaining Support Systems

The challenges experienced by military families caused the National Guard to develop networks at the federal, state, and local community level. Integrated networks provide a baseline of support allowing families to prepare for future deployments and the nation to continue to rely on an all-volunteer force. Budgetary pressure from sequestration and a general reduction in funding threatens this network. The Yellow Ribbon Reintegration Program has shown the National Guard that systems can be modified, but should not be eliminated.

4.5.2   Physical Sites Support the Geographically Dispersed

While Military One Source and Army One Source provide valuable services to service members and families, neither service provides the high touch skills required to develop long-term local therapeutic relationships with the vast number of local communities throughout the nation. In many instances, Military One Source and Army One Source refer SMVFs to the network of local FACs for support. An organization called Veterans Community Connections concluded, based on a 2015 San Diego Chamber of Commerce study of returning veterans, "Respondents overwhelmingly reported that current online or web-based resources do not provide them and their family enough personal information to meet their needs in transitioning from military to civilian life" (Veterans Community Connections, 2015, p. 3). FACs are also the primary resource for identifying community-based resources that support the Military One Source Community Directory.

4.5.3   SAMHSA Policy Academies Were High-Return Events

SAMHSA hosted policy academies for almost all states. These academies often were the launching points for states to form statewide coalitions addressing veteran and military family issues. State National Guards sent senior decision makers, often the Adjutants General themselves, to these events. SAMHSA has since hosted implementation academies to assist states in following up on their initiatives. We firmly believe this is a definitive best practice that should be used in the future.

4.5.4   Partnership Integration Was an Ongoing Process

With the multitude of nonprofits and other organizations operating in the family program lane, the National Guard at the national and state level continue to identify new partners to improve and expand resources or address gaps for military families. These relationships continue to develop over time as organizations learn each other's capabilities. Personnel turnover and changing needs of the population emphasize the need to maintain network relationships over the long term and to routinely communicate program information necessary to provide the right services at the right time.

No single agency, non-governmental organization (NGO), or private organization has the full manpower, resources, and authority to provide support service to all veterans, service members, and their families. As Sloan Gibson, the Deputy

Secretary of the VA said in May, 2015 at the Warrior Community Integration Symposium in Augusta: "…if I'm partnering with the right people and the right organization, and I focus on what my partner needs while we're working to serve those who have served us, the world is our oyster. We can accomplish anything" (Gibson, 2015).

4.5.5 *Centralized Support Structure with Decentralized Execution of Services Provides a More Efficient and Economic Delivery of Services*

States are in a position to allocate resources where they determine they have the most impact. In addition, state Family Program Directors provided oversight and provided state-level organization for the overall Family Support Program. Each state organized the assets differently to meet the unique needs to their particular physical, political, and demographic situation. These best practices were then shared among the states through the National Guard Joining Community Forces platform.

4.6 Recommendations

4.6.1 *Maintain Budgetary Funding Levels for National Guard Family Support Programs*

Continued reductions in forces will place high demand on the readiness of the Reserve Component. The National Guard continues to recruit service members to meet these demands but also realizes the need to retain families. Currently funded programs are needed to provide a baseline of support. However, repeated Congressional continuing resolutions impact reliable funding sources and timely letting of contracts. This affects program delivery and impacts the level of trust that geographically dispersed families place in the reliability and sustainability of these programs.

4.6.2 *Federal Statutory Authority for National Guard to Conduct Outreach to Maintain Networks of Support for the Geographically Dispersed*

No DoD organization is designated as the lead agency to develop support networks to reach geographically dispersed service members and families. The National Guard is uniquely positioned to lead best practice efforts such as JCF. Best practices should be used to create a nationwide concept for developing these networks.

4.6.3   Continued Funding of Accreditation

Accreditation provides a method to validate that National Guard programs are effective in meeting their goals. It also provides a methodology to maintain the professionalism of National Guard family program personnel. This is a low cost, high payoff methodology for ensuring that funds expended are being used to support our military families.

4.6.4   Simplify Methodology for Public/Private Partnerships

The National Security Strategy validates the importance of public/private partnerships. DoD, however, lacks specific regulations and guidance focused on developing said partnerships. This approach is not conducive to encouraging an organization to develop a public–private partnership. The VA recently developed an agencywide policy for public–private partnerships that passed the General Council's muster and appears to encourage personnel to further develop both national and local partnerships. This methodology should be analyzed and vetted for possible adoption by the DoD.

4.6.5   Continue to Expand upon Community-Based Programs

The success with which service members and their families are integrated into their civilian communities directly contributes to a sustainable, viable, all-volunteer force. Volunteerism is the American way of sustaining its military. Out of over 240 years, the United States has only relied on conscription for 35 of those to fill the ranks. Volunteering, raising a hand and taking an oath to support and defend the Constitution of the United States, is an American tradition, and a defining moment for everyone in the all-volunteer force. The willingness of the nation's daughters and sons to sustain this tradition is a direct reflection of how they see the free society—civilian communities and government-embracing veterans and their families upon their return from service.

The National Guard is the natural link between the military and our communities. Almost every state has a process to address military and veteran issues. These vary from state chartered nonprofits to collaborative counsels. DoD, however, lacks a formal policy to provide national/state oversight, strategic outreach, and identify performance measures and gauge relevant outcomes. A program such as JCF would provide policy, structure, branding, and consistency of services.

Possible goals for integrating these efforts might include:

– Provide policy, structure, branding, and consistency of services across the 54 states, territories, and DC.

- Analyze trends, eliminate gaps in programs, and improve local community awareness.
- Implement a "no wrong door approach" to improve access for geographically dispersed.

Leverage the "brick and mortar" system of armories to strengthen and add depth to programs and services.
Broaden reach of current White House, DoD, and Service Programs

- Foster a community network that is sustainable and relevant.

Facilitate governmental/non-governmental, nonprofit, corporate partners and local citizen collaboration.

Government at all levels must proactively participate in this construct by increasing access, sharing data and information, and finding ways to effectively partner with private sector. Several states have taken the lead as part of our Joining Community Forces outreach plan. Changing the transition outcomes for the returning veteran will come from better cross-sector coordination and not from the isolated intervention of individual organizations. Substantial progress can be made if nonprofits, state governments, businesses, and the public are brought together around this common core agenda. Cross-function collaboration will provide the horizontal integration necessary for a national, state, and local (level) no-wrong-door capacity… That remains our vision.

References

Bureau of Labor Statistics. (2014, March). *Unemployment rate for veterans edges down in 2013.* Retrieved from https://www.bls.gov/opub/ted/2014/ted_20140325.htm

Brown, R. A., Marshall, G. N., Breslau, J., Farris, C., Osilla, K. C., Pincus, H. A., Ruder, T., Voorhies, P., Barnes-Proby, D., Pfrommer, K., Miyashiro, L., Rana, R., & Adamson, D. A. (2015). *Access to behavioral health care for remote service members and their families.* Santa Monica, CA: RAND Corporation. Retrieved from https://www.rand.org/pubs/research_reports/RR578.html.

Carter, P., & Kidder, K. (2015). *Charting the sea of Goodwill.* Washington, DC: Center for a New American Security. Retrieved from https://www.cnas.org/publications/reports/charting-the-sea-of-goodwill.

Department of the Army. (2014). *Army Command Policy, AR600-20 6 Nov 14, 5-10.b.3.a* (p. 51). Washington, DC: Department of the Army. Retrieved from http://www.apd.army.mil/pdffiles/r600_20.pdf.

Department of Defense. (2012). Instruction (DoDI) 1342.22 "Military Family Readiness". Retrieved from www.esd.whs.mil/Portals/54/Documents/DD/issuances/dodi/134222p.pdf

Gibson, S. (2015). Remarks at the 2015 Warrior Community Integration Symposium, Augusta, Georgia. Retrieved from https://www.va.gov/opa/speeches/2015/05_22_2015.asp

Office of the Deputy Under Secretary of Defense, Installations and Environment. (2017). *Frequently asked questions.* Retrieved from http://www.acq.osd.mil/housing/faqs.htm#3

National Security Strategy. (2015). Retrieved from https://www.whitehouse.gov/sites/default/files/docs/2015_national_security_strategy.pdf

Office of the Secretary of Defense. (2014). *Quadrennial defense review*. Arlington, VA: Department of Defense. Retrieved from http://www.defense.gov/pubs/2014_Quadrennial_ Defense_Review.pdf.

Veterans Community Connection. (2015). *Supporting Research. Summary of Veterans Community Connections Study, conducted by Market Enhancement Group*. San Diego, CA: Veterans Community Connections. Retrieved from http://media.wix.com/ugd/dcdc77_45f18d3e84624 b1d833e4521826873d3.pdf.

Warrior and Family Support Office. (2012). *Keeping Faith with Our Military Families*. Arlington, VA: Office of the Chairman of the Joint Chiefs of Staff. Retrieved from http://www.jcs.mil/ Portals/36/Documents/CORe/Keeping_Faith_with_Our_Military_Family.pdf.

Chapter 5
Confluence: Merging Reintegration Streams for Veterans and Military Families

Jillian Bourque, Christopher Forsythe, Brian Gilman, Christian Johnson, Robin Johnson, Sean Jones, Michael Lawson, and Jason Schmidt

5.1   Introduction

Clausewitz, the iconic Prussian theorist, famously differentiated the unchanging nature of war from the changing character of warfare. He made the observation that certain elements—violence, uncertainty, chance, reason—are enduring, while other elements—tactics, techniques, technology, level of intensity—will vary from conflict to conflict. We make a similar observation about the challenges of veteran transition and reintegration. Some elements of transition and reintegration are enduring—uncertainty, difficulty of re-acculturating into civilian life—while other elements may change based on the veteran cohort—economic conditions, service delivery models, veteran educational level, changing veteran demographics, etc. Some veteran needs are universal while others are based on the unique situation of the individual veteran and his or her family.

Veteran reintegration is not a post-9/11 phenomenon. Since the Revolutionary War, American service members have returned to their homes, communities, and livelihoods once the fighting was over. Similarly, some elements of transition and reintegration are common to all conflicts while other elements may change based on

J. Bourque • C. Forsythe • C. Johnson (✉) • R. Johnson • M. Lawson
Department of Defense, US Army, The Pentagon, Washington, DC, USA
e-mail: jillian.r.bourque@us.army.mil; christopher.forsythe@us.army.mil;
christian.j.johnson@us.army.mil; robin.angela.johnson@us.army.mil;
michael.lawson1@us.army.mil

B. Gilman
Department of Defense, US Marine Corps, The Pentagon, Washington, DC, USA
e-mail: brian.gilman@usmc.mil

S. Jones • J. Schmidt
Department of Defense, US Air Force, The Pentagon, Washington, DC, USA
e-mail: sean.s.jones.1@us.af.mil; jason.schmidt.1@us.af.mil

© Springer International Publishing AG 2018
L. Hughes-Kirchubel et al. (eds.), *A Battle Plan for Supporting Military Families*, Risk and Resilience in Military and Veteran Families,
https://doi.org/10.1007/978-3-319-68984-5_5

the character of the conflict and the generation who participated in the conflict. Fortunately, many of today's veteran-serving organizations, nonprofits, and community service providers have made great strides recognizing that one size does not fit all when it comes to meeting the evolving needs of our veterans and their families. While most veteran issues can be categorized broadly into the "reintegration trinity"—employment, education, and well-being—it is important that stakeholders recognize the unchanging nature as well as the changing character of veteran reintegration. It is equally important that all stakeholders understand the imperatives for prioritizing veteran reintegration. First, America has a social contract to care for those, and their families, who have defended the nation. Second, there is a civic imperative; today's veterans not only represent talent for America's workforce that can help create a vibrant economy, but are civic assets that can help build strong communities for a vibrant society. Finally, prioritizing veteran reintegration helps to sustain the all-volunteer force. Since its inception in 1973, when President Nixon ended the draft, the all-volunteer force has been America's qualitative military edge. It is not the advanced technology or the exceptional training that makes America's military the best in the world, it is the quality of the professionals that make up the all-volunteer force. It is, therefore, a national security imperative to sustain the all-volunteer force. By focusing on veteran reintegration today, we will inspire future generations to volunteer for military service.[1]

Over the last few years, the authors of this white paper have collaborated with veteran-serving organizations, community service providers, thought leaders, and other stakeholders in every corner of the country, from small communities to our nation's largest cities. We have observed public, private, and nonprofit efforts that have brought our nation near an inflection point: a confluence of collective efforts of the government, private, nonprofit, and philanthropic sectors that has created sustained momentum in the veteran space. Take, for instance, the 2015 Department of Labor report of historic lows for veteran unemployment rates, to include the post-9/11 cohort of veterans (Department of Labor, Bureau of Labor Statistics, 2016). This is a positive indicator of the efficacy of collective action among stakeholders in the veteran space, although the recent economic upturn is also relevant.

---

[1] The terms "reintegration trinity" and "well-being" are used broadly here; the authors fully acknowledge the complex nature of veteran reintegration and understand that veteran needs do not always fit neatly into these three categories. Generally, well-being elements include career, community, financial, physical, and social. For a good examination of the multidimensional nature of veteran wellness as it relates to successful reintegration, see, for instance, Berglass, N. and M. C. Harrell, *Well After Service: Veteran Reintegration and American Communities*, 2012; Schell, T. L. and T. Tanielian [Eds.], *A Needs Assessment of New York State Veterans: Final Report to the New York State Health Foundation*, 2011; and Werber, L., A.G. Schaefer, K.C. Osilla, E. Wilke, A. Wong, J. Breslau, and K.E. Kitchens, *Support for the twenty-first Century Reserve Force: Insights on Facilitating Successful Reintegration for Citizen Warriors and Their Families* [Santa Monica, Calif.: RAND Corporation, 2013]. For additional sources of veteran reintegration literature, visit University of Southern California's Center for Innovation and Research on Veterans and Military Families, http://cir.usc.edu/publications (accessed 19 April 2016); and Purdue University's Military Family Research Institute, https://www.mfri.purdue.edu/publications/reports.aspx (accessed 19 April 2016).

As we approach this change in the environment, now is the time to identify long-term goals to sustain the momentum. There is still much work ahead, as more than 200,000 veterans will continue to transition to civilian communities annually for at least the next 5 years. We do believe, however, that we are nearing an important inflection point where we have achieved sustainable momentum that ensures the "Sea of Goodwill" does not turn into an "ocean of apathy" (Carter, 2012, p. 22). It appears the evolution of the veteran landscape mirrors other sectors marked by collective action. Indeed, multiple factors likely drive integration and consolidation in the veteran ecosystem—for example, competition for limited resources and the realization that organizations can increase their efficacy when they partner with and leverage the strengths of other organizations. In short, what we have seen from most stakeholders is encouraging and we are optimistic about the future with regard to reintegrating veterans and families back into civilian communities.

The purpose of this chapter is threefold: to briefly highlight some recent veterans' initiatives among the myriad stakeholders across the veteran space—in the government, private, and nonprofit sectors—that have set the conditions for an inflection point; to analyze recent trends; and to offer recommendations to help institutionalize the momentum achieved over the past several years. This chapter is not a roadmap that offers answers or a detailed way-ahead to the myriad transition and reintegration issues.[2] Simply, it is an opportunity to encourage continued dialogue about veteran reintegration issues. The impending inflection point makes this a good time to reassess the state of the veteran space based on our environmental scans across the country. This chapter also highlights some innovative examples on transition and reintegration efforts by veteran-serving organizations, nonprofits, community service providers, and other stakeholders. Although this chapter mainly focuses on initiatives that benefit members after they leave the military, we fully realize that successful veteran reintegration must start further upstream. Attention must be given across the continuum of service—from military service to transition to reintegration back into civil society; DoD's recent implementation of the Military Life Cycle acknowledges this fact. The chapter concludes by listing several recommendations to challenge stakeholders in the veteran space over the next 10 years.

5.2   Recent Initiatives: A Veteran-Centric Approach Begins to Take Shape

While conducting environmental scans during recent years, we noted several innovative examples and positive trends in the veteran space. Now is a good time to highlight some of the encouraging efforts, from national level and below, that aim

---

[2]Author's note: We acknowledge this chapter focuses on the employment component of the "reintegration trinity" and does not adequately address all of the efforts across the vast veteran space. There are numerous progressive efforts across many sectors—e.g., higher education, the justice system, and community mobilization—that are not included within the scope of this chapter for practical reasons.

to better facilitate the transition and reintegration of veterans and their families. Starting with the actions of government stakeholders, below we list some of the key efforts that show cause for cautious optimism in the veteran space.

Following reports of systemic problems with management and scheduling within the Department of Veterans Affairs (VA), Secretary Robert A. McDonald redoubled efforts to improve customer service for veterans since his confirmation in July 2014. As part of Secretary McDonald's effort to transform the department, the VA conducted research using human-centered design methodology to improve service delivery that results in a more veteran-centered experience. One specific initiative is the MyVA Community model. The overarching goal of this initiative is to connect veterans with service providers, community leaders, education centers, job training/ employment services, and other leaders in the community. Realizing that veteran reintegration is a national challenge that ultimately requires community solutions, MyVA Community is intended to act as a catalyst that brings together stakeholders from the national, state, and local levels to provide better outcomes for veterans and their families. Connecticut was the first state to stand up a MyVA Community in summer 2015. As of this writing, there are over 50 communities across the United States and the VA plans to extend that to over 100 communities by the end of 2016 (VA – Navigation, 2016a, 2016b).

Another initiative under the auspices of the MyVA transformation is the Veterans Economic Communities Initiative, launched in spring 2015. Designated economic liaisons for this initiative assist transitioning service members and veterans in learning new, high-demand skills to enhance their employability and increase economic security and prosperity for themselves and their families. The key to this initiative's success is leveraging public-private partnerships that connect veterans to community-based resources related to education, training, and economic growth. The Veterans Economic Communities Initiative encourages collaboration with the Department of Labor (DoL), the Small Business Administration, nonprofit organizations as well as local business leaders and educators. By the end of 2016, the Veterans Economic Communities Initiative has launched in 25 communities across the United States, with plans to launch 25 more in the coming months (VA—Veterans, 2016b). Through the VECI and MyVA, VA has committed to growing partnerships through new memoranda of understanding and to expanding current agreements to reach more than 15,000 veterans and family members. Per Christi Collins, Office of Transition, Employment and Economic Impact for the VA, as of this writing, these expanded partnerships have reached approximately 22,265 service members, veterans, and their families (personal communication, March 3, 2016).

One of the highlights of the first-year initiative was the fall 2015 Vet Camp hosted by Texas A&M University, attended by veteran-serving organizations, veteran employers, campus resources, veterans, service members, and their families. The event showcased the Veterans Employment Center (VEC) to student veterans and all companies/organizations in attendance. In Los Angeles, Mayor Eric Garcetti's 10,000 Strong Hiring Summit connected over 1000 attending veterans with over 100 employers and 100 veteran-serving organizations. In addition to familiarizing over 60 hiring managers with the VEC, this event enabled veterans to network with prospective employers and led to new VEC registrations. Finally, Bunker Labs in Chicago, an entrepreneurship incubator for veterans, provided an overview of VA's new Learning Hub initiative and launch of the Veterans Economic Communities Initiative (VECI). The event highlighted opportunities for veterans with education and training through the Learning Hub and partnership with The Bunker.

With these efforts, the VA embraced a more comprehensive approach to facilitating the reintegration of veterans and their families. Rather than focusing exclusively on providing benefits and administering healthcare for veterans, the VA's efforts through MyVA Communities and the Veterans Economic Communities Initiative seek to align public, private, and nonprofit resources and opportunities in the local communities based on the individual needs of the veteran.[3] The potential that these initiatives have to energize community-level collaboration, link veterans and their families to hyperlocal opportunities and resources, and provide a mechanism for newly transitioned veterans to navigate the vast veteran-support landscape is profound. Their success will depend on the willingness of local, state, and federal governments, private organizations, funders, and nonprofit organizations to truly align their altruistic rhetoric with their actions and put the well-being of veterans and their families ahead of the needs and desires of individual organizations. Ultimately, the efficacy of these initiatives hinges upon smart policies and strong leadership from all stakeholders.

5.3   DoD Adopts a Life Cycle Model of Military Service

While the VA is the lead department for the well-being of veterans and their families, other government agencies contribute significantly. DoD's primary mission is to deter war and protect our nation, but the department has increased its efforts to prepare transitioning service members for their reentry into civilian life. In 2011, Congress passed a bipartisan bill to address the veteran unemployment rate which led to the President signing the Veterans Opportunity to Work to Hire Heroes Act. In addition to providing tax credits for businesses that hire veterans, this legislation resulted in the redesign of DoD's transition curriculum overseen by the Transition to Veterans Program Office (TVPO). The new curriculum, Transition Assistance Program-Goals, Plans, Success (TAP-GPS), prepares transitioning service members to find employment, return to school, or even start up their own business. Additionally, in October 2015, each of the services implemented the Military Life

---

[3] U.S. Department of Veterans Affairs, *VA 2017 Budget Request: Fast Facts* [Washington, DC: U.S. Department of Veterans Affairs, 2016], http://www.va.gov/budget/docs/summary/Fy2017-FastFactsVAsBudgetHighlights.pdf (accessed March 4, 2016). While the VA is expending more effort on culture-changing initiatives, like MyVA, to better serve veterans and their families, it is important to note that the vast majority of its budget is obligated for traditional healthcare. The VA 2017 budget request is $182.3 billion, 95% of which is slated for medical and mandatory benefits programs.

Cycle which requires military members to conduct goal-planning for their post-military lives at certain touchpoints throughout their career. The implementation of the Military Life Cycle potentially signals an evolution in our military service culture that encourages service members to think about–and plan for—their post-military goals early and often.

While some may argue that a one-week course is insufficient to adequately prepare transitioning service members for today's workforce, any fair consideration of the value of Transition GPS must acknowledge its true purpose. Transition GPS is designed to provide transitioning service members and their families with tools that will enable their successful reintegration into civilian society.[4] Service members and their families must effectively wield these tools and in the circumstances when their available tools are insufficient, actively seek out the myriad of additional tools that are available through the public, private, and nonprofit sectors. In order to maximize the intended benefits of Transition GPS, it is paramount that DoD find ways to work effectively with the VA's MyVA initiatives and nonprofit organizations to create mechanisms through Transition GPS that will enable transitioning service members to connect, prior to transition, with the resources and opportunities that await in their communities.

Recognizing that many veterans naturally possess entrepreneurial skills, DoD implemented—as part of the interagency effort that revised and expanded the Transition Assistance Program—an entrepreneurship education and training course, known as Boots to Business (B2B), which is one of three Transition-GPS elective training tracks. The program is administered by the US Small Business Administration (SBA) in cooperation with the Institute for Veterans and Military Families (IVMF) at Syracuse University and SBA's other nonprofit partners (e.g., Veteran Business Outreach Centers (VBOCs) that provide business assistance services). B2B provides transitioning service members with the foundations for starting their own business to include lessons on drafting business plans and gaining access to start-up capital. Boots to Business was purposefully designed as a two-phase, hybrid program that introduces individuals to the vocation of business ownership, and then provides them with the technical skills to launch an entrepreneurial venture. Phase 1 is a two-day orientation workshop that basically helps transitioning service members answer the question, "Is business ownership the right pathway for me, and/or my family?" Phase 2, which is 8 weeks long, employs an applied skills-training model to prepare entrepreneurial-minded individuals to successfully act on their intention to launch or grow a business venture. To measure the program's

---

[4] While TAP-GPS does include an education track, the bulk of the curriculum is employment-centric. This is understandable as the program was redesigned in response to high veteran unemployment rates, Congressional bipartisan bills, and the Veteran Employment Initiative, Executive Order 13518 from 2009. Perhaps a more holistic approach is needed, one that addresses the "reintegration trinity" of employment, education, and well-being. A TAP-GPS requirement, transitioning service members must complete several Career Readiness Standards to be determined as prepared for a civilian career. Instead of focusing on being "career" ready, perhaps a more comprehensive approach would require transitioning service members to meet "*Civilian* Readiness Standards."

effectiveness, the SBA and IVMF developed a program of assessment and evaluation to capture pre- and post-training level of entrepreneurial intention, motivation, and efficacy among the B2B participants. Additionally, SBA and IVMF developed short- and long-term metrics focused on technical-skills transfer, venture creation, and venture sustainability and growth. The initial assessment is that the Boots to Business program is effective and the metrics are consistent with or exceed the performance levels of similar introduction and orientation business-ownership programs offered to other student cohorts (non-military students) by higher education and/or private-sector programs. For example, 93% of Boots to Business survey respondents indicated they were "somewhat" or "very" likely to have the skillset required to start a business after completing the program, as compared to 55% who indicated they were likely to have the skillset required to start a business prior to participating the program. Since its first full year in 2013, Boots to Business has trained over 35,000 transitioning service members and spouses. More recently, this public-private partnership led to a spin-off course, Boots to Business Reboot, open to veterans of all eras, service members (including National Guard and Reserves), and their spouses. Like its predecessor, this two-day entrepreneurial course is also instructed by the Small Business Administration and its business advisor partners.[5]

Signaling an understanding that strong military families are the backbone of a ready, resilient force, in 2010 the White House issued Presidential Study Directive-9, making military family support a national security policy priority. The resulting interagency report, *Strengthening Our Military Families: Meeting America's Commitment,* highlighted four priorities to better address the unique challenges of military families, to include preparing military spouses for career opportunities (White House, 2011). In response to this report, DoD launched the Military Spouse Employment Partnership program as part of the broader Spouse Education and Career Opportunities initiative. In short, this initiative prepares military spouses though education and training programs (e.g., goal setting, marketing skills, licensing, and credentialing) and connects them with prospective employers. To date, the Military Spouse Employment Partnership includes more than 300 partners who have hired over 90,000 military spouses (Defense Media Activity, 2016).

In recent years, DoD has implemented several initiatives that facilitate transitioning service members' ability to receive valuable training in preparation for post-military careers. Credentialing Opportunities On-Line, allows service members to obtain professional certifications and licenses at little or no cost. Recognizing that service members obtain valuable education, training, and experience during their military careers, this credentialing program allows members to obtain industry-recognized credentials that not only benefit them in their current job but also prepare them for future success in the civilian sector.[6] Another fairly recent innovative program is the DoD SkillBridge Initiative. Under SkillBridge, industry partners

---

[5] For more information on Boots to Business, visit SBA's web site at: https://www.sba.gov/offices/headquarters/ovbd/resources/160511 (accessed April 5, 2016).

[6] In FY2015, the services funded over 55,000 civilian occupational credentials according to the Office of the Assistant Secretary of Defense (Readiness).

provide training—including apprenticeships and internships—to transitioning service members within 6 months of separation from active duty. Participating companies include General Motors and Microsoft as well as several labor unions, like the United Association of Journeymen and Apprentices of the Plumbing and Pipefitting Industry who implemented a Veterans in Piping training program. In addition to the invaluable opportunity for transitioning service members to develop industry-specific career skills, SkillBridge Initiative creates unique opportunities for them to connect with private sector organizations well prior to their transition from military service.

As the federal government's lead agency for employment and training services, DoL is uniquely positioned to facilitate veterans' reentry to the civilian workforce through the work of DoL's Veteran Employment and Training Services. Veterans can access priority service at approximately 2500 American Job Centers across the country and through the American Job Centers, access tailored employment support from Local Veterans Employment Representatives and Disabled Veteran Outreach Specialists. Randall Smith from the Veterans' Employment and Training Service, U.S. Department of Labor, notes the department has provided training and employment services to over 3.5 million transitioning service members which speaks to the reach and potential impact of DoL's efforts to create meaningful career opportunities for veterans (personal communication, March 17, 2017).

5.4   Public-Private Partnership Models Emerge

While the federal government's efforts to support and enable transitioning service members and veterans have improved over the last 5 years, the government cannot meet every need of each veteran and family member. Recognizing this, corporations, philanthropic organizations, and nonprofit organizations—big and small—have stepped up to create veteran opportunities and provide support where government cannot.[7] These efforts have created a marketplace of veteran support which responds to the forces of supply and demand, disruption, and innovation. This marketplace, however, is characterized by fragmentation, strident competition, and complexity. As a result, veterans and their families are often challenged to navigate this marketplace effectively and the organizations that comprise the market are challenged by the need to raise long-term sustainable funding, measure and evaluate the impact of their efforts in a meaningful way, and to amplify their impact through partnerships and collaboration.

---

[7] As highlighted in a recent CNAS report, "the true engine of economic opportunity for veterans is the private sector, not government." It makes sense, then, that the private sector take the lead in certain areas like employment since the private sector hires 98% of the civilian workers in America. Phillip Carter et al., *Passing the Baton: A Bipartisan 2016 Agenda for the Veteran and Military Community* [Washington, DC: Center for a New American Security, 2015], 16, http://www.cnas.org/sites/default/files/publications-pdf/CNASReport_PassingtheBaton_151104_final.pdf (accessed March 7, 2016).

Despite these challenges, multiple organizations in the veteran marketplace are deploying locally focused referral and support networks of like-minded organizations that can serve as a single point of entry for veterans and their families to access the opportunities and services available to them effectively and efficiently. Examples of these efforts include the Institute for Veteran and Military Families' America Serves networks, America Warrior Partnership networks, the United Service Organizations Transition 360 Alliance, and the United Way's Mission United networks.[8] While each of these models differs in the details of their implementation, they share similar characteristics: ease of access and navigation for veterans and their families; collective support through effective referrals and follow-ups; an emphasis on measurement and evaluation; and public-private partnerships. At the time of this writing, some of these networks are exploring the feasibility of expanding their reach to entire states or regions.

In the communities where these networks have been deployed, veterans and their families can find a single point of entry from which they are able to access wraparound services and support that will enable them to create and access opportunities that otherwise may be beyond their grasp. Unfortunately, these networks have not and perhaps will not proliferate into every community to which our veterans return. When combined with—or even better, partnered with—the MyVA initiatives discussed above, however, they have the potential to positively impact the transition and reintegration of a majority of veterans and their families. With sufficient support by funders and truly meaningful partnerships within the veteran services marketplace, this potential can be realized.

5.5   The Private Sector Emerges as a Force Multiplier

Finally, efforts by the corporate and nonprofit sectors to create post-service employment opportunities for veterans and their spouses are improving the outlook dramatically for veterans to find meaningful post-service careers that will provide long-term financial well-being and a renewed purpose for our veterans and their families. These efforts are addressing four fundamental issues that determine the ability of our veterans to find meaningful careers following military service. First, they augment the tools provided to transitioning service members in Transition GPS and elevate them from novice job-seekers to highly competitive candidates who are well-informed, skilled, and able to maximize technology and professional networking to find meaningful post-service careers. Second, they enable employers who

---

[8] For more on these efforts, visit: Institute for Veterans and Military Families America Serves, http://vets.syr.edu/americaserves-a-community-discussion-on-investing-in-collective-impact-strategies-supporting-americas-transitioning-servicemembers-veterans-and-their-families/; America's Warrior Partnership, http://americaswarriorpartnership.org/; USO Transition 360, https://www.uso.org/programs/uso-transition-360-alliance-overview; and United Way Mission United, https://www.unitedway.org/blog/mission-united-connects-veterans-with-critical-help

recognize the value in hiring veterans through the research, development, and proliferation of best practices for recruiting, hiring, and retaining veterans. Third, these efforts counter ill-informed and harmful veteran stereotypes and, instead, help shape a national narrative that more aptly portrays veterans as civic assets who will make their communities, companies, and organizations better, more effective, and more competitive. Fourth, they create job opportunities for our veterans and their families that improve their economic situation. These corporate commitments are substantial and initial indications suggest they are making a real difference in the lives of our veterans.

We believe the efforts outlined above have created the conditions to improve veteran transition and reintegration writ large. While this tipping point is imminent, it is not yet within our grasp. Much work remains. The remainder of this chapter discusses our views of the goals and conditions that must be achieved.

5.6 Recommendations and Conclusion

In 1961, President Kennedy delivered the "moonshot challenge" speech to Congress that catalyzed the United States to land a man on the moon by the end of the decade. It is in the same spirit that we challenge stakeholders with this aspirational goal: every veteran reintegrates successfully back into civilian society and is well positioned to pursue security and prosperity for themselves and their family. With the impending inflection point, now is a good time to reimagine the veteran transition/reintegration space 10 years from now. To that end, we offer several considerations in pursuit of the aspirational goal above.

1. **Foster high-trust relationships among stakeholders.** The veteran space is a competitive marketplace. As a result of this competition, trust, transparency, and the willingness to partner and work together for the betterment of veterans are significant challenges. It is necessary that government, funders, and nonprofit leaders develop innovative approaches to incentivize collaboration and partnerships among veteran-serving nonprofits. This paradigm shift could be achieved through collective grantmaking that incentivizes collaboration and collective impact. Indeed, grantmakers play a key role in funding veterans' initiatives. Grantmakers, however, are more than just funders—they are critical partners in shaping strategy and programs that bring functional fields and communities together to tackle complex veteran and military family issues. They foster connections and set the conditions to allow collective impact initiatives to flourish. The success of effective collective grantmaking partnerships depends on the grantmaker's ability to align interests, cultivate relationships, and to fund the costs of collaboration.[9] Another potential trigger

---

[9] For a practical treatment on the importance of trusting relationships, read Stephen M.R. Covey's *The Speed of Trust: The One Thing that Changes Everything*. New York: The Free Press, 2006.

for this paradigm shift could be creating a mechanism (or expanding an existing platform) for the customers in this marketplace—veterans and their families—to pick the winners and losers in the market. The ability for veterans and family members to rate publicly the services provided by veteran nonprofits and community service providers could provide the needed incentive for organizations to work more effectively with each other. Ultimately, grantmakers can catalyze collective impact that will better support initiatives and provide a stable platform for success in meeting the needs of veterans and military families throughout the country (Bartczak, 2014).

2. **DoD Leadership should signal an expectation, through effective policies, that the military services and OSD will partner effectively with veteran-serving nonprofits to create opportunities for veterans and their families.** DoD leaders should also signal an expectation that legal counsel will help commanders find a way to do this effectively within the law and regulations. The predominant culture within the Department and within the services is one that emphasizes protecting transitioning service members and DoD from private sector exploitation—but at the cost of precluding mechanisms to connect transitioning service members to private-sector opportunities. That culture must be flipped on its head. Instead, we should instill a culture that proactively connects transitioning service members to private-sector contacts and resources to effect a successful transition and reintegration.

3. **Increase DoD data sharing among trusted partners.** A hallmark of the most effective veteran-serving nonprofit organizations is their collection and utilization of data that characterize the targeted veteran population in terms of demographics, skills, geographic distribution, and needs. The collection and analysis of these data enables veteran nonprofits, community service providers, and their partners to identify trends and emerging requirements, as well as align the delivery of services and the allocation of resources against the greatest challenges that the targeted veteran population faces. DoD's Defense Manpower Data Center collects and aggregates key personnel data that, if made available to the private sector, would significantly enhance veteran nonprofit access to relevant data about the veteran population they serve. In aggregate form, these data reveal no personally identifiable information while providing a wealth of information that can be used to great effect by the private sector and interagency partners in developing and delivering programs and services to transitioning service members and veterans. For example, researchers could use DoD data to conduct longitudinal studies to measure the outcomes of reintegration programs more accurately.[10] In addition to enabling interagency partners,

---

[10] Cynthia L. Gilman, JD, *The Veteran Metrics Initiative (TVMI): Learning What Works for Veterans and their Families* [Bethesda, MD: Henry M. Jackson Foundation for the Advancement of Military Medicine, Inc., 2013], http://rwtf.defense.gov/Portals/22/Documents/Meetings/m19/041tvmi.pdf (accessed February 29, 2016). The Veterans Metric Initiative, led by the Henry M. Jackson Foundation, is an example of a research effort that proposes to measure evidence-based outcomes of veteran reintegration programs.

veteran nonprofits, and community service providers to more effectively design and deliver services and programs, the regular DoD release of aggregate transition-related personnel data would signal a firm commitment by DoD to work collaboratively with interagency partners and the private sector to improve the reintegration outcomes of our veterans and their families.

4. **Maximize community collaborations.** As institutions often have scarce resources, there are typically other organizations within their area who can help provide some of these resources. It would be beneficial for academic institutions to embark on community partnerships with at least two or three other organizations in their area to provide the necessary support services to their students. This includes local business looking to hire veterans who might collaborate to build out internship or networking opportunities, a local facility that provides mental healthcare that specifically addresses the needs of military-connected individuals, and/or a local veteran/military support organization that helps connect service members or veterans to other local support services.

5. **Establish a national structure characterized by functional cooperation, cross-sector collaboration, and an integrated network.** This enables a no-wrong-door capacity that allows our country to reintegrate veterans and their families effectively as a matter of course. This would ensure service members, their families, and survivors would receive the support they need, regardless of the community to which they return.[11]

6. **Establish a U.S. Interagency Council on Veteran Reintegration.** This entity would foster collaboration among all stakeholders, ensure program integration and strategic alignment, promote information sharing, and encourage public-private partnerships, to improve the transition and reintegration of veterans and their families. This would help to knock down any barriers between organizations and effectively knit together the myriad veteran-support efforts.

7. **Improve measurement and evaluation of Transition Assistance Program outcomes, with special emphasis on "at risk" populations. DoD collects statistics on TAP, measuring each military service's compliance with legislative and policy requirements.** These metrics measure the *output*. However, they do not necessarily equate to successful veteran reintegration. Rather, it is necessary to determine the *outcome* of the individual efforts exercised through TAP. As currently executed, TAP allows the military service insufficient flexibility to focus on their "at risk" populations, those at greatest risk of not successfully reintegrating into the civilian sector. With unique demographics for each service, the "at risk" population composition varies. When the time is right—at the point when outputs are maximized and conditions become relatively stable—consideration could be given to adjusting TAP policy requirements to

---

[11] Efforts are already underway to make this recommendation a reality sooner than later. In November 2015, VA Secretary McDonald announced a strategic alliance with the Bob Woodruff Foundation to establish a "single front door" to better connect veterans and their families to services and programs in their communities, http://www.va.gov/opa/pressrel/pressrelease.cfm?id=2740 (accessed 10 March 2016).

afford more flexibility to the military service. Additionally, most realize the importance of using data-driven metrics when making resource-prioritization decisions. As such, we could isolate the TAP requirements and measure each individually for effectiveness. These metrics would allow the services to properly align resources to their "at risk" populations and help to inform policymakers when reevaluating TAP requirements. DoD, however, may not be best positioned to measure the effectiveness of TAP. As the *outcome* will actualize after the service member has transitioned, perhaps DoL or VA could take responsibility for gathering this information then sharing the data with the DoD. This step would highlight areas of sustainment and improvement regarding service member transition and reintegration across the interagency. Furthermore, once effective metrics have been established, they could also be used to measure the outcomes for the programs in the private and nonprofit sectors as well.

8. **Establish transition and reintegration programs and solutions that are multigenerational.** While our nation has transitioned service members for 240 years, "It is worth noting that, by default, the first Gulf War and the Post-9/11 wars—and related contingency operations beyond Operation Enduring Freedom, Operation Iraqi Freedom, and Operation New Dawn—are among the first functional tests of the all-volunteer force since its institutionalization in 1973" (Zoli, Maury, & Fay, 2015, p. 14). Data are being collected and multiple academic institutions are studying the social phenomenon of both the all-volunteer force and the impacts after the nation experienced the longest conflict in history. Indeed, it is paramount that we capture the lessons learned today in order to develop effective programs for future generations of veterans. As we near the end of the millennial generation, do we need to reemphasize the value and cost of the all-volunteer force to the generation we are intending to recruit in 2026? For example, 91 percent of Americans have never served and studies show that fewer and fewer of the millennial generation are willing to serve in the armed forces.[12]

9. **Organizations that serve veterans and military families could "take the pledge" not to reinforce the negative narrative that casts veterans as victims in order to increase awareness and attract funding.** Currently, there is a popular, dueling narrative that characterizes veterans as either victims or heroes. Unfortunately, this binary narrative fails to capture the majority of veterans that fall somewhere in the middle of the spectrum. Instead of solely focusing on extreme cases, organizations could offer a more balanced narrative that recognizes the fact that most veterans are civic assets who will strengthen the communities, companies, and organizations that embrace them. The sign of a

---

[12] A 2010 report by DoD's Joint Advertising, Market Research & Studies suggests that the propensity for military service among America's youth declines for myriad factors, including the declining number of US veterans who positively affect recruitment, and increasing educational attainment by America's youth. This decline in military propensity will likely continue to present recruiting challenges for the all-volunteer force. http://jamrs.defense.gov/Portals/20/Documents/Youth_Poll_20.pdf (accessed 10 March 2016).

mature sector is the ability to tell both narratives simultaneously and understand they are not mutually exclusive or contradictory. Ultimately, a balanced narrative that portrays veterans and their families as civic assets can help close the civil–military gap.

10. **Recognize that military service and reintegration are challenges not only for service members but also for their families.** Family members make it possible for service members to do their work, and the care and well-being of family members directly impact service member performance and retention. Conversely, the consequences of deployments can be substantial for families. Stakeholders could focus on ensuring successful outcomes for family members in the areas of employment, education, well-being, and social functioning.

5.6.1   Conclusion

Undoubtedly, military conflicts will persist into the future, requiring the nation to sustain a ready, capable all-volunteer force. But once these volunteers take off their uniform, it is equally imperative that we have set the conditions which facilitate their successful transition and reintegration back into civilian society. It is also important to realize that while some needs are enduring and universal, other needs will vary from cohort to cohort based on the changing social, economic, and demographic profiles of veterans. Regardless of the unchanging nature or changing character of veterans' needs, a strategically coherent and collective effort by all stakeholders—government, private, nonprofit, philanthropy—will best position our veterans and their families for success. Our observations over the past few years have given us reason for cautious optimism. The cumulative effects of the myriad cross-sector efforts have put us on an optimal trajectory. Granted, there is still much to do to improve veteran reintegration, but recent trends are encouraging as we near a consequential point of sustained momentum. Acknowledging this inflection point is important and necessary…but insufficient. Ultimately, stakeholders will need to act collectively to optimize veteran reintegration. The future of the all-volunteer force depends upon it.[13]

The authors would like to thank all committed supporters for their continued efforts, and to encourage all to keep setting the conditions for the successful reintegration of our veterans and their families—because our nation's military families deserve nothing less.

---

[13]Author's note: We used the word "stakeholder" consistently throughout this chapter since it is commonly quoted within the veteran space; going forward, perhaps we should endeavor to replace "stakeholder" with "shareholder" in the veteran transition and reintegration lexicon. Shareholder conveys *ownership of*, more than simply *interest in*, veteran reintegration.

References

Bartczak, L. (2014). The role of Grantmakers in Collective Impact. *Stanford Social Innovation Review*, 2014. Retrieved from https://ssir.org/articles/entry/the_role_of_grantmakers_in_collective_impact

Carter, P. (2012). *Upholding the promise: A strategy for veterans and military personnel in the next four years*. Washington, DC: Center for a New American Security.

Defense Media Activity. (2016). *DoD Military Spouse Employment Partnership Reaches Milestone*. Retrieved from https://www.defense.gov/News/Article/Article/681788/dod-military-spouse-employment-partnership-reaches-milestone/

Department of Labor, Bureau of Labor Statistics. (2016). *2015 employment situation of veterans summary*. Retrieved from http://www.bls.gov/news.release/vet.nr0.htm

Department of Veterans Affairs. (2016a). *Navigation, advocacy, and community engagement (NACE): MyVA community model*. Retrieved from http://www.va.gov/nace/myVA/index.asp

Department of Veterans Affairs. (2016b). *Veterans economic communities initiative*. Retrieved from http://www.benefits.va.gov/veci/veci.asp

White House. (2011). *Strengthening our military families: Meeting America's Commitment*. Washington, DC: The White House. Retrieved from https://www.whitehouse.gov/sites/default/files/rss_viewer/strengthening_our_military_families_meeting_americas_commitment_january_2011.pdf.

Zoli, C., Maury, R., & Fay, D. (2015). *Missing perspectives: Service members' transition from service to civilian life*. Syracuse, NY: Institute of Veterans and Military Families.

Chapter 6
Ready or Not, Here It Comes: Navigating Congress and Caring for the Wounded and Their Family Members During War Time

William T. Cahill

The observations, opinions, conclusions, and/or recommendation contained in this chapter are the author's alone and should not be construed or otherwise interpreted as those of his current or former employer(s). Any factual mistakes or errors are not intended to misrepresent events described from personal recollections.

6.1 Background

Capitol Hill, Washington DC is best known as the place where 535 elected Members of Congress meet to debate proposed changes in law and set budgets (in the form of spending and taxes) for operating the Federal Government. Less well-known is that there are thousands of staff members who serve in either the personal office of an elected member or as a "professional staff member" on one of the dozens of standing committees and subcommittees of the U.S. House of Representative and U.S. Senate. In general, personal office staff focus more on issues of importance to an individual member and the district or state he or she represents, whereas committee staff focus more on advising members with respect to the specific policy issues related to the committee's jurisdiction. From 1997 to 2007, I was privileged to serve in various roles as a professional staff member with the U.S. Senate Committee on Veterans' Affairs. My focus was predominantly on the legislation, statutes, and policies governing operations of the Department of Veterans Affairs (VA) health care system. My perspectives, observations, and opinions stem from my experience advising Senators and collaborating with the dedicated men and women who lead the VA and its health care programs.

W.T. Cahill (✉)
Georgetown University Law Center, Washington, DC, USA
e-mail: Cahill703@gmail.com

© Springer International Publishing AG 2018

79

L. Hughes-Kirchubel et al. (eds.), *A Battle Plan for Supporting Military Families*, Risk and Resilience in Military and Veteran Families,
https://doi.org/10.1007/978-3-319-68984-5_6

Prior to September 11, 2001 the U.S. military and its Congressional supporters had been admirably focused on the needs of the military family. In the era of an all-volunteer force, the military followed the axiom: recruit a service member, retain a family. The issues of importance to the family of service members were the same issues that occupied the minds of all Americans: good schools, safe neighborhoods, decent pay, and quality health care. During the 1990s, Congress focused on making improvements to all of these areas in concert with the military leadership.

To improve the quality of base housing, the Department of Defense (DoD) partnered with a national builder to construct more attractive homes for military families. To improve educational opportunities for military children, DoD focused time and attention on collaborating with local communities to ensure good schools were available near bases. Perhaps the most significant new public-private partnership to impact military personnel was the expansion of private sector health care options in the military health system. Multiple Base Realignment and Closure Commissions undertaken between 1988 and 1995 had closed or slated for closure nearly 100 military bases, and with them numerous military medical facilities (Lockwood & Siehl, 2004). After a decade of testing the best ways to expand private sector care for the military, DoD awarded its first TRICARE managed care support contracts in 1997. The new and improved TRICARE program would become a key feature in later debates over separating from military service those wounded in action.

During this same time period, the VA also underwent significant changes in delivering services to its beneficiaries. In particular, VA and Congress worked to expand veterans' access to care with changes to both the types of facilities operated by the Veterans Health Administration (VHA) and the scope of care offered to veterans. The changes were heavily influenced by a paper published in 1996 by Dr. Ken Kizer, who served as Under Secretary for Health at VA, called "Prescription for Change" (Kizer, 1996). Dr. Kizer outlined VA's intention to expand access to care for veterans by spending more on operating outpatient clinics in communities all over the country, and less on institutional care delivered in a hospital setting. In response to Dr. Kizer's vision, Congress passed the Veterans' Health Care Eligibility Reform Act of 1996 (Public Law 104-262, 110 Stat. 3177. Oct. 9 1996), which fundamentally expanded the scope of VA's health care services to veterans. Previously, VA health care was focused on addressing the individual illnesses and injuries resulting from service-connected conditions. The Eligibility Reform Act expanded the mission of the Veterans Health Administration (VHA) to address the full spectrum of health care needs for enrolled veterans, service-connected or not. Following these changes, VA devoted the savings generated from its lower cost of care to a major expansion of its medical footprint all across the country.

Then came September 11, 2001. Following that fateful day, the movement of troops, the logistics of providing them the right equipment, and the readiness of military forces to respond took priority on Capitol Hill and certainly within the walls of the Pentagon. With that, at least for a time, the needs of military families, which had garnered so much focus and attention during the previous 15 years, took a back seat to the prosecution of the war efforts. VA's mission, however, changed little. On September 12, 2001 there were still millions of veterans from previous wars and conflicts relying on the VA health care system. The general age cohort of those veterans (primarily men who fought during World War II, Korea, and Vietnam), their health care needs, and their families were still the same. So too was the VA's responsibility to care for them. And while the war had changed the focus of the nation, it had not immediately changed the responsibilities of VA.

6.2 VA Becomes Relevant to the War

It wasn't until a sizable population of wounded warriors returned home from the battlefield that the pendulum of focus began to swing back towards the need for health care services, benefits, and family support to handle the injuries inflicted by the Global War on Terror. Questions soon arose surrounding the readiness of DoD and VA to care for the injured and their families. As challenges in both departments became clearer to political leaders on Capitol Hill, policy makers (and the two agencies) began trying to address the inadequacies. With two distinct systems (DoD and VA), overseen by six different committees in Congress, the first several years following 9/11 demonstrated that the respective roles of DoD and VA in caring for the injured (and their family members) were anything but clear. The lack of clarity was, quickly, coupled with scandals in both DoD and VA, leading to policy fights and oversight hearings by Congress to focus attention on caring for the wounded, ill, and injured. As is often the case, the spotlight on failures laid the foundation for changes in policies and programs focused on the family members of those whom the nation sent off to war. But, even today, it is still only a foundation.

Proactively establishing clearer expectations about when DoD's responsibilities end, when VA's begin, and how that transition occurs should be the focus of policy makers, advocates, beneficiaries, and budgeteers now—prior to the outset of the next major conflict—much like housing, education, and health care benefit design was in the 1990s. Those discussions should take into consideration the fact that at the start of any war, DoD has the political attention; motivation; flexibility; people; and, most importantly, money to care for the wounded and their families. Therefore, DoD should do it.

Expecting VA to manage that work immediately upon the start of a combat action ignores the reality that VA will not even know what is needed until sometime after the first deployments occur. Following the first troops rotations, it will take time to adjust the focus of a system that simply cannot drop its current workload in favor of a new one. VA needs be provided ample time and funds to simultaneously concentrate on its current patient base, and their families, while making room, literally and clinically, for the needs of its future beneficiaries.

6.3 Congressional Advocacy Is Necessary. But where to Start?

The House of Representatives and the Senate are environments dominated by "turf" and "tenure." That is not necessarily negative. It just is. Responsibilities for the development of policy, agency and program funding, and oversight of those programs and agencies are scattered among more than 180 Congressional committees and subcommittees in the House and Senate. Committees all have Chairs (from the majority party) and Ranking Minority Members (from the minority party), as does each subcommittee of a committee. Those Chairs and Ranking Members have vested interests in doing "something" and whatever they do needs to fit within the confines of their committee or subcommittee's scope and jurisdiction. That is how political reputations are built and maintained.

While it is true that the seniority system does not always determine who is elected Chair or Ranking Minority Member of a committee or subcommittee, there is still a very strong bias towards electing as Chair of any full committee the member of the majority party who has been on the committee the longest. There are exceptions to this bias, but these remained rare on Capitol Hill in the early post-9/11 period. Senators John Warner (R-VA), Arlen Specter (R-PA), Ted Stevens (R-SC), Carl Levin (D-MI), John D. Rockefeller IV (D-WV), and Robert Bird (D-WV) led the Armed Services, Veterans' Affairs, and Appropriations Committees, respectively, in the Senate. In the House of Representatives, Bob Stump (R-AZ); Chris Smith (R-NJ); C.W. "Bill" Young (R-FL); Ike Skelton (D-MO); Lane Evans (D-IL); and David Obey (D-WI), respectively, served in those positions. With the exception of Representative Smith, who was elected in 1980 and born in 1953 and Rep. Evans, elected in 1982 and born in 1951, all of these distinguished members were elected prior to 1980 and all were born before the United States entered World War II. Each was a well-respected member of Congress who had come to their position of power after serving on those committees for decades.

In theory, the committee structure has a number of benefits. Chief among them is that it allows members to focus on certain subject matter policies (for example, military or taxes) instead of trying to learn everything government does. This fact, coupled with longevity driving the election of committee Chairpersons, means that most leaders of committees have spent many years becoming subject matter experts on issues within the jurisdiction of the committees they lead. Additionally, the committee structure allows members to become well-versed in the operations of the agencies subject to the jurisdiction of their committees. This provides the experience needed to question results and hold Executive Branch managers and political appointees accountable.

As with most things in politics, though, there are inherent negative consequences. Most notably, the committee structure can at times create a dynamic where members see a problem only through the lens of their respective committees' jurisdictions. If they are not on the committee responsible for the problem being raised, the response is that they cannot help (this is often a response given to national advocacy groups or organizations, but rarely to hometown constituents). Alternatively, members may seek ways to "carve" an issue important to them into legislative solutions technically within the jurisdiction of their committees. Those two mindsets make it difficult to focus on the kinds of comprehensive policies that are needed to better coordinate services between and among differing agencies of government when those agencies are subject to the jurisdiction of different committees in Congress.

Such was the case in the years following September 11, 2001 in the development of policies and the conduct of oversight in areas impacting wounded service members, those transitioning out of the military, and their families. There was DoD, with its facilities, budget, and policies, all under the watchful eye of the Armed Services and Defense Appropriations Subcommittees. Then there was VA, answerable to the Veterans' Affairs and the VA Appropriations Subcommittees. While the two pairs may have some overlapping members, as organizational institutions, they rarely meet.

In many ways, the results of these challenges can best be seen in the case of a single Army soldier who was injured by an Improvised Explosive Device (IED) early in 2004. His case was the first real indication I had as a staff member on the Senate Committee on Veterans' Affairs that things simply were not working well. Problem was, I did not know for sure where the fault should lie.

When this soldier first came to Capitol Hill with his wife and an advocacy organization's representative, I was the first person with whom he visited. At that time, coming to see me seemed perfectly rational because he was no longer in the military. He was a veteran and the majority of his concerns and complaints were about the medical treatment he was receiving from the VA Health Care system. However, what is readily apparent, in hindsight, is that my focus was on how VA was caring for him and where they were failing, not really considering that the root cause of his problems most likely stemmed from the fact that Congress never considered, let alone decided, when the military's responsibility for treating the injured and caring for their families ended, and when VA's responsibility to assume those duties subsequently began.

When this brave young man was first injured, it was clear that DoD had primary responsibility to stabilize him on the battlefield and transfer him to a military medical facility for his treatment. The Department of Defense (DoD) flew his wife to Germany to be near to her husband as he fought for his life. Then DoD flew them back to the United States to receive more treatment at Walter Reed Army Medical Center. At this point, all was seemingly in order. [As an aside, it bears noting that the military's performance of these functions during the War on Terrorism led to the highest battlefield injury survival rate in U.S. history; Wilson, 2010.]

While at Walter Reed, the Army continued to pay this young soldier and his spouse continued to receive the benefits that come with being part of the active force. However, not long after arriving state-side, it was determined that military medicine was unable to provide the full panoply of services he required. Given the significance of his injuries, it was also pretty clear that he was unlikely to return to active duty. As this point, he was discharged from the Army and transferred to the VA Health Care System. His first stop was a nursing home unit at a VA Medical Center (VAMC) several hours from Walter Reed. As soon as he arrived at the

VAMC, his wife knew things were going to be completely different. The first clue was that his new roommates were World War II Veterans. In fact, most of the patients at the VAMC were elderly residents of the nursing home unit for reasons ranging from the need for everyday palliative care to poststroke rehabilitation. None of them, however, had recently been injured by a roadside bomb.

In some ways, the military's decision to discharge this soldier made perfect sense. He was badly injured, having suffered an amputation and a traumatic brain injury. Historically, the wounded were transferred to the agency established "to care for him who shall have borne the battle" for recuperation and recovery. But, I can attest to the fact that, at this time, few on Capitol Hill had considered what the discharge would mean to his income, housing for his family, or how it would impact the support structure necessary to provide caregiver services when his young wife had to return to the workforce. In fact, very few of us (myself included) had spent much time considering whether VA was truly ready to accept young, traumatically wounded patients into its system. In short, from my perspective, there was little discussion about the "life consequences" of discharge from the military for this era of wounded service members.

As the war progressed, and the injured multiplied, it became clear that no committee or group of members had sat down to thoroughly consider the nation's overall policies for caring for the wounded. Issues such as: who should be responsible and why, when should wounded service members be discharged quickly from military service, and under what circumstances should the military take the time to conduct a Military Evaluation Board proceeding to determine whether the injuries are something from which the service member can recover and return to active duty, and what are the strategic military considerations for making those decisions and what would be the impact of those decisions on service members and their families? To some degree the problem still plagues us today.

Congress, as an institution, is certainly aware of the consequences (both positive and negative) of the committee system. But, there is little acknowledgement of the deficiencies, let alone any effort made to correct them. Instead, there is only a recognition of its existence and how one must operate within it. That is to say, as a member or staff, you solve the problems you can solve within the Congressional structure you have. As previously noted, Congress provided little guidance to determining when DoD responsibilities to care for the wounded ended and when VA's began. Perhaps no situation highlighted the challenge caused by that lack of clarity more than the revelation of the conditions that existed for wounded service members "recovering" at Walter Reed Army Medical Center. The troubling environment in which service members lived at the time was well documented in a February 19, 2007 article in the Washington Post written by reporters Dana Priest and Anne Hull (2007).

Congress and the Pentagon responded with great alarm and concern. Hearings were called by the Senate Armed Services Committee, generals were relieved of command, and President Bush appointed a commission to make recommendations on the care and treatment of America's Wounded Warriors. The Commission would be chaired by former Senator Robert Dole (R-KS) and former Secretary of Health and Human Services, Donna Shalala. The military had to fix this problem.

To those of us who served as Congressional staff, the issues presented by the reporters' piece were much deeper than the condition of the facilities of Walter Reed or the medical staff's failure to review patient records and provide disability ratings in a timely manner. The questions some of us on the VA Committee were asking ourselves included: why is the military responsible for continuing to treat wounded service members for prolonged periods of time, is any service branch even equipped, from a staffing perspective to do that, or did we just assume that, like the military always does, "they'll figure it out." Perhaps even more existentially, we wanted to know why there were two disability adjudication systems for service members. Why were they not going through VA's program called "Benefits Delivery at Discharge" (BDD) and then transitioned to VA in a timely manner? Was the problem that service members did not trust VA to provide quality care and services? Or were service members and their families simply not ready to "give up" their military careers?

Many in Congress began wondering whether the compensation system in the military was influencing the desire of those in uniform to make every effort to obtain a disability rating that came with military retirement. What we quickly saw was that military retirement brought with it access to the TRICARE program, which covered not just the service member but also his or her spouse and minor children. Equally important, it preserved access to the Military Health System. This is distinct from VA, which typically covers only the veteran (and in rare instances a spouse and minor children) and generally does not afford beneficiaries an opportunity to access Military Treatment Facilities. These and other questions led us to focus on where or when DoD and VA were truly failing versus where or when the agencies were simply failing to meet the evolving needs and expectations of service members, veterans, and their families in the midst of largest US military engagement since Vietnam.

Gordon Mansfield served in the VA during this turbulent time, first as an Assistant Secretary for Congressional and Legislative Affairs and then as Deputy Secretary and ultimately Acting Secretary. Secretary Mansfield was a wonderfully affable man with a warm heart and a big smile, who I first encountered during his tenure as Executive Director of the Paralyzed Veterans of America. Secretary Mansfield was also a combat wounded paraplegic, whose heroism in Vietnam after being shot in the back twice, earned him the Distinguished Service Cross (McDonough, 2013). In short, he had firsthand experience dealing with many of the challenges now being faced by seriously wounded service members and their families.

Secretary Mansfield was pained by the perception that VA was unprepared to deliver needed care and treatment to wounded service members and also care for their families. During one conversation he and I had on the topic, he shared with me a story about meeting a soldier in the waiting room of a VA Medical Center who had been recently been discharged from the Army. The soldier had spent one of his last few days in the Army being honored on the field of a professional baseball stadium by nearly 40,000 fans. The veteran, he noted, seemed melancholic to be out of the military and was now just among the many veterans sitting in a VA waiting room. Moreover, his spouse was frustrated that her husband was no longer receiving the level of attention he had previously been provided. Secretary Mansfield observed that VA cannot compete with Yankee Stadium. Moreover, he shared his belief that the perception of inferior customer service and attention was possibly true. But, it was also possible it was an evolution of transition to VA where celebrity visits are less common and the clinical focus is more often on helping veterans manage the lifelong impact of traumatic injuries. He strongly believed that VA provided veterans world-class health care. Unfortunately, not enough people outside of VA believed that, which was becoming a growing problem.

In 2005, then-Major, now Lieutenant Colonel (Ret.) and U.S. Senator (D-IL), Tammy Duckworth testified before the Senate Committee on Veterans' Affairs. Her experience highlights one of the reasons for the perception of inferiority in VA care. Major Duckworth was grievously wounded when her helicopter was struck by a rocket propelled grenade in Iraq in 2004. In the resulting crash and explosion, she lost both of her legs and partial use of her right arm (Duckworth, 2005). Setting aside her military experience and heroic recovery, Major Duckworth was an extraordinary and compelling witness, who convincingly demonstrated that in the area of prosthetic care and technological advancement, DoD's quality and capabilities had far surpassed VA. And, it had done so without much awareness on the part of the Veterans' Affairs Committee.

For many years, VA held a reputation as a forward-leaning, research-focused organization in the field of prosthetics. VA officials routinely touted the agency's involvement in the development of the "Seattle foot" as far back as 1985. That invention is credited with forever changing the landscape of prosthetic devices. Yet, here sat a decorated female helicopter pilot who had lost both of her legs in combat pointing out to the Veterans' Affairs Committee how fantastic DoD, including the prosthetics team at Walter Reed, had been in providing her with the most advanced products available. Her simple observation was that no one understood the types of injuries suffered by combat veterans like military medicine. She noted "[t]he VA will have to face the challenge of providing care at the high level set by the military healthcare facilities. This is a challenge that the VA can meet if it is given enough resources and if it listens to disabled service members and puts forth the effort to meet our needs" (Duckworth, 2005). The message to the Committee and the public was clear. No longer were VA researchers proactively focused on injuries that might be experienced by the next generation coming back from a war and how to treat them. Instead, VA's research efforts and dollars were predominately devoted to the ailments and diseases of elderly from previous conflicts.

Even with an immediate shift after the hearing, a change in focus for VA research would take time. As late as 2006, during a hearing of the Senate Committee on Veterans Affairs, Dr. Jonathan Perlin was touting VA's cutting edge research on cardiac defibrillators, diabetes, hypertension, and chronic disease. Fortunately, however, during that same hearing, VA also showed that it was beginning to prioritize research the improve care and treatment for the illnesses and injuries from the more recent wars. Nearly 5 years after the start of the war in Afghanistan, the VA system was finally beginning to respond to the medical consequences.

6.4 Making Progress... Slowly

While it may seem as though Congress spent too many years discovering problems and not enough time solving them, such is actually not the case. Victories came in the form of small and incremental changes. The first of those was enactment of the Traumatic Service Members Group Life Insurance program in May 2005. Just a few months prior to the legislation's enactment, advocates from the Wounded Warrior Project® brought forward to the Chairman and staff of the Senate Committee on Veterans' Affairs three traumatically injured service members. All of the men noted that the greatest fear they had while serving in combat was not that they would be killed—although that was certainly a fear—but rather that they would return home severely wounded and need to adjust to life with those new realities, likely unable to assist with the needs of their family. These veterans were not focused solely on the long-term challenges of severe injury (a topic which fits more squarely in the jurisdiction of the Veterans' Affairs Committee), but they were also concerned with the impact the injuries had on their families. They knew that VA administered a benefit for active duty service members that provided cash benefits to policy beneficiaries (typically a spouse and/or children) in the event a service member dies on active duty. Known as the Servicemembers Group Life Insurance (or SGLI), active duty service members are automatically enrolled for the benefit upon joining the military. Following enrollment, service members pay premiums each month based on the level of coverage ($50,000–$400,000) desired. The advocates sought to update the scope of coverage provided by SGLI to include benefits for traumatically disabled service members.

As noted previously, there was little disagreement in Congress that the military is the organization responsible for the care and treatment of an injured service member immediately following the injury, including the provision of support to his or her family. Yet, here was the Veterans' Affairs Committee Chairman, Larry Craig (R-ID) being asked to add a VA benefit to cover unmet needs confronting these still active duty service members. It can be argued that the Chairman of the Veterans' Committee should have approached the Armed Services Committee and discussed what he had learned. He could have asked for joint hearings or a meeting of the members of the two committees to discuss the perceived (and likely real) shortcomings in the benefits made available by the DoD to those who are severely injured. He did neither. Instead, he approached Senator Ted Stevens (R-AK), Chairman of the Senate Appropriations Committee, himself a Veteran of World War II, and advocated for legislation creating the Traumatic Servicemembers Group Life Insurance (TSGLI) program to be included in the so-called "Supplemental Appropriations bill" that was nearing passage on the floor of the Senate. Chairman Stevens agreed to support the legislation as an amendment to the appropriations bill. And on May 5, 2005, TSGLI become the law of the land. Unfortunately, other needed policy changes would not come so easily.

Another key improvement to support military families took more than 5 years to understand and "get right." That was the provision of caregiver assistance. VA, as an agency, had long supported policies and programs recognizing that those severely injured in service to the nation may require long-term assistive care. Typically, that service is provided through a contract arrangement with a home health agency near a veteran's home, which sends a licensed, trained, and insured caregiver to provide services. If the parent or spouse of a veteran wanted to be paid for providing assistance, VA was not necessarily opposed. However, from VA's perspective, that did not change the requirement to be licensed, trained, and work under the supervision of an agency. While such a stance might seem extreme, VA had long believed it was important to maintain the line between paying for health care services rendered by a licensed and trained provider, and simply paying friends or family members of severely disabled veterans to stay home with them. To VA, it was imperative for the protection of the veteran.

Further, and perhaps equally important, it generally was not—and still is not—VA's mission to provide care or services for the spouse, minor children, or family members of a veteran, with limited exceptions in the case of health benefits and some education benefits for the spouses and minor children of severely disabled veterans. Of course, VA also provides adaptive housing, automobile, and clothing allowances for severely disabled veterans. But, while one or more of those benefits may be helpful to the spouse or child of a veteran, the primary purpose is to assist the veteran. Yet, the longer spouses, parents, and other family members served in the role of primary caregiver for severely wounded service members (now veterans), the clearer the picture became of what life would require of them over the long run. The picture was one constant need for care provision to the veteran… but it was also one that would require assistance for caregivers in order to be sustainable. Without such assistance, it was not realistic to think family members could perpetually sustain the levels of effort required to care for wounded veterans in the years to come. It would be exhausting and possibly unbearable financially, emotionally, and physically. When the needed support became unsustainable, the impact would fall squarely on the veteran.

Thankfully, in 2010, despite the concerns of some advocates and the cautious (and perhaps reasonable) opposition of VA, Congress passed the Caregiver and Veterans Omnibus Health Services Act of 2010. The bill provided a range of benefits to a primary family member, caregiver so designated by the veteran. In a nod to the legitimate quality concerns of VA, the program requires that the caregiver receive some training. Meanwhile, in a nod to the realities these caregivers face, the program also provides benefits, such as a monthly stipend, travel expenses (including lodging and per diem while accompanying veterans undergoing care), access to health care insurance, (if the caregiver is not already entitled to care or services under a health care plan), as well as mental health services and counseling. Passage of the bill was a tremendous victory for advocates who, historically, had found VA a fairly insular agency with a more limited mission in the provision of services to family members. Now, the aperture is open and the key is to capitalize on the momentum built by that effort.

6.5 Recommendations for the Future

Recommendations for improving the response of members and staff to the outbreak of a war in the future must take into consideration that Congress, as an entity, is a conservative organization. It is not conservative in the sense that everyone favors lower taxes and less government, but rather in the sense that it does not change easily, either organizationally or operationally. With that in mind, recommendations for improvements that would require substantial or even modest changes to the organization of Congress or its operations are, in my mind, at best a fool's errand and at worse too long-term to prioritize here. Instead, my recommendations focus on accepting the organization and operations as they are and suggesting ways to achieve faster and more focused outcomes from the start of any conflicts. My recommendations focus on establishing clearer lines of responsibility and better coordination between the agencies responsible for caring for wounded, ill, and injured.

First, Congress should make clear (and advocates should focus on the fact) that DoD is expected to lead the way in caring for wounded, ill, and injured service members for a substantial period of time following the start of any major conflict, while VA begins coordinated engagement with DoD to prepare for the eventual transition of those service members.

Second, DoD should be charged with caring for any seriously wounded service member and their families for an established duration (for example, 24 months) following a serious injury.

These two recommendations may seem simplistic. But, in my view, both would greatly reduce the confusion and blurred lines of responsibilities experienced immediately following September 11, 2001. Additionally, they would help Members of Congress, staff, and committees focus their energies and attention on areas of responsibility within their respective committees. In these cases, the immediate needs of those injured would fall to the Armed Services Committees and Defense Appropriations subcommittees to oversee and fund. Whereas preparing for the future needs of those injured (after the fixed duration of time) would fall to the Veterans' Affairs Committees and VA Military Construction Appropriations subcommittees.

Additionally, outlining responsibilities more clearly and establishing fixed durations of time should improve communication and coordination between and among the members and staffs of differing committees. That's not to say there is poor communication now. To the contrary, in my decade of service on the Senate Veterans' Affairs Committee, I had countless conversations with my counterparts on the Senate Armed Services Committee. However, many of those discussions were prompted by the need to resolve "issues of the moment" rather than thoughtful coordination based on an understanding of committee and agency responsibilities. Maybe the clearer lines of responsibility will not change this. But, as noted above, it will clarify responsibilities among committee members and their staff.

Finally, this change would align the expectations of troops and their families with the proper targets in Congress for advocates. Notwithstanding the fact that much of the general public might see VA as the agency required to care for "him who shall have born the battle," for many troops and their families, they expect that "their Army" or "their Corps" will take care of them if they are injured in battle. Quickly moving injured troops out of the military and into the VA would likely greatly trouble service members who see military medicine as "their system." As then-Major Duckworth pointed out in her testimony before the Senate Committee on Veterans' Affairs in 2005, "I would like to take a moment to stress the unique nature of the military healthcare system. While civilian professionals are an important component in that system, there is no substitute to being treated by, and recovering with fellow Soldiers. Only a fellow service member can understand the stresses and wounds of combat." There, anything seen as an abdication of responsibility or a breakdown in the trust between military leaders and enlisted men and women could, literally, lead to a breakdown in the willingness of young men and women to volunteer to fight. Making it clear that DoD is the responsible entity would meet the expectations of the troops and their families.

One of the unfortunate realities of politics is that elected officials often believe that in order to effect positive change at an agency of government, they must first demonstrate that the agency is failing. Highlighting failures creates the momentum needed to rally support for the proposals a member of Congress has for making changes. Unfortunately, that has sizable downstream impacts on the public's belief in the institutions of government. In the case of VA, it meant pointing out that the agency wasn't ready to treat the veterans of Iraq and Afghanistan—in order to get them ready to treat those veterans. Not exactly confidence inducing. For all of these reasons, I strongly recommend Congressional policy and legislation that clearly denotes that the military is primarily responsible for caring for injured troops and their families for a fixed period of time at the start of a conflict and, in all case, at least 2 years following an initial traumatic injury.

My third recommendation is not one of policy change, but rather advice for advocates that goes hand in hand with my recommendations for an early focus on DoD as the source for care. Advocates should focus on DoD. It is the agency with the money.

In any conflict, Congress can more easily justify spending on the military through the DoD appropriations budget than spending on any other agency. The public supports our troops, even when they do not always support the justification or cause of a war. It takes money to launch new programs or make improvements to existing ones and DoD has the money or they will get it.

My recommendation is not based solely on the fact that it is easier, politically, to give money to DoD (although in my opinion that is true). But, more importantly, Congress tolerates trial and error from the military far more than it does from any other agency. As noted above, in testimony before the SVAC in 2006 (Perlin, 2006), VA revealed that it was just beginning to focus a portion of its research dollars on the wounded of the current war. Yet, in 2007 alone, the Defense Appropriations Committee provided $50 million to the brand new Defense Centers of Excellence for Psychological Health and Traumatic Brain Injury. And by 2009, the amount had grown to over $210 million. Congress had provided nearly a quarter of a billion dollars for brain research and psychological health trials to an organization that did not exist in 2006. That's just reality.

Fourth, I recommend advocates focus attention on the updating VA benefits to allow for the provision of more services to family members of veterans. I mentioned earlier that DoD recruits service members and retains families. This forces DoD to spend ample time considering the services, programs, and benefits needed in order to retain service members and ensure that their spouses and children can have a reasonable and enjoyable life during their collective time in the military. VA sometimes sees itself as playing a role in that continuum and sometimes does not. Too often in the area of health care, members of Congress, VA, and to some degree Veterans Service Organizations see VA as an agency devoted to caring only for veterans, not their families. The challenge, as any family member of a severely wounded service member will tell you, is that it takes tremendous efforts on the part of family members to care for a veteran in need of that service. Those efforts can involve stress on family members, children, and even parents. As a system, VA needs to begin to turn its operations towards one that better recognizes that when a service member is injured, the whole family is impacted. And VA's response—with Congressional backing—must be geared towards that reality long-term.

Finally, I recommend that Congress focus some attention on delivering a benefits structure for care support that allows individual circumstances to dictate the needed response. By that, I do not mean that programs geared towards specific injuries (spinal cord injury, PTSD) are not needed. But, I do mean that the family support structure can be an evolving concept for any American (single, married, married with kids, no kids, living with parents, etc....). That is also true for a service member. As such, when a service member is facing an injury that will require a lifetime of support, in some manner, the benefits structure needs to be flexible to allow for the changing circumstances that the Veteran will confront over a lifetime. Any structure for lifetime support should be flexible enough to recognize that a service member may be single when injured, married when discharged, divorced a few years later, and cohabitating with a significant other for an extended period of time without being re-married far into the future. Or some variation of all of those. VA will increasingly see single parents, same sex couples, and those who spend the rest of their lives living with friends and family members. The need for support won't change. Only the circumstances in which the support is required.

Congress should not attempt to design a litany of programs that take each of those circumstances into consideration. There should be a menu of services and/or benefits to which an injured service member is entitled. From among that menu, what is needed can be accessed and what is not required need not be provided.

6.5.1 Conclusion

As noted at the outset of this chapter, many of the most important improvements to programs and services that impact families in the military took place in the 1990s. The most obvious of these were changes to base housing and the health care benefit available to spouses and children (TRICARE). These changes took place in an environment that allowed time for discussion and focus on Capitol Hill and in the agencies. That type of opportunity is once again, thankfully, upon us. Now is the time to begin raising questions about which agency has primary responsibilities for caring for the wounded and their families in a time of war and for how long. When should transitions begin to VA and what should VA have available to assist family members so that the transition is a welcome one and not a step down in service?

Advocates for family members need to approach Congress understanding how the Committee structure works and focus their efforts on the members who sit on the committees that oversee the agencies that need the attention. Concentrate on creating a framework now for the environment and structure that the next advocates, at the outset of the next conflicts, will encounter. It will be time well-spent.

References

Duckworth, T. (2005). Opening Statement: Hearing of the Senate Committee on Veterans' Affairs. May 17.

Kizer, K. W. (1996). *Prescription for change: The guiding principles and strategic objectives underlying the transformation of the veterans healthcare system.* Washington, DC: Department of Veterans Affairs. Retrieved from https://www.va.gov/healthpolicyplanning/rxweb.pdf.

Lockwood, D., & Siehl, G. (2004). *Military base closures: A historical review from 1998–1995.* Washington, DC: Congressional Research Service.

McDonough, M. (2013) *Gordon H. Mansfield, top Veterans Affairs official and advocate for disabled soldiers, dies.* Washington Post.

Perlin, J. (2006). *Opening Statement: Hearing of the Senate Committee on Veterans' Affairs: April 7, 2006.*

Priest, D., Hull, A. (2007). Soldiers face neglect, frustration at Army's Top Medical Facility. *Washington Post.*

Public Law 104-262, 110 Stat. 3177. Oct. 9, 1996.

Wilson, E. (2010). *Official Notes Health System's 'Amazing' Impact.* Armed Forces Press Service.

Chapter 7
An Advocate's Lament: Creating a Strong Voice to Support Military Families at War

Joyce Wessel Raezer

7.1 Introduction

Immediately following the attacks of September 11, 2001 (9-11), and the start of the wars in Afghanistan and Iraq, Members of Congress, policy makers in federal agencies, and state officials eagerly stepped up to show their support of our troops and address the challenges military families faced as mobilizations increased and the military poised for war. But, most legislators knew little of existing troop benefits, what programs might have the greatest impact, or fix emerging problems for military families at war.

Enter military advocacy organizations. As war began, military associations with strong grassroots connections expanded their outreach beyond their traditional legislative and policy contacts and took advantage of the public desire to help troops and families in time of war. Advocacy for military families in the post-9/11 environment was a complex, often-frustrating task in which patriotic appeals could open doors to decision-makers, but sometimes were not enough to spur the most productive action. Military family life went on in many ways after 9/11 just as before; family advocates still had to sustain the bedrock infrastructure of military personnel and family compensation, benefits, and support. New challenges brought new solutions and new advocacy voices, but also unintended consequences that made connections to the grassroots and a broader network of decision-makers more essential for family advocates.

This chapter explores the military family advocacy trajectory after 9-11, sharing insights that may help future military family advocates prepare for the next crisis. Advocacy is about preparation—anticipating the consequences of events, engaging and listening to the grassroots, doing one's homework to create options, and building

J.W. Raezer (✉)
National Military Family Association, Alexandria, VA, USA
e-mail: JRaezer@MilitaryFamily.org

© Springer International Publishing AG 2018
L. Hughes-Kirchubel et al. (eds.), *A Battle Plan for Supporting Military Families*, Risk and Resilience in Military and Veteran Families,
https://doi.org/10.1007/978-3-319-68984-5_7

networks of partners to help further one's cause. Stories from the last war cannot fully prepare a military or an advocate for the next one. Short-burst reactions to a catastrophic event such as 9-11 demand one kind of advocacy focus and energy; war that spans more than a decade creates more complex circumstances and needs. The specific efforts cited in this chapter are included as illustrative examples of the types of actions that led to success, but also as cautionary tales.

7.2 Who Were the Advocates?

The pre-9-11 military advocacy world was populated by a variety of military and veteran organizations, most founded to meet the specific needs of their members, not necessarily the entire community. The leading champion of benefits and policies to protect service members, military retirees, veterans, and their families was and is remains The Military Coalition. Founded in 1985, the Coalition is composed of more than 30 military and veteran focused membership-based organizations, representing all seven uniformed services. Individual Coalition members may have advocacy interests that include military equipment or strategy, but the Coalition remains focused on personnel benefits (health care, pay, family support, retirement, survivor support) for currently serving troops, retirees, and veterans, as well as their families and survivors.[1]

In 2001, only one Coalition member focused solely on advocacy on behalf of military families, the National Military Family Association (NMFA). The story of military family advocacy is, therefore, the story of NMFA, both in the pre-9-11 years and for most of the years afterwards. Founded in 1969 by military spouses concerned over the lack of benefits for surviving spouses of military retirees, NMFA's information, case work, and advocacy have always served all families, regardless of whether they are association members. NMFA's 200-member Volunteer Corps, most of whom are military spouses, connects the organization to military families at the grassroots level, raising issues from military communities needing to be addressed at higher levels.[2]

---

[1] For more information on The Military Coalition, its members, and history, go to: www.themilitarycoalition.org.

[2] I first encountered NMFA in the early 1990s when my Army husband was assigned to Fort Knox, Kentucky. I was a member of the school board, elected by parents whose children attended the Department of Defense Schools on the installation. NMFA helped us navigate a difficult dispute with the Department of Defense Education Activity (DoDEA) that threatened our ability to provide the advice and counsel to school administrators prescribed by law. When my husband received an assignment to the Pentagon in 1995, I became a Government Relations volunteer with NMFA. I went on the payroll in early 1998—joining the Association's paid staff of six—and became Government Relations Director in 2000, after the retirement of my mentor Sydney Tally Hickey, who had orchestrated NMFA's advocacy response to Desert Storm. I remained in that position until early 2007, when I became the Association's fourth Executive Director in 5 years. So, this military family advocacy story is a personal one, but one enhanced because of the strong network of dedicated advocates with whom I've been privileged to work.

Operations Desert Shield and Desert Storm in 1990 and 1991 gave NMFA a test run on how to advocate for military families in times of war and provided important lessons learned to guide its post-9-11 Board and staff. During Desert Storm, NMFA leveraged its relationships with senior military spouses, its grassroots volunteer connections, and the press to encourage increased military Service support of families of deployed troops, including those of National Guard and Reserve members affected by sudden call-ups, and raising awareness of the needs of the many families who left their installations to go back home to family after their service members deployed (Hallgren, 1991).

7.3 Who is Paying Attention in Times of Peace?

As in many other periods of relative peacetime, the military disappeared from the public view after the end of Operation Desert Storm and throughout most of the 1990s. These years were a time of uncertain troop morale brought on by the post-Cold War downsizing, a sense pay and benefits were eroding, and increased missions to places like Bosnia and Kosovo. Military retirees, especially those eligible for Medicare, mobilized to fight for expanded health care access as the military health system constricted and implemented the new TRICARE benefit. Military advocates pointed to a growing gap between military and private sector pay, grudgingly acknowledged even by the Department of Defense (DoD).[3]

Spurred by military advocacy organizations and, in some cases, by uniformed military leaders concerned about the future of recruiting and retention, Congress passed a series of provisions as part of the annual defense bills in 1999 and 2000 aimed at improving morale and enhancing military readiness. These included the creation of a Women's, Infants, and Children (WIC) nutrition program for military families overseas in the FY1999 National Defense Authorization Act (NDAA, P.L. 105-261). The most significant response to the growing concerns about the morale and readiness of the force can be found in the FY 2001 NDAA (P.L. 106-398). The law included a provision to set military pay raises for the next 5 years at the level of the Employment Cost Index (ECI), the measure of private sector pay growth, plus .5% to eliminate the gap between military and private sector pay. It also contained the most significant federal health care benefit expansion since the institution of

---

[3] The 9th Quadrennial Review of Military Compensation, begun in the waning months of the Clinton Administration and released in early 2002 after the 9-11 attacks, warned of future recruiting and retention challenges and acknowledged gaps in the current military compensation structure: "Military and civilian pay comparability is critical to the success of the All-Volunteer Force. Military pay must be set at a level that takes into account the special demands associated with military life and should be set above average pay in the private sector.... New data and analyses by the 9th QRMC suggest that military pay—particularly for mid-grade enlisted members and junior officers—has not kept pace with compensation levels in the private sector. Today's force is more highly educated than in the past and the current pay table may not include a high enough premium to sustain this more educated force."

Medicare in the creation of TRICARE for Life, which provided Medicare-eligible military retirees with a health benefit that would follow them wherever they were for the rest of their lives.

These benefit changes represented a high point for military advocates. But, the concept of family support remained a hard sell. When advocates—whether from associations or from family program staff in DoD—talked about family needs, the first question they heard from Congress or from military line leaders in the Pentagon was, "And how does this relate to service member readiness?" Sometimes, even when a readiness link was made and a need identified, the fix did not happen rapidly. It took more than 5 years for advocates to persuade Congress to enact the WIC Overseas legislation and another 2 years for DoD to implement it. The creation of TRICARE for Life was the result of years of retiree mobilization, association persistence, pilot programs, and reports. Wheels often had to squeak a long time before Congress made a fix.

7.4   The World Changes and New Challenges Emerge

In peacetime, a grindingly slow legislative process can often be accepted as the status quo if short-term emergencies such as floods, fires, and hurricanes are addressed promptly. But, war creates an urgency that brings new opportunities and new hazards to advocates. Almost immediately after the 9/11 attacks, military family advocates discovered those challenges. The first military people searching the internet for help on September 12th and 13th were families of the newly mobilized National Guard and Reserve members, now facing the realization that being a military family meant more than having their service member go off to drill 1 weekend a month and 2 weeks in the summer.

Advocates, as well as the government's family support providers, discovered they had much to learn about these new military families—and they needed to learn it quickly. Lessons learned from Desert Storm soon proved inadequate. Local and national press saw the call-ups of the Guard and Reserve as an interesting angle to the stories about the nation's 9/11 response. Communities far from New York City and Washington, DC, might not have had a resident die in the attacks, but they saw their Sheriff's deputies, high school teachers, small business owners, friends, and neighbors called up to do cleanup and recovery efforts at attack sites or to guard airports, bridges, military installations, and government buildings. And then there was the internet—families searched it for help, the press searched it for stories, and advocates learned to use it to supplement their own grassroots connections about what families needed and to advance the issues they believed demanded more attention.

What were the issues? Where would isolated, dispersed National Guard and Reserve families find support? How would the military wade through the myriad of mobilization statuses to ensure service members called up for duty had correct orders and got their pay on time? What was needed to help National Guard and

Reserve families transition from the mobilized service members' employer-sponsored health plans to TRICARE in places where medical providers had limited knowledge of the military health system?

And what about the active duty families of the All-Volunteer Force? Many already felt strained by the multiple peace-keeping deployments of the late nineties. How would they handle wartime deployments of indeterminate length and frequency? What did they need and what should they expect from their leaders to become ready to meet the challenges of the new realities of war in a new century?

7.5   A Battle Plan for Future Military Family Advocates

The move to war footing posed challenges for military and veteran advocacy organizations just as it did for military families. But, the lessons outlined below learned by post-9-11 advocates through hard-fought efforts and a bit of trial and error can be the start of a battle plan for military family advocacy in future challenging times.

7.5.1   Make Military Family Research a Priority—In Peace and War

No one stood at the door of the airplanes taking the first Marines and Soldiers to Afghanistan in October 2001 and surveyed them about how healthy they were and what concerns they had about their families. No one circulated through the crowds of family members asking about their current state of physical or mental health, how their kids were doing in school, or what support services they were using. The lack of good baseline data on military family well-being or on the "typical" course of development for service members and families put advocates, family support providers, and future researchers at a disadvantage that ultimately may have hurt families as well. Why? Because they had no data to tell them how families were doing before the war, advocates could not fully answer the question: "How has war affected military families?"

Desert Storm was too short to generate research on military families. Research from the Vietnam era reflected a different population than the All-Volunteer family force that fought in the post-9/11 wars. Some government surveys, such as the Army's Survey of Army Families and DoD's Survey of Active Duty Spouses, were available to outsiders. Research entities such as RAND would occasionally be asked by government clients to conduct and publish research on specific issues affecting military families, but most of these projects were of small populations and did not touch on many of the issues that became important as military families experienced repeated deployments.

Because good advocacy starts with anticipating needs and devising solutions, advocates and family program providers need the best information possible about military families to be effective, to argue for the right set of policies and benefits, and to direct resources where they are most-needed. One upside to the length of the wars in Afghanistan and Iraq was that more researchers entered the space, the government became a sponsor for and funder of family research, and nonprofits found ways to make their more informal information-gathering efforts more sophisticated. Government had the resources to sponsor large-scale research projects, as well as the capability to sponsor longitudinal studies. But, government funders remained most interested in research that informed service member readiness. As the wars lengthened, academic researchers became motivated to conduct research on deployment effects, behavioral health, child well-being, and the effects of visible and invisible injuries on service members. Many, however, had limited knowledge of the military and often struggled to identify relevant projects or interventions or to recruit military family participants.

Nonprofits had access to military families, but usually lacked the financial and staff resources to conduct or sponsor major research projects. Their interactions with military families through their programs, surveys, and other outreach did help them identify emerging issues of concern that could be explored by government or academic researchers. Advocacy groups discovered making connections with researchers to promote more study on critical issues affecting military families was just as important as shepherding legislation through Congress.

In the absence of relevant family research, NMFA urged both the DoD and Congress to make military family research a priority. It also supplemented its informal information-gathering methods with surveys and focus groups conducted by NMFA staff and volunteers, its access to families enabling it to take the pulse of military families quickly.

In early 2004, NMFA launched the first effort by either the government or a private entity to assess on a broad scale the state of military family support since 9/11. The resulting report from its survey of 2500 military family members and military family support staff, *Serving the homefront: An analysis of military family support from September 11, 2001 through March 31, 2004*, highlighted that many programs and services were in place to strengthen and support military families, but were doing so inconsistently and, in many cases, failing to reach out to families who needed the services the most. Families were resilient, but their strength was wearing down as the high pace of operations continued. The report emphasized the need for better coordination among the individual military services and between the active and reserve components, for resources to provide more robust counseling services, and for government facilitation of research on military families, especially on the needs of children during high operations tempo and on the dynamics of service member return and reunions with families during and after multiple deployments (NMFA, 2004).[4]

---

[4] In late 2005, NMFA published results of a follow-up survey, the *Cycles of Deployment* Report.

As the war progressed, new organizations in the advocacy space began their own surveys. Some, like the Iraq and Afghanistan Veterans of America (IAVA) and Wounded Warrior Project (WWP), surveyed their members annually. Others, like Blue Star Families, reached out to a wider audience and enlisted the help of fellow associations to encourage members of the community to participate in the survey. The larger organizational surveys became more sophisticated as organizations hired staff trained in research methods or worked with university partners such as the Institute for Veterans and Military Families at Syracuse University or the Military Family Research Institute at Purdue University. While there remain no apples to apples comparisons between surveys of different organizations—indeed, in some cases, not even between surveys conducted from 1 year to the next by the same organization—advocates found surveys enhanced their visibility with key audiences, including the press, Congressional leaders, and DoD and VA officials. More importantly, survey findings gave advocates ammunition to pursue legislative change. Legislation leading to the Post-9-11 GI Bill, provisions for in-state tuition for military families, and support for caregivers of the wounded would not have happened if organizations had not collected input from their constituents via their surveys.

Advocacy groups are not research entities and advocates using survey and program participant data should be prepared to encounter criticism that the information gathered is "anecdotal" and not hard data acquired in more "scientific" studies. So-called anecdotal information should never be the only "data" in an advocate's arsenal, but there is a use for it. A survey population representative of the demographics of the force provides more context than smaller snapshots of a narrower slice of the community. A good story always helps to personalize a complex issue when used in the appropriate context and only when the advocate can support the story with other facts.

Advocacy organizations supported researchers' efforts by encouraging them to explore emerging issues of concern and by helping to find family participants for their studies.[5] Usually, their only request of a researcher asking for help in finding military family participants was a request to see the findings. Early academic studies generally focused on small samples and narrow topics related to deployment or family separation. Advocates became increasingly frustrated at the lack of large-scale longitudinal data about military family well-being in time of war and urged DoD to prioritize research on how families, especially military children, were dealing with multiple deployments.

By 2007, NMFA got tired of waiting for someone else to sponsor large-scale family research and so approached RAND to explore the possibility of studying the effects of deployment on military children and to measure how effective its

---

[5] For example, in 2004, the first year of its Operation Purple® camps, NMFA allowed Dr. Angela Huebner, a researcher from Virginia Tech University, to conduct focus groups with military teens attending several of the camps. Huebner's research became the first to be published about military kids and deployment (Huebner & Mancini, 2005; Huebner, Mancini, Wilcox, Grass, & Grass, 2007).

Operation Purple® camps were in helping them. For a relatively small nonprofit, the decision to pay a research entity to conduct a study on its behalf is a tough one and a departure from the usual advocacy trajectory. With the goal of using the research to support its advocacy, NMFA selected RAND because of its reputation and credibility among military leaders and others in the military community.

NMFA and RAND started with a small pilot study with a couple of hundred Operation Purple campers and their parents in the summer of 2007 (Chandra, Burns, Tanielian, Jaycox, & Scott, 2008). Working with RAND in 2008 to finalize the processes to be used for a larger study to follow 1500 children and their at-home mothers over 1 year, NMFA staff simultaneously began looking for funding for such an ambitious plan. They convinced two foundations—and the NMFA Board—of the urgency of the research proposal. At any time during that process, if DoD had announced its intent to move forward with its own longitudinal study of military families and deployment, NMFA would have found other ways to use its time and donors' money. But, they did not and so NMFA and RAND embarked on the journey that became *Views from the homefront: The experiences of youth and spouses from military families*, published in 2011 (Chandra et al., 2011).

Research is useless if advocates fail to do anything with it. NMFA and RAND built an outreach plan around both the release of the final report and a peer-reviewed article that had been published in Pediatrics in 2010 (Chandra et al., 2010). The plan included Congressional testimony and presentations at various professional conferences by the RAND researcher and NMFA staff, briefings for senior DoD officials and senior military spouses, and a briefing for the staff of First Lady Michelle Obama. To introduce a wider audience of organizations, educators, health care professionals, military family support personnel, and others to the research findings and to use these findings to help chart its next steps, NMFA held a 2-day summit in May 2010. Knowing Mrs. Obama was looking for a venue to announce White House initiatives to support military families, NMFA worked with her staff to secure her as the keynote speaker, which provided exactly the right audience for a call for broad collaboration on behalf of military families from government, nonprofits, and the private sector (Obama, 2010).

Armed with the research, the input from its summit participants, and a call to action by the First Lady, NMFA put together a resource kit for community providers and others supporting military families. Using the research to inform the resources, NMFA chose to create the toolkit in response to summit participants' feedback that military families did not suffer from a lack of resources, but rather a lack of knowledge by both families and the people who wanted to help them about what was available and most effective (NMFA, 2011).

The key for advocates and program providers trying to prepare for the next crisis is the existence of a military family research network, promoting ongoing research on the totality of military family life, so that a baseline of data and a plan for acquiring and disseminating new knowledge exist. Ideally, some of that research should be longitudinal, like the DoD Millennium Cohort Family Study, to provide a sense of how families change over the course of their military journey.[6] Research should not just look at weaknesses, but also at sources and predictors of strength.

One essential task of a broader network of those interested in the perpetuation and continued relevance of military family research must be to build more flexibility and speed into the research agenda and processes. Government must be a player in the promotion, funding, and dissemination of research, but government moves slowly. For example, shortly after RAND ended its work on NMFA's research project, it began a project for DoD that had been in the talking stages for several years. The 3-year longitudinal study of 2700 families (service member, spouse, and child) with data captured at pre-deployment, deployment, and post-deployment periods was what many advocates and family support personnel—in DoD and out—had asked for. But, by the time it was funded, reviewed, conducted, analyzed, and released, the largest deployments to Iraq and Afghanistan were over. The unfortunate time lag was noted by RAND as a caveat to its findings (Meadows et al., 2016).

A strong research network should have a role for multiple communities of interest: academia, think tanks, government agencies, private and government funders, and the end users and disseminators, which include family support personnel and the advocates. Discussions between these groups should be ongoing, perhaps following a model like the Research Symposia sponsored occasionally by Purdue University's Military Family Research Institute.[7] Opening these research discussions to government entities and nonprofits can help disseminate research findings, but also allow researchers to think about policy and program implications of their findings. Input from advocates' nonprofit surveys and programs can help researchers identify new issues or populations needing deeper study.

The military advocacy loop is: families raise a concern, advocates voice the concern to Congress or someone who can make a change, a change is made, and the advocates tell families of the change and how their voices were heard. Inserting researchers into that loop adds depth to advocacy and connects research to action.

7.5.2 War is the Quickest Way of Finding Out What Doesn't Work

Thanks to advocates' early surveys and their grassroots connections, they, military leaders, and Members of Congress soon learned that protections and programs put in place during Desert Storm or implemented during peacetime did not fully address military family needs during a multi-theater prolonged war. Fixing an existing program or process is sometimes more difficult than starting a new one. Many times, advocacy groups became aware of issues like inconsistent powers of attorney

---

[6] The Millennium Cohort Family Study is a DoD research project at the Deployment Health Research Department: https://www.familycohort.org/. It enrolled its first panel of spouses of service members participating in the DoD Millennium Cohort Study in 2011.

[7] For example, see: https://www.mfri.purdue.edu/newsroom/view-news.aspx?newsitemid=95.

acceptance, families losing access to safety net programs, wounded service members' problems with coordinated health care, or inadequate command support of unit families before the leaders responsible for them were.

After advocates identified the source of a problem, they then had to convince program proponents a problem existed. They also had to know when to push for a quick fix to a problem grabbing the headlines and when to take a more strategic approach. Times of crisis often lead to bad legislation or hastily developed programs, which then lead to other negative consequences. Trust relationships between advocates, military leaders, Members of Congress and their staff gatekeepers based on an appreciation of an advocate's expertise and a leader's desire for long-term solutions can help avoid the unintended consequences of political expediency.

In the aftermath of Desert Storm, the services had required some sort of unit-based family support/readiness system. Volunteer-led and as active or inactive as the commander and unit volunteers wanted to make them, most networks tended to gear up if the unit or ship was deploying and then slow their activities when the unit was home. If units—either active or reserve component—had not deployed in the 1990s, family support groups were less organized or even non-existent.[8]

For decades, support systems for families in Europe had focused on helping families become acclimated to living abroad, not on how to help American families overseas deal with the deployment of their service member to a war zone elsewhere. On 9/11, many installations in Europe were in the last phases of the post-Cold War downsizing. Now short-staffed family support centers and DoD Schools were asked to find resources to help families of those at war even as their installations prepared to close. Spouses and children, often living in isolated housing areas with few support programs or amenities, faced a dilemma—do we stay here in a foreign country so that we can stay in touch with the unit or do we go back to the states where we will have help from our loved ones but be more isolated from information about our service member?

Family care plans generally worked—a lesson learned from Desert Storm when many had not—but some families had to make difficult choices about who would care for their children. Military demographic changes since Desert Storm compounded the situation—more dual military members (service members married to other service members) meant a higher probability both parents would have to deploy and would need different, longer-term caregiving solutions. The issue of child custody became more complicated because many service members had not addressed deployment in their custody agreements. Angry custody battles often played out not just in the courts, but also in the media and in Congress, where some Members, to the dismay of military family advocates, pushed for federal solutions to an issue under state jurisdiction.

---

[8] Immediately after the 9/11 attacks, the Army's ceremonial "Old Guard" unit, stationed at Fort Myer, VA, adjacent to the Pentagon, was tasked with cleanup and the removal of bodies. Said one Old Guard spouse (and NMFA employee) worried about her service member and desperate for information and a connection to other spouses, "Nobody thought the Old Guard would need a Family Support Group."

One of the major areas of advocacy focus after 9/11 was over pay and benefits for the members of an all-volunteer force at war. The rank and file and their families appreciated the increased compensation, to include special combat deployment pays, reflecting the increased demands of service and the military's recruiting and retention challenges in war. But, changes in compensation also brought unintended consequences for military families needing continued access to other federal safety net programs, such as food stamps and free and reduced price school lunches.[9]

As the first Marines deployed in 2001, some families with severely disabled children learned their service members' combat pay would drop their children from the Social Security Administration's Supplemental Security Income (SSI), which is the gateway to additional services in many states. For example, one family who contacted NMFA received approximately $400 in additional deployment allowances, but stood to lose services, supplies, and medical care for their disabled 3-year-old worth $8000 a month. The problem: Social Security counted special pays and allowances as unearned income when calculating a person's eligibility for SSI, thus weighting the allowances heavier than basic pay. It took until early 2003, after advocates and families raised the issue with Members of Congress, for the Social Security Commissioner to issue an emergency regulation exempting deployment pay to a combat zone from the SSI eligibility calculation.

Building trust with key government leaders and maintaining that relationship even as Congressional staff, political appointees, and senior government staff come and go is key for advocates who will be called on to lead efforts to fix an identified problem. But, advocates must remember that the government, or even a single department such as DoD, is not a monolithic entity—and figuring out who owns the solution to a problem can be a challenge.

7.5.3 *If You Want America to Understand Military Families, Educate the Press First*

Advocates often received help in discovering unintended consequences, a failed program, or inadequate benefit from members of the press. Successful advocates create collaborative relationships with the press prior to an emergency, enabling them to be proactive contributors to a compelling story that leads to a problem solved. Sometimes a cold call from a reporter can work out well when questions lead to a story advancing an organization's agenda. More problematic is a story that could be helpful but that comes as a surprise. Then the advocate must slip into reactive mode and spend valuable time tracking down information or family stories to prepare for other reporters who want in on the story or a Congressional staffer wondering if the issue requires a legislative fix.

---

[9] In the Consolidated Appropriations Act of 2005 (P.L. 108-447), Congress first created the combat pay exclusion for food stamp eligibility. Later it codified the same protections for free and reduced price school lunch eligibility.

After 9/11, like many of those new National Guard and Reserve military families, members of the civilian press Googled "military family" and found NMFA and other advocates. As family advocates developed trusted relationships with individual members of the press, these reporters continued to contact them as the wars unfolded, deployments continued, and new issues emerged. Before these relationships could become productive, however, advocates first had to educate the press about who the families of the troops heading off to Afghanistan and Iraq were. Advocates found many members of the press, like other civilians, still thought of the military in the context of the old Vietnam-era draftee force. Under this stereotype, the military was made up of a lot of young single men and only officers and senior enlisted had families. One essential tool for advocates in this "Military 101" educational effort was the DoD annual Demographics Report. By sharing key data from this report, advocates helped reporters understand that half of the military is married, almost half of military children are younger than age 6, that an increasing number of service members were married to other service members, and that more women were serving and moving up the ranks.[10]

Reporters also needed good information about military benefits and military life in general. Many, for example, still thought most families lived on military installations and almost all military kids attended DoD schools. Advocates frequently had to dispel two opposite narratives: one that depicted almost all enlisted military families as impoverished recipients of welfare programs who were unable to access any help from the military and another that portrayed military families as pampered beneficiaries of a paternalistic government system that provided free health care, child care, housing, and groceries.

Accurate information about the current generation of military families helped focus reporters on actual issues and not on topics the stereotypes they held made them suspect were issues. What advocates want most from the press is a true portrayal of military families' lives to solve the real issues these families face. What the press wants most from advocacy organizations is access to military families. Reporters new to military subjects usually had no contacts in the military installation public affairs offices. Security concerns closed off some communication channels between the military and the press. Family members were often reluctant to identify to a broad audience that they had a service member deployed.

The ideal situation for an advocate is connecting a reporter with a family, but also having a member of an organization's staff being interviewed to put the individual story into a broader context. Sometimes that is easier said than done. NMFA reached out to its volunteers to develop a list of families willing to talk with reporters about their deployment experiences. Advocates also asked family members who contacted them with a particularly poignant problem representative of a larger issue if they would be interested in speaking with the press. Sometimes a match could be made, but often the criteria laid out by the reporter—the male spouse of a female National

---

[10]To access the most recent Demographics Report, go to: http://download.militaryonesource. mil/12038/MOS/Reports/2015-Demographics-Report.pdf.

Guard Soldier from Ithaca, New York, whose deployment to Iraq was extended and then was injured—were too hard to match.[11]

Despite the complications, trusted members of the press can be the most effective tool advocates can wield in educating the rest of America about the needs of military families. Advocates should not be shy about pitching stories, offering topics for reporters to investigate. They can leverage their relationship with trusted reporters to advance a legislative or policy agenda. They can aggressively insert their talking points into conversations with reporters searching only for a family member to interview. Advocates who are themselves family members should not use their own family story all the time, but pulling bits and pieces of it can make the issue seem more personal to a reporter.

In their interactions with the press, advocates must always be sensitive about the kind of narrative they are helping to create about military families. The press normally reacts to crisis, with a tendency to show weakness rather than strength. So, stories about families back home dealing with multiple deaths in a unit or military kids struggling with deployment get more interest than research showing most children are resilient and doing OK.[12] Therefore, advocates must always be mindful of the danger of creating an incomplete or inaccurate narrative or one that somehow disempowers or sends a negative message to families. This is not just an issue for advocates in their dealings with the press—it also applies to charities' solicitations to donors and advocates' messages to Congress. How can advocates accurately portray both the challenges and the strengths of military families in the hope of making life better without portraying them as victims without strengths, resources, and hope?

7.5.4   Put On Your Own Mask Before Helping Others

To be most effective over the long term, advocates must build a sustainable organizational capacity and ensure the well-being of the people they depend on to implement their advocacy strategy. These tasks become more important during times of crisis. When the post-9/11 deployments started, advocacy organizations' blueprint for action was lessons learned from Operation Desert Storm—a short war. And so,

---

[11] I am not making this example up. A reporter from New York asked me to find such a soldier.

[12] One of the toughest interviews I ever had resulted in a USA Today story written by Greg Zoroya (2006, October 19). Zoroya had a long history of covering military issues and usually contacted us when doing a story related to families. I happened to be visiting Fort Hood, Texas, when Zoroya contacted me asking for a comment about the deaths in units deployed from there. He knew the monthly memorial service had just taken place. Imagine my surprise when he asked if I knew anyone who attended the memorial service and imagine his surprise when I said I had as the culmination of a week visiting the post. A good reporter knows when to allow a source to be on the record and when not. The challenge for the advocate is knowing how much to share. This story captured well what I felt was important to say, but waiting for the story be posted is always an anxious time.

just as they had done in Desert Storm, advocates ran on adrenaline. But you can only run on adrenaline for so long. A cumulative sapping of time and energy took its toll on military family advocates as the wars progressed with no end in sight. Deployments, injuries, and deaths among the organizations' families increased the commitment of staff and grassroots volunteers, but affected their spirit and focus. The volume of activity, the multiple channels now required to communicate, the many entities that needed to be educated before they could act forced an expansion in the scope of military family advocates' work that demanded a different kind of organizational support infrastructure. There remained so much to do, but an over-whelming sense no one could do it all.

Military family organizations, by the very nature of who they are and who they serve, had to intensify their advocacy activities at a time when the people they depended on to conduct that advocacy were feeling the full effects of war. Firsthand experiences of staff and volunteers whose spouses and adult children deployed to war zones added to the credibility of organizations' advocacy message and made the fight for better family support more personal and sometimes more emotion-laden. Volunteers, who were now forced to balance unit family support obligations and family demands, often scaled back or stopped their engagement with the organiza-tion. This loss of volunteer support at the grassroots level could have disadvantaged NMFA's advocacy and support role at a time when it was needed most. While con-tinuing to recruit new active duty spouse volunteers, NMFA also found ways to maintain communication with its existing volunteers even as it tried to limit its requests of these busy military family members.

Recognizing the importance of expanding volunteer networks outside a tradi-tional installation focus, NMFA recruited more National Guard and Reserve spouses and their family support personnel into its Volunteer Corps. To accommodate the addition of Guard and Reserve family issues to its advocacy agenda, NMFA scaled back its involvement in retiree issues, keeping its public voice tuned to the concerns of currently serving active duty and National Guard and Reserve families. NMFA looked to its partners in The Military Coalition active on retiree issues to carry the water on them.

Advice to pace yourself is not practical if an organization lacks the capacity to allow individuals to do so. In times of war, nations incur debt to have the tools to fight the war. Association boards must plan for ways to surge support where needed. That is not easy for a nonprofit to do—associations do not have the borrowing capacity of the federal government. But, when military families need strong advo-cates supporting them, association boards must find ways to be prepared to intensify that fight and to support its people charged with the advocacy mission.[13] They must

---

[13] If I were facing the situation again, I would encourage my Board to dig into reserves to hire more Government Relations and Communications staff earlier, to provide more staff support services and benefits—to include access to our own Employee Assistance Program (which we did not get until 2015)—and would put in place a staff sabbatical program like that of our partners at the Military Officers Association of America. Robust staffing is the key to making a sabbatical pro-gram work—an employer must ensure those not on sabbatical wouldn't be overwhelmed by pick-ing up extra responsibilities.

be flexible and creative in supporting staff members dealing with a family member's deployment, injury, or, unfortunately, death. Military spouse employees with young children at home needed more flexible hours, more options to work from home, and co-workers willing to cover more evening events or association-related travel. Association employers of National Guard and Reserve members gained many first-hand stories to support their advocacy, but had to accommodate deployments of members of their staff, as well as support the families left behind.

7.5.5   Be Ready to Take Advantage of Opportunities

In the swirl of challenges facing advocates in war come opportunities waiting to be seized. The first opportunity in the wars in Afghanistan and Iraq came through the surge of patriotism after 9/11. Ordinary Americans as well as governments at all levels wanted to do all they could to support the troops. They wanted to extend that support to the families of those troops. Despite events that did not always show the military at its best, such as the Abu Ghraib prisoner abuse and torture scandal, public support for military families remained strong, generating more donations for military charities and making a wider audience sympathetic to advocates' messages.[14]

In war, small windows of opportunity can emerge to speed an advocate's legislative agenda. Once such opportunity came in April 2003 as Congress was readying the Supplemental Appropriations Bill to fund the new operations in Iraq war as well as in Afghanistan. As they reviewed lessons from Desert Storm and from the past year and a half of conflict in Afghanistan, NMFA staff saw an opportunity repeat one of its legislative victories from Desert Storm: increasing the Family Separation Allowance (FSA). The FSA, set at $100 since Desert Storm, is paid to any service member on orders away from their family to help with higher expenses incurred while a service member is deployed, such as phone cards, care packages, and increased child care and home repair costs. When a staffer for Senator Richard Durbin (D-IN) asked what they could do quickly and easily in the appropriations bill, NMFA suggested increasing the FSA. The Senator included a provision, which passed, raising the allowance to $250, retroactive to the beginning of the fiscal year.[15]

The military decision to fight these wars as a true **All-Volunteer, total force** and the resulting large deployments of National Guard and Reserve members meant every Member of Congress now had troops deployed and families struggling at

---

[14] For more information on the Abu Ghraib story, see: https://en.wikipedia.org/wiki/Abu_Ghraib_torture_and_prisoner_abuse.

[15] Congress made the increase permanent in the FY 2005 NDAA (P.L. 108-375). NMFA continued to push when it could for automatic annual increases in the FSA based on the Cost of Living Allowance (COLA) and hopes future advocates will note it will probably take another war to spur the next increase.

home—not just transient active duty families, but the members of the local civic organizations, their campaign volunteers, and their local donors. And, to the surprise and delight of military family advocates, the issues these Members wanted to help with were, for the most part, not the usual military equipment and big procurement contracts Members of Congress often seek for their districts, but the people issues: health care, employment, behavioral health, family support. In most cases, neither these Members nor their staffs knew a lot about military pay, benefits, or family support programs. They reached out to advocates when they received constituent questions and wanted to help. Did a law need to be changed? Who in the Pentagon could fix this? Where can this family go for help? How can Congress help?

This interest in the well-being of National Guard and Reserve members and their families, as well as in the medical readiness of reserve component troops, led Congress to expand TRICARE programs for National Guard and Reserve, resulting in the creation of TRICARE Reserve Select in the 2004 NDAA (P.L. 108-136). Members of Congress concerned about access to behavioral health services pressed both DoD and physicians at home to expand provider networks, long a goal of military family advocates. They passed legislation to mandate more outreach to providers in the civilian communities experiencing National Guard and Reserve deployments, but also used their Congressional bully pulpit to encourage doctors in their states to accept TRICARE patients. These efforts did not just help National Guard and Reserve families, but also military retirees; active duty members, such as recruiters, assigned far from installations; and active duty families who could not obtain care in military hospitals because of the deployment of military providers.

But, advocates should not just look to Congress for opportunities. In the wake of the massive call-ups of National Guard and Reserve members, more states sought to support military members and their families. Several created relief funds, often funded through voluntary contributions from state residents on their tax returns, to assist families of the deployed with unexpected household repairs, utilities, and other expenses.

As crass as it may seem to say, war can also provide opportunities to advance issues beyond deployment and war-related support. Many states increased their assistance to active duty families, easing in-state tuition eligibility, providing for unemployment compensation for military spouses forced to quit their jobs when their service member received orders to move, and voting to join the Interstate Compact for the Education of Military Children to ease student transitions from one school to another. Advocacy groups had worked these issues in the states for several years, often with little success. Appealing to the patriotism of state leaders desiring to support troops and their families in time of war broke some of these issues out of the committees in which they had languished or prompted new champions to embrace these changes. In some states, patriotism combined with the desire to make their military installations more resistant to Base Realignment and Closure (BRAC) decisions by appearing more military-friendly—an advocacy opportunity, nonetheless![16] There is no guarantee the next conflict or military emergency will come with such an outpouring of public support or, even when initial support is there, that it can be sustained. As the end of the Bush Administration neared, the country had been at war for 7 years. War and the families of the people serving in those wars were no longer at the top of the nation's consciousness. Advocates and military families were tired and in need of a boost of support, which they soon received from the new Obama administration. Joining Forces, the initiative created by First Lady Michelle Obama and Dr. Jill Biden, gave advocates the opportunity they needed to revitalize efforts by corporate America, nonprofits, state governments, and others to enhance support for military families. Nothing can match the power of the White House bully pulpit for giving hope to exhausted advocates, spurring the creation of new partnerships, energizing government to expand support, and reminding all Americans of the service and sacrifice of our troops and their families.

7.5.6   Old and New Can Learn From Each Other and Model Collaboration

Existing advocacy organizations were not the only ones taking advantage of opportunities to advance their cause. As the challenges of war brought out the best of this nation's charitable spirit, many Americans directed more of their charitable giving toward military and veteran charities. Others saw the advantages of creating a new charity to support their efforts. Much has been made of the explosion in the number of military-related charities—usually pegged at around 40,000—in the wake of 9-11 (Carter & Kidder, 2015). While only a few of the new groups among that 40,000 ever engaged in advocacy, it took time for these new advocates and the pre-9-11 organizations to figure out how to develop productive working relationships.

At the founding of each of the pre-9-11 military and veteran organizations were members of a specific segment of the military community who saw a need to band with others like them, who shared a similar service experience. The new organizations emerging during the wars in Afghanistan and Iraq were also born out of the needs of their generation, formed from the belief an unmet need or a gap in support services or advocacy existed only they could fill. Advocates already in the space should expect a new generation will start their own groups rather than joining what another generation built. The challenge is how to deal with the entrance of new players without being insulted they did not join your group, dismissing them as unnecessary, or fearing them as competition. It is not always easy.

---

[16] The DoD provided critical support to these efforts by in a sense becoming an advocate through the creation of the DoD State Liaison Office (DSLO) in 2004. The DSLO works with states to address key issues affecting military families that fall under state jurisdiction. For more information, go to: http://www.usa4militaryfamilies.dod.mil/MOS/f?p=USA4:HOME:0.

Early in a war or time of change, legacy organizations can have a huge advantage over new groups because they have an infrastructure, history, and connections. But, they can also be at a disadvantage because their established organizational structure may make them less nimble or their reputation for serving a specific constituency can make them seem out of touch. Legacy organizations can spout the history of a legislative fight and provide the reason why a proposal didn't make it into law. New organizations bring enthusiasm and impatience and say, "That was then—this time we'll win!" The groups formed after 9-11 brought new skills to the fight, showing others how to successfully use social media to further advocacy or online communication to build connections between members. Successful advocacy needs an understanding of history, but it can also benefit from the passion and fresh perspective of those who are newly arrived to a fight. The trick is for both the old and the new to use their specific advantages, but ultimately find a way to work together.

The pre-9/11 military advocacy environment had been dominated by The Military Coalition (TMC) and its member organizations, plus a handful of nonmembers such as the American Legion and the Disabled American Veterans. These organizations' advocacy agendas and organizational benefits were geared to the characteristics and needs of their specific memberships.[17] TMC members had perfected processes for collaboration and were trusted resources for Members of Congress. They could easily reach out to the Hill when new challenges emerged for their members. In developing their advocacy agendas, most established military and veteran organizations took advantage of their chapters and annual state and national conventions to follow a complex process to develop the issues their national advocacy teams would pursue. The resolution processes used by these traditional organizations certainly created buy-in from members and projected credibility in these organizations' advocacy positions. But, the process could sometimes delay raising new and emerging issues at the national level. As the speed at which events affected military families intensified after 9/11, older groups such as NMFA and new advocates with a more flexible, staff-driven issue development process could address emerging concerns more quickly than those with a more rigid resolution system.

Legacy organizations facing the emergence of new organizations reacted in multiple ways. Some embraced the entrepreneurial spirit and grew their own outreach to and support of the generation fighting the wars and their families. For NMFA, that meant expanding its concept of what it meant to be a military family advocate. Entering the program space with its military spouse scholarships and Operation Purple® camps was a big step for the Association and one some Board members and staff approached gingerly. They worried about the financial commitment and whether engaging in programs would diminish its advocacy standing. But, the programs helped expand NMFA's visibility among military families, helped it raise funds from donors who traditionally shied away from supporting advocacy, and ultimately helped deepen its advocacy message by generating more information about the military families it served.

---

[17] NMFA was one of the few that allowed anyone to join—its board welcomed civilian supporters of the military—and did not limit its assistance or eligibility for its programs to members.

Legacy organizations, like government officials and the press, must be careful not to fight the last war or to let the experiences of previous generations of service members, veterans, and families color their reactions to the expectations of the new generation at war. Sometimes, the experiences from a previous war can bring out sympathy for the new generation. NMFA heard from the spouses of the Vietnam generation who offered to mentor and support young military spouses. To a woman, these spouses said they did not want the new generation of spouses to experience the isolation they felt. But, there were other cases when earlier generations—who were heavily represented on the Boards and senior staff of the legacy organizations—discounted the needs of the new generation. Young veterans and families forced legacy organizations to reexamine positions on a variety of issues, including expanding family support services beyond the installation fences; women in combat; Don't Ask, Don't Tell; sexual assault response; and military spouse employment support.

As the wars progressed, many legacy organizations worked to balance the needs and influence of their older members with the desire to be relevant to the new generation. Traditional Veteran Service Organizations began hiring young veterans just out of the military or Guard and Reserve members who were still on call for deployments. Other old-guard groups also created programs and special outreach initiatives. The Military Officers Association of America (MOAA) began its efforts to reach out to the currently serving population before 9/11 and changed its name from The Retired Officers Association in 2002. As part of its outreach to younger officers, they offered free digital memberships and created special initiatives supporting military spouses.

Given new organizations will always emerge to meet either real or perceived needs, legacy organizations have an obligation to initiate the outreach and say, "For the good of the community, we need to find a way to collaborate." That collaboration between old and new can lead to powerful results. Probably the best example is the work by the Iraq and Afghanistan Veterans of America (IAVA), TMC associations, and the American Legion to secure the passage of the Post-9/11 GI Bill. Founded by post-9/11 veterans in 2004, IAVA launched a new type of advocacy and new association membership model. With a lean organization, IAVA founders created free online memberships—no dues, no chapters. Veterans who signed up became part of a community of their peers. In their outreach to the American public, IAVA focused on raising the visibility of these new veterans.[18] Their first advocacy issue, to which they dedicated all their energy, was to seek legislation creating an enhanced GI Bill, comparable to that provided to veterans of World War II.

IAVA mobilized its grassroots and encouraged veterans to come to Washington, DC, often at their own expense, to start the conversation for enhanced GI Bill benefits for those serving in the Afghanistan and Iraq Wars. With the input of old and new groups, freshman Virginia Senator James Webb (D-VA) introduced the Twenty-First Century GI Bill legislation in early 2008. The entire Military Coalition quickly signed on as well, anxious to move beyond its original goal of simply updating the

---

[18] See the powerful ad IAVA produced with the Ad Council: https://www.youtube.com/watch?v=fDbqLul97Fg.

existing Montgomery GI Bill. The result of this impressive multi-organization collaboration that also gained administration support was the passage of the Post-9/11 Veterans Educational Assistance Act of 2008 in June 2008 (P.L. 110-252).

Collaboration between old and new can result in impressive legislative wins, but sometimes not everyone's members benefit from the victory—at least right away. As the issues facing the wounded gained more national attention, several organizations worked together to increase support for the spouse, parent, or other caregivers of wounded service members and veterans. A key victory was the passage of the Caregivers and Veterans Omnibus Health Services Act of 2010 (P.L. 111-163), made possible through the work of new organizations such as the Wounded Warrior Project (WWP) and IAVA (by then a member of The Military Coalition) along with NMFA, other TMC members, and organizations such as Paralyzed Veterans of America. Groups supporting the current generation of wounded and their caregivers came armed with stories from the population they served. Caregivers' stories of a lack of respite care reduced family income because they had been forced to leave their jobs, and inadequate training for some of the tasks they had to perform as they cared for their warrior helped to shape the provisions of the legislation and secure its passage. One issue dampened the success for many groups. The new law and the benefits it brought only applied to caregivers of post-9/11 wounded veterans because of the high price tag of those benefits. Members of legacy groups disabled in previous conflicts and their caregivers did not begrudge younger veterans and caregivers the support provided in the law, but were upset the law did not include all.

Not all advocates will be organizationally based. The scope of the wars and the complexity of some of the issues facing service members and families caused the rise out of the grassroots of a vocal and often very effective group of individual advocates. In some cases, these were the family members of the wounded or parents of a special needs military child, who began their advocacy by championing better care for their family member, but then became known by the senior officials and Members of Congress they engaged in their individual struggles. Many eventually became mentors for other families. While some created support organizations or online communities, many chose to remain independent voices for their cause. One unique, highly respected advocate for the wounded and their caregivers started as a Congressional staffer. As she encountered the wounded who approached her office for help, Meredith Beck developed a knowledge of government agencies and officials who could cut red tape or connect the service member, veteran, or caregiver with what they needed. She developed expertise in complex issues, such as what happens when a wounded 24-year-old becomes eligible for Medicare. Sometimes working for support organizations and sometimes working independently, but with those same groups, she helped others learn the details necessary to support those who had fallen through the cracks. Advocates should never ignore the gifts of individuals like Meredith—unbound by organizational constraints, they can help point the way toward change and can be the catalyst for collaboration.

7.5.7   Focus Pays Off

IAVA's campaign to win the Post-9/11 GI Bill is a powerful example of what advocates can do when they make the decision to devote all their energy to a single, important cause. Diverting staff time and visibility from other priorities and hoping nothing else important emerges can make the decision a difficult one, especially for organizations with a full plate of issues, but advocates should always be aware of the power that comes from a focused campaign.

In the rush to mobilize and then deploy National Guard and Reserve members to war zones, "dental readiness" became the symbol of the lack of health preparedness in the Guard and Reserve, especially after Guard members reported having teeth pulled instead of more extensive work done so they could deploy with their units. The Enlisted Association of the National Guard of the United States (EANGUS) made the cause of better health care readiness for Guard members its priority. In every meeting with Congressional Members or staff and every encounter with DoD and military health care officials, the EANGUS Executive Director pounded away at the health care readiness issues. The result? The creation of TRICARE Reserve Select in the FY 2005 NDAA (P.L. 108-375), which provided for subsidized health care coverage for Guard and Reserve members so they could obtain the preventive care they needed to remain ready.

In 2005, NMFA focused its efforts on the horribly named "death gratuity," the payment made to the surviving next of kin of active duty deaths to cover immediate expenses after the deaths. Congress raised the payment amount from $6000 to $12,000 at the beginning of the war, but as deaths in Iraq and Afghanistan increased, calls came to increase both the death gratuity and the benefit paid under the Servicemembers' Group Life Insurance. In early 2005, DoD proposed raising the amount of the gratuity to $100,000, but only for deaths occurring in combat zones. The proposal meant, for example, that the family of a service member killed in a vehicle accident in Iraq would receive a higher death benefit than one who died in a vehicle accident while training to deploy. In response, NMFA began a campaign to secure an increase for all active duty deaths, reminding leaders that the survivor benefit package should not create inequities by awarding different benefits to families who lose a service member in a hostile zone versus those who lose their loved one in a training mission preparing for service in a hostile zone. To the family, the loss was the same.

Prior to a hearing of the Senate Armed Services Committee, which included witnesses from the DoD and senior military leaders from each Service, NMFA worked with committee staff on questions about the proposal and were heartened to hear the military Service leaders testifying urge caution in creating a distinction between types of deaths (Shane, 2005, February 2). In every meeting on the Hill, NMFA staff was instructed, no matter what the intended subject of the meeting, to bring up the issue of the inequitable treatment of survivors under the DoD proposal. NMFA conveyed the stories of family members whose service members had died of training accidents and illnesses while at their home installations, pointing out the inequity.

Initially these efforts were not enough; the first legislative change in the death gratuity, passed as part of the Emergency Supplemental Appropriations Act for Defense, the Global War on Terror, and Tsunami Relief, 2005 (P.L. 109-13), raised the payment to $100,000, but only for deaths in combat zones. NMFA and its allies continued to work the issue in the press and with Members of Congress and were rewarded by language in the FY 2006 NDAA (P.L. 109-163), which applied the increased death gratuity to all active duty deaths, retroactive to September 11, 2001. Focus paid off.

7.5.8   It's Never Just About the War

During the 16 years after 9/11, there were:

- Four Presidential elections and nine Congresses—the 107th through the 115th—with four changes of party control in the Senate and three in the House of Representatives
- Six Secretaries of Defense
- Five studies of military pay and benefits: the 9th Quadrennial Review of Military Compensation, Defense Advisory Committee on Military Compensation, the 10th and 11th Quadrennial Reviews of Military Compensation, the Military Compensation and Retirement Modernization Commission
- Three TRICARE health care contract changes
- Two recessions
- One government shutdown and 4 years of budget sequestration cuts and threats of cuts
- Eight Harry Potter® movies
- Hurricanes, floods, tornados, droughts, fires

When a war starts, all everyone wants to do is help those troops who are deploying and the families they've left behind. As a war progresses, issues become more complex. And, as much as advocates will want to keep everyone's focus on the crisis at hand, other issues—military and not—will divert attention and sap energy. While war hangs over every aspect of military family life like a dark cloud, regular life continues. Military families will still move approximately every 3 years, babies will be born, kids will change schools, spouses will look for jobs, families will want bargains in their commissaries and quick appointments when their kids get sick. And, new members of the military and their families will experience war and deployment for the first time.

The challenge for the advocate is to anticipate how the unintended consequences of war will affect the other aspects of military life and work to strengthen military families at war. In a long war, advocates must be prepared to convey a continued reminder of urgency. They must not only fight to secure the benefits and support needed by the families of a wartime force, but also to sustain benefits, policies, and support they fought so hard to achieve. Sometimes the advocate's job is to fight the same battle over and over again. During the decade-plus of war after 9-11, perennials advocates faced included: commissary funding, child care center construction, TRICARE fees, and the size of military pay raises.

Advocates must look for the opportunities to obtain improvements in pay, benefits, and support programs that will outlive the war and help families over the long term. They cannot just dwell on current needs of their families, but also how those needs will change over the years as a consequence of the war. Wartime medical advances in Afghanistan and Iraq kept many troops alive who would have died in previous conflicts. But, the survival of so many severely injured service members brought new challenges to their families, the government, and communities that will continue to unfold for years. Issues of caregiving will change as both the veteran and caregiver age. Little is known on the long-term effects of a parent's wartime injury on children. Evidence is emerging on disease progression among wounded veterans, to include the early onset of dementia and other conditions.

The emergence of new consequences of war years after the war makes it essential that the advocate have a response for anyone uttering the words "peace dividend." Most advocates for military people would have shaken their heads in disbelief if they had been told in 2003 that a budget shutdown, across the board pay cuts, and downsizing of the number of troops would have occurred while our military remained at war. Nevertheless.

7.6   Some Closing Thoughts

Many themes run through the post-9/11 military family advocacy story even as it continues to unfold. Understanding these themes can help you, the advocate, be ready to step up efforts when necessary for the next crisis. Preparation for the unexpected or predicting where unintended consequences might emerge is not easy, but an advocate can work in peacetime to develop needed expertise and put in place processes that will help in a crisis. But, no matter how well-prepared, an advocate will discover things will go wrong in unexpected ways, new issues will emerge, and new populations will need to be served.

The crush of issues and the needs of those you serve can seem overwhelming and so, advocate, set boundaries for yourself and your organization. But, have a process that forces you to assess whether the issues you are pursuing within those boundaries are the right ones for the times and that allows you to readjust those boundaries when you find you must pursue a cause no one else is pursuing. If you are an advocate working on behalf of an organization, get your Board on board. The preparedness and flexibility you build in yourself must also be built into your organization and that cannot happen without a responsive and plugged-in Board. By their very nature, nonprofits have the potential to be more nimble than large government entities. They can get things started—research or new programs—and be models for action while the government moves through its various wickets before responding with funding or new policies and initiatives.

Nurture relationships with other advocates, the government professionals who serve the people you support, Congressional staffers, the press, the research community, and donors who believe in your work. Cast a wide net in your search for partners, cherish the ones who have been your allies in bad times, and never be afraid to reach out to organizations and advocates joining your cause for the first time. Be a mentor, model collaboration, but never be afraid to go it alone if you believe something is worth the fight.

Understand that your work will never be just about the war or crisis you face and that the rest of America may want to fight the last war rather than addressing the challenges you see on the horizon. The rest of America will also lose interest in your cause before you do. Strong public support helps, so use whatever bully pulpits—press, Congress, even the White House—are available to you to raise awareness about the people you serve.

Take care of yourself. When people offer to help, let them. Celebrate the victories, however small, and always keep a reminder of a time when you made a difference handy to get you through a bad day.

References

Carter, P., & Kidder, K. (2015, December). *Charting the sea of goodwill*, 1. Washington, DC: Center for a New American Security.

Chandra, A., Burns, R. M., Tanielian, T., Jaycox, L. H., & Scott, M. M. (2008, April). *Understanding the impact of deployment on children and families: Findings from a Pilot Study of Operation Purple Camp Participants*. Santa Monica, CA: RAND Center for Military Health Research.

Chandra, A., Lara-Cinisomo, S., Jaycox, L. H., Tanielian, T., Han, B., Burns, R. M., & Ruder, T. (2010, January 1). Children on the homefront: The experience of children from military families. *Pediatrics, 125*(1), 16–25.

Chandra, A., Lara-Cinisomo, S., Jaycox, L. H., Tanielian, T., Han, B., Burns, R. M., & Ruder, T. (2011). *Views from the homefront: The experiences of youth and spouses from military families*. Santa Monica, CA: RAND Corporation.

Department of Defense. (2002). Report of the 9th Quadrennial Review of Military Compensation, Vol. 1. xxiii. Washington, DC: Office of the Under Secretary of Defense for Personnel and Readiness.

Hallgren, M. (1991, January). President's Annual Report. *National Military Family Association Newsletter*, 6.

Huebner, A., & Mancini, J. (2005, June). *Adjustment among adolescents in military families when a parent is deployed*. Final report submitted to the Military Family Research Institute and Department of Defense Quality of Life Office, Washington, DC.

Huebner, A., Mancini, J., Wilcox, R., Grass, S., & Grass, G. (2007). Parental deployment and youth in military families: Exploring uncertainty and ambiguous loss. *Family Relations, 56*(2), 111–121.

Meadows, S. O., Tanielian, T., Karney, B. R., Schell, T. L., Griffin, B. A., Jaycox, L. H., Friedman, E. M., Trail, T. E., Beckman, R., Ramchand, R., Hengstebeck, N., Troxel, W. M., Lynsay, A., & Vaughan, C. A.. (2016). *The deployment life study: Longitudinal analysis of military families across the deployment cycle*, xx. Santa Monica, CA: RAND Corporation.

National Military Family Association. (2004). *Serving the homefront: An analysis of military family support from September 11, 2001 through March 31, 2004*. Alexandria, VA.

National Military Family Association. (2005). *Report on the cycles of deployment: An analysis of survey responses, April to September 2005*. Alexandria, VA.

National Military Family Association. (2011). *Finding common ground: A toolkit for communities supporting military families*. Alexandria, VA.

Obama, M.. (2010, May 12). *Remarks by the First Lady at National Military Family Association Summit* [Speech transcript]. Retrieved from https://obamawhitehouse.archives.gov/the-press-office/remarks-first-lady-national-military-family-association-summit

Shane, S. (2005, February 2). Senate panel on benefits for survivors hears critics. *New York Times.*

Zoroya, G.. (2006, October 19). Surge in military deaths weighs on families. *USA Today*, 1A.

Part II
Industries, Associations and Education

Chapter 8
Supporting Military Families: Learning from Our Past to Create a New Future in Business

Sherrill A. Curtis, Vivian Greentree, William Baas, and Bob Cartwright

8.1 The Evolution from Reactive Patriotism to Strategic Engagement

This chapter explores the integral role of employers in supporting military families, and its evolution over the recent, unprecedented, 16 years of war. It is a chronicle of the authors' discoveries, research, and insights, based on their extensive human resource and business management experiences within the public, non-profit, and private sectors. Each author has either personally experienced, or connected one-on-one or in groups, with transitioning military members and their families regarding the variety of topics addressed within these pages. Their collective experiences include: military service; military to civilian career transition; serving as a reservist while holding a full time position in the private sector; pursuing GI Bill benefits; military spouse; member of a Fortune 500 talent acquisition team; creating award-winning best practices and employer training programs to source, hire, and engage veterans and military spouses; career coaching and job seeker training for over 2000 career transitioning service members and their families; and delivering over 40 years

S.A. Curtis, ACC, SPHR, SHRM-SCP (✉)
Curtis Consulting Group, LLC, East Rutherford, NJ, USA
e-mail: sherrill@curtisgroupllc.com

V. Greentree, Ph.D.
First Data, Washington, DC, USA
e-mail: vivian.greentree@firstdata.com

W. Baas
Comcast Corporation, Philadelphia, PA, USA
e-mail: Williambaas@comcast.net

B. Cartwright, SPHR, SHRM-SCP
Intelligent Compensation, LLC, Pflugerville, TX, USA
e-mail: bob.cartwright@intelligentcomp.net

© Springer International Publishing AG 2018
L. Hughes-Kirchubel et al. (eds.), *A Battle Plan for Supporting Military Families*, Risk and Resilience in Military and Veteran Families,
https://doi.org/10.1007/978-3-319-68984-5_8

of human resource, workforce management guidance to hundreds of large, mid, and small-size businesses representing a broad range of industries. It is our aim that business leaders will use this information to create career transition experiences and workplaces to better serve future generations of service members and their families.

To our nation's credit, since the attacks on 9/11, the employer perspective has expanded from understanding how to support military and veterans in transition, to include support for military families. Noteworthy for the X, Y, or millennial generations of readers, it was not until 1973 that the USA converted to an all-voluntary military force. This significant change set a different tone for those serving, as well as for the country. Today, those who enlist to serve do so, at least in part, because they feel compelled to be a part of the defense effort for our country. We have come to realize that *how* our country treats these volunteers, *and* their families, through every aspect of support efforts, benefits, and services, impacts the longer term viability of the USA remaining an all-volunteer military force. And, perhaps nowhere is that more clear than when a service member transitions from active duty and looks to find a career with a civilian employer.

The ongoing development of positive dialogue within corporate America ultimately sparked a perspective shift from compliance and doing the right thing to proactive engagement and creation of shared value—because it was also the right thing to do for the health of the business. Ten years ago, even five years ago, the unemployment rate for veterans returning from Iraq and Afghanistan, female veterans, and Gulf War II era veterans was higher than the national average as reported by the Department of Labor (DOL). Ideas and solutions emerged to not only impact the employment rate; but also to create a talent and human capital case for hiring veterans and their spouses. A new energy developed around military hiring programs. Organizations that were considering military talent acquisition programs asked: "Are we effectively doing all we can to tap into this key talent pool?" Employers assessed the attributes veterans bring to the workplace such as: teamwork; ability to deal with stress, ambiguity and change; ability to be both a leader and a follower; drug free; reasonable salary expectations; and security clearances. Their response was: "This is the type of employee I want to have in my organization!" Organizations began to step up to deliver civilian sector employment opportunities for this diverse, ready-to-succeed talent pool whenever possible.

Business mantras of "We Support Our Troops" developed into a more thoughtful, measured, and proactive approach of support through targeted employment programming enhanced benefits and programs designed for active military, transitioning service members, and their families. From J.P. Morgan Chase creating the 100,000 Jobs Coalition (now Veteran Jobs Mission), to the U.S. Chamber of Commerce Foundation's development of Hiring Our Heroes (among other efforts nationally and locally, both virtually and in-person) the private sector effort to hire veterans was in full swing.

During the latter part of the war's first decade, strategy dialogues evolved to include: organizational branding, website presence, non-traditional talent outreach methods, interview and performance management training, job design flexibility, and more effective administration to close the gaps in benefit programs. Essentially, employers shifted from "it's the right thing to do," to "we are creatively structuring our efforts to ensure veterans are a successful part of the organization's sourced talent pool." Employers began to work in coordination with the public sector to reduce the veteran unemployment rate, concurrently committing to specific veteran-hiring objectives. They also set aside talent wars by collaborating together asking solution-focused questions such as: "How do we share talent? How do we act as a responsible part of the American employment landscape?"

As positive outcomes accumulated, employers intensified their strategies and efforts by challenging themselves with probing questions: "What more can we do? How can we increase our role? How can we retain veterans we hired at our organization?", and "What do we need to do to be leaders in this space?" Many organizations with long-standing veteran employment programs, representing household names and icons of industry have understood how to source, hire, and engage this talent pool for years. However, those just starting up their military programs had to reconfigure a host of internal reporting systems and in some cases, create entirely new ones. As they became more aware of this newly available talent pool through a national focus on veteran unemployment rates, these employers began to adapt their talent planning, outreach and support methods along with benefit programs, learning from, and mirroring, the best practices of those who were already doing it right.

Organizations began offering training programs for transitioning military and leveraging government-funded Work Opportunity Tax Credit (WOTC) incentives. We saw a rise in the creation of Military Affinity and Employee Resource Groups (ERGs), as well as expanded use of Employee Assistance Programs (EAPs) within HR departments. Award programs were created to highlight "above and beyond" compliance efforts by employers who chose to close the benefits and service gaps for veterans, and especially guard and reservists; extending their outreach to support military spouses and families (e.g., the Families and Work Institute's Work Life Legacy Military Award).

However, there was still a long way to go. Employers and military-affiliated candidates alike discovered that systems for accessing job opportunities, career transition, benefits, resource and service information, though well intentioned, were often inefficiently siloed and/or ineffectively delivered. In particular, confusion and frustration were strongly experienced during military demobilization, in the Transition Assistance Program (TAP; now Transition GPS), and during the civilian hiring processes. Communication and follow-through gaps, combined with the lack of understanding and military and civilian business culture differences, left many veteran job seekers frustrated. Concurrently, many potential employers were discouraged at the lack of coordination among federal, military, and state resources to help them tap into the veteran talent pool.

In the larger context of playing an active role in reducing the military unemployment rate, employers also realized they needed to continue to explore and extend supportive solutions beyond simply hiring. As the conflicts abroad continued, and one deployment turned into several (and longer) tours for many service members, the domino-style after-effects began to appear. Organizational leaders, especially

Human Resource professionals, continued to explore solutions through strategic questions such as: "How do we bring that need forward into our organizations and translate it into meaningful policies, programs, partnerships and collaborative initiatives?"; "How may we better connect with, and understand, the needs of our military-affiliated employees?"; and "How do we ultimately retain and provide a clear path for our military-affiliated employees?". In response, Employee or Affinity Resource Groups (ERGs/ARGs) and employee surveys expanded to include questions and analytics aimed at understanding military-affiliated employees.

Questions at management team planning meetings began to delve deeper, addressing less comfortable topics such as: "How can we respond to pay and benefit gaps, especially for guard members and reservists?"; "What is the effect of hiring someone who may have Post-Traumatic Stress (PTS), require deployment, or may need to relocate?"; and "How do we offer non-intrusive assistance to ease the stress of our employees with family members either serving overseas, or those with service-related disabilities?" As more questions arose, it became clear that developing the most effective solutions would require a multi-pronged, strategic approach incorporating new (or refreshed) policies, combined with training, communication, and personalized delivery options.

Benefits professionals revised their vetting processes for third-party Employee Assistance Program (EAP) providers, requiring vendors to validate the availability of behavioral health staff trained on how to respond with cultural competence to military-related issues. These issues included: reintegration challenges (i.e., child behavioral issues due to multiple, periodic parental absences; and combat-related PTS issues for returning service members or for military spouses experiencing PTS transference) as well as company benefits and health care plan navigation, with an understanding of service-related disabilities, and knowledge of Department of Defense (DoD) resources such as the Exceptional Family Member Program (EFMP). Interview and management training addressed legal issues related to asking applicants or employees about injuries, characterization of discharge, potential deployments, or if a military spouse might be required to relocate. For many organizations, this meant developing internal policies that go above and beyond legal requirements, and providing military awareness training to ensure that managers and recruiters understood their roles.

Employers learned that many variables in addition to compensation and benefits affect the fabric of military family life. Along with the more common fears about safety, there are other, more complex, issues faced by military families, ranging from: becoming a new parent with an absent spouse; child care; elder care; singly managing an out-of-state move while working; quickly finding a job in a new town; living far from a support network; and sourcing the right school system. The latter being especially difficult for military parents with special needs children. Other issues that can directly affect job search and performance relate to the social aspects of: establishing new friendships; creating a safety net of day-to-day support; and dealing with feelings of isolation. For military spouses, the combined effects of these military-related challenges can be overwhelming. Syracuse University's Institute for Veterans and Military Families 2016 study cites the cumulative impact of these issues on unemployment, career progression, and ultimately, economic security (Bradbard, Maury, & Armstrong, 2016).

Whether the employee is a veteran, guard member or reservist, or the working spouse of an active duty member, it is clear that like all employees, concern for the well-being of their family is paramount. Exemplifying this point is the sentiment of thanks expressed by guard members or reservists who nominate their employer for the annual Secretary of Defense National Freedom Award through the Employee Support of the Guard and Reserve (ESGR) program. Over and over again, nominators share sentiments such as knowing that their employers are watching out for, and staying connected with their families allows them to focus on their mission and goals for the country. Employer contributions towards creating peace of mind for the person serving are considered essential, and immeasurable. Award-winning strategies include a variety of replicable, low-to-no cost options for businesses of any size that provide continuity, and support, for their military-affiliated employees.

Syracuse University's Institute for Veterans and Military Families (IVMF) stated well the twenty-first century employer goal regarding veterans and military families (Institute for Veterans and Military Families, 2012, p. 6):

> "Employers can help to provide veterans with stable households and families to return to after their service by supporting their family's economic and personal wellbeing. Supporting military families as they navigate complex benefit systems, restructured child and elder care, attend military separation and reunion events, and possibly care for injured veterans helps military members focus on their duties with the knowledge that they have stable homes, to which they may return."

8.2   Defining Twenty-First Century Military and Family Needs

Before defining support strategies or implementing programs, employers must first understand who comprises today's military, and the needs of military families. Modern warfare redefined the profile of a service member, veteran, guard member or reservist, and the military family. In contrast to previous generations of service members, twenty-first century service members are more likely to: deploy multiple times and for longer durations than their previous counterparts; be married; and have children. A key aspect affecting home life for today's military families is a different battle experience from that of prior wars. According to the U.S. Department of Veterans Affairs National Center for PTSD, 60–80% of soldiers who have blast injuries may also have traumatic brain injuries (TBI) resulting from continued exposure to blasts and IEDs (improvised explosive devices; Summerall, 2017). Additionally, the prolonged periods of multiple (and longer) deployments interfered with household routine and stability for military couples, and their family units. Research reveals the effects can manifest in behavioral and communication changes for military children and relationship distress in adults, affecting social and professional interactions (National Center for PTSD, 2016).

Multiple relocations, short-term and some long-term activations, profoundly affected military families. Careers of military spouses were often put on hold, while their job search process became tenuous as many worried about biases because of their potential for future relocations, breaks in their employment, or frequent partial employment changes (i.e., altered schedules). The military spouse employment transition between states was especially difficult in instances of specialized certifications and licenses that were not transferable from state to state, requiring additional time and expense to secure the requirements in the new home base state. Additionally, childcare challenges complicated military spouse employment efforts. Such challenges included limited access to on-installation childcare, quality of accessible care, and available hours of coverage. The gender profile of the modern-day military also shifted as the number of women serving on active duty increased. The increase in women serving also increased the number of dual-military households. As of 2015, women made up 14.5% (213,000) of the active duty Armed Forces; and 190,000 women served in the Reserves and National Guard (Office of the Under Secretary of Defense, Personnel and Readiness, 2016). Conversely, many men took on the role of the civilian working spouse, often with childcare responsibilities.

Women veterans, as a growing percentage of veterans looking for civilian employment, represent an opportunity for employers looking to increase the number of women in their leadership roles. In 2015, women veterans seeking civilian jobs also leveraged educational opportunities at a higher rate than male veterans, resulting in 33.8% achieving at least a Bachelor's Degree, as compared to 28.1% of non-veteran women (National Center for Veterans Analysis and Statistics, 2017). This shift provided an expanded, highly qualified, talent pool for employers seeking to increase the presence of women on their teams and in key leadership roles. However, in spite of the education and experience levels of women veterans and female military spouses, underemployment remains high. IVMF survey results, published in 2014, reports "90% of female military spouse respondents of active duty service members were underemployed" (due to their) higher levels of education (33%), experience 10%), or both (47%)" (Maury & Stone, 2014).

When analyzing what is needed to address these expanded needs of a more diversified military population against existing services and resources, employers must reflect on long range issues including: "What may we eliminate, build upon or create to reset the strategy for successfully serving our military-affiliated employees—now and in the future?; "Does our leadership reflect diversity?"; "Do our talent screening processes and hiring initiatives consider education and experience relative to the inclusion of female military veterans and spouses?"; "Do we have the right confidential EAP services and in-person coaching or group support programs in place?"; "Are we creating opportunities for connecting and professional progression?"; "How is our physical environment set up to be inclusive of those with disabilities?"; and "Is job design, replacement and succession planning allowing flexibility for the relocating family, deployed family member or at-home spouse?".

Ultimately, organizations that provide creative solutions to these challenges will win the talent that drives success over their competition.

8.3 Responses and Strategies

Overall, two fundamental sets of resources were necessary to support the success of military families in the labor market. The first was purposeful employment programs and the second was benefit programs offering sustainable solutions for optimum health, including both behavioral and physical health, as well as overall well-being for every member of the military family.

By 2012, employers could choose from a plethora of veteran hiring resources ranging from web-based virtual recruiting services to traditional in-person job and career fairs. In addition to job postings from the 100,000 Job Coalition (now the Veteran Jobs Mission) members, many veteran hiring resources offered touch points between employers and veteran job seekers by industry or by state. Job fairs were produced by for-profit and non-profit organizations, as well as national organizers (i.e., Hiring Our Heroes, delivered through the U.S. Chamber of Commerce Foundation), technical and trade organization training programs (i.e., Helmets to Hardhats), and the Yellow Ribbon Program for the college bound.

Though these efforts were intended to support career transitioning veterans, challenges arose that impacted the ability to create meaningful connections between prospective employers and job seekers. Organizers struggled with drawing high levels of veteran participants. Employers strove to meet qualified, ready-to-start candidates and veterans experienced frustration when directed to visit a company's website. Recruiters were not able to translate the veterans' skills into specific civilian job skills. Initially, job fairs did not include military spouses as targeted candidates. Over time, employers aiming to improve their support of military families recognized that effective hiring strategies should include targeted sourcing, benefits, and work options (i.e., telecommuting and flexible schedules) that are attractive to military spouses.

The experiences of job and career fair stakeholders improved over time, after addressing some of the earlier challenges that affected job seeker participation and development of meaningful connections. Such challenges included: buy-in from military leadership regarding the importance of longer networking lead time necessary for service members to source civilian careers; training organizational staff and third-party recruiters about military-equivalent skillsets and experiences to include in job descriptions; and education for all parties that aligned expectations of what can be accomplished at a job fair. In order to foster mutually beneficial interactions with veterans, Human Resource professionals developed a broad range of integrated solutions that addressed needs related to veteran hiring, engagement, overall health, and well-being. Employers also introduced education and training for their existing workforce about the characteristics, skills, and value of veterans, and military spouses, as job seekers and co-workers.

Education for both sides of the interview desk heightened awareness and understanding for both employers and transitioning service members of their respective cultural differences based on realities and data rather than myths and perceptions. One particular area that impacted trust between employers and veteran job applicants was misaligned expectations during the civilian hiring process regarding how it differs from the military process that follows explicit protocols. This expectation gap included misconceptions among transitioning service members that civilian employers are like the military when it comes to clearly defined career progression paths. Many job-seeking veterans participating in career coaching or transition workshops expressed their frustration with experiences of: being "left in cyberspace" after submitting a resume; not receiving timely employer communications in response to inquiries or follow-up; or being told to visit a company's website by organization representatives at job fairs. Conversely, employers, career coaches, and job developers also reported experiencing frustration when liaising with veteran job seekers who became unresponsive to e-mail or phone communications, or who could not be available within three months for a start date.

Because these are business etiquette issues, which vary by industry and company, for both employers and applicants, communication remedies are best aligned to each organization's larger talent acquisition model. Organizations with the bandwidth to commit dedicated staff adjusted their recruiting practices and on-boarding processes to provide consistent, personalized candidate communications, and follow-up. Facilitators of briefings, job search seminars, and workshops educated veteran job seekers about the differences between the military and civilian job search processes. Many organizations created required, periodic training for line managers, supervisors, and anyone in a hiring or performance management role. Such training provided learning opportunities about how to effectively interview, manage, and engage military-connected talent in the workplace.

As awareness of the importance of retention began to emerge, employers worked closely with the Employer Support of the Guard and Reserve (ESGR), a DoD program developed to promote cooperation and understanding between Reserve and Guard members and their managers. ESGR representatives provided employer training on the rights of members of the National Guard and Reserves, along with guidance for creating effective employer processes to manage leaves of absence related to periodic training, deployment, and readiness to return to work. Employers that demonstrated compliance could sign a Statement of Support signifying their commitment to guard and reservist employees. The ESGR offered training and personalized assistance for members of the National Guard and reservists experiencing difficulty navigating compliance regulations with their employer. They also offered training and support to Human Resource and line managers to ensure they too felt supported and had accurate information to ease the stress of deployment and reduce potential non-compliance experienced by employers with regard to military leave.

Diversity and inclusion programs for managers and staff were updated to include awareness and understanding of the military community. These programs also highlighted the value added by military talent to private sector organizations. Issues addressed included: effects of multiple deployments, reintegration, relocations, managing daily life with a background of anxiety while a spouse is deployed, and alignment of expectations around pay, benefits, and job performance. Employee Assistance Program (EAP) vendors refocused their self-education efforts about Department of Veterans Affairs (VA)-provided and state-enhanced benefits in order to refer military-affiliated employees to appropriate resources.

Employee Resource Groups (ERGs) were another way organizations that began to offer peer support, networking and professional development opportunities for military-connected employees. These groups also provide valuable training and information on topics such as: career progression, professional development, and managing transition challenges and daily stress.

National non-profits established program goals that resulted in an increased impact of their services delivered at the local community level. Their wide variety of resources and programs served as an additional resource fulfilling unmet needs by the government as well as employer provided benefits and services. That outreach strategy leveraged the scale of services, while maximizing connections between local resources and military-affiliated employees, which also contributed to building community capacity.

The use of Federal Personnel Exchange Programs, such as the Army's Training With Industry (TWI), grew, producing positive results and shared value for both private sector organizations and active duty service members. Similar to an internship program, Exchange Programs place active duty service members in Fortune 500 organizations for a specified period of time. Upon program completion, service members return to their military role for a minimum 4-year period. These programs help service members gain skills in the civilian sector while giving an employer an early look at talent and exposure to leveraging the skillsets these service members bring from the military. Service members gain career-relevant day-to-day experience in the civilian workplace along with a greater awareness and understanding of civilian business culture. Private sector employers experience the value of a veteran's knowledge, skills, and abilities.

8.4   Results and Insights

Over time, we discovered how to better understand the value of military skills and experiences and then relate them to jobs in the civilian sector. MOS (Military Occupational Skills) translation, in relationship to job descriptions and resumes, became part of the ongoing employment discussion that led to increased understanding for interviewers and applicants. Incorporating the translation of military experience into the job description, accepting applicable military experience relevant to private industry experience within position descriptions, and resume development processes eased the task of matching candidates with military experience to appropriate civilian jobs. Online military skills translation solutions, coupled with employer and military job seeker training, took time to develop, implement, then trust and utilize.

Both employers and military job seekers could more readily ascertain which military experiences and technical skills related to certain civilian jobs while also appreciating the soft skills veterans brought with them. Some organizations (i.e., United Parcel Service) connected with military veteran job seekers through their own websites and application processes by including a military transition guide or video shorts on their website that describe specific military transferable skills correlative with open positions. Free resources, many developed and provided by mainstream resume and job search sites, (i.e., military.com and LinkedIn), also resulted in substantially increasing the opportunity for veterans and employers to find one another.

When the Veteran Jobs Mission reached their original goal of 100,000 military hires much earlier than expected, they established more ambitious hiring goals. As the overall economy improved, and our nation experienced a decrease in veteran unemployment rates, competition increased to hire veterans and the dialogue expanded to discussions of retention, internal mobility, and even entrepreneurship. This created opportunities for some veterans to receive multiple job offers from some of the best-in-class organizations in the country. It also prompted the private sector to focus on providing meaningful career opportunities for transitioning military service members and their spouses in more holistic ways. This spirit of cooperation continued to expand beyond the original core of hiring programs to include emphasis on retention and entrepreneurship as organizations identified the value of veterans as co-workers, organizational leaders, and business owners in the marketplace. Entities such as the Coalition for Veteran Owned Business (CVOB) and Bunker Labs arose to provide resources for veteran entrepreneurs and provide access to corporate supply chains.

Veterans' success within the private sector continued to increase as organizations developed their military affinity group programs. Many programs included opportunities for military-affiliated employees to volunteer with community-based services or connecting with, and mentoring, newly hired veterans and military spouses within the organization. According to Comcast employee opinion surveys, veterans participating in military affinity resource groups are more engaged, less likely to look for another job, happier and more satisfied, much more positive than others when it comes to dealing with stress, ambiguity, and change. At First Data, surveyed employees rated "knowing that [the company] has a commitment to you as a military-affiliated employee and that [you] have advocates/support (including the Military Affinity Group)" as a top factor affecting their career success.

One of the more surprising aspects of private sector engagement in military hiring was the transcendence of corporate rivalry as the spirit of cooperation for sharing veteran talent and programming quickly spread. For example, Northrop Grumman's Operation IMPACT (Injured Military Pursuing Assisted Career Transition) focused on assisting severely wounded service members as they transitioned from the military to a private sector career. The Network of Champions (NoC—a group comprising private sector employers, non-profit organizations, and federal agencies with a shared commitment to support veterans) expanded the service members' ability to locate career opportunities within the network's organizations.

8.5 Continuous Process Improvement

Over the past 16 years, employers have made considerable progress in improving support for their current and potential military-affiliated employees, while benefiting from service members' transitions into their organizations. There have been many successful efforts; some will benefit from further adjustment; others are not yet fully developed. Human Resource professionals in particular have the opportunity to play a key role in the development of strategies, policies, and programs that effectively and efficiently serve the career transition needs of veterans and military-affiliated families. However, as with any core value (i.e., diversity, sustainability), top down modeled buy-in combined with integration throughout the organization is vital to creating successful programs.

This section offers a variety of options for employer engagement in developing and delivering the right-fit solutions to fulfill the goal of providing meaningful career opportunities for veterans and their spouses. From simple, quick actions to deep dive, long-term commitments, there are options and solutions to fit every organization from small to medium and large.

8.5.1 Preparing to Hire and On-Boarding

Society for Human Resource Management (SHRM) survey research indicates that the first three to six months of employment are the most critical; with organizations losing an average of 17% of their new hires during the first three months of employment (Maurer, 2015). Seasoned human resource professionals understand the impact of these statistics on productivity, engagement, and retention. By proactively developing and delivering comprehensive, well communicated, and measurable pre-hire and on-boarding processes, the organization can yield high dividends. This approach is especially beneficial for military-affiliated talent, and even more vital for employees having their first civilian-career experience.

Job Descriptions and Translating MOS

Utilize the myriad of free online translation tools to correlate job descriptions with skill sets developed during military service. Initially focus on current open jobs, followed by high yield positions, then expand to translate the remaining jobs. Similar to utilizing education to experience equivalents for civilian jobs, organizations should define and include the "military experience equivalent" in a job description, citing the required military role, level, and years of experience. This diversity and inclusion approach allows service members with the relevant type and years of experience, without a degree, an opportunity to successfully compete in the recruitment process.

Provide Interview Training

It is crucial that anyone with responsibility for interviewing, or participating in hiring decisions, understands how to evaluate military experiences and skills that correlate with the organization's job functions. Having this knowledge and understanding will ease the interview process for both the interviewer, and the veteran, ensuring good fit hiring opportunities are not missed.

Taking into consideration the number of jobs, positions, and hiring team size, Human Resource professionals may choose to: 1) review an MOS translated job description one-on-one with a hiring manager or supervisor; or 2): implement a formal group training with a hiring team. Both approaches ensure a consistant understanding of the MOS translation in relationship to the job description's list of preferred knowledge, skills, and abilities. Human Resource professionals also have opportunities to clarify MOS definitions, address any innacuracies, and explore potential interview questions (using correlative military terms) with hiring managers/teams before beginning the interview process.

Be Alert for Opportunities to Build the Talent Pipeline Aligned with the Organization's Geographic Footprint

For example, consider if participating in national hiring events will fulfill the organization's hiring goals as well as state-specific efforts. Increasingly, many states hold state-of-the-veteran convenings that bring together in-state resources such as non-profit partners, state leaders, and community-based resources. These events may be worth attending in states where employers have large employee populations. Establish local talent pipelines by developing relationships with military installations, colleges, state level workforce agencies, and student veteran organizations (SVOs).

Military Family Friendly Branding

Put your brand front and center for military talent to take notice. In addition to the Careers page, include the commitment to hiring, promoting, and supporting the needs of military talent and their families on the About Us, Values, or Philosophy page(s) of the organization's website, Include success stories (creating the "similar to me" approach to attract candidates) along with profiles of current military-affiliated employees.

Small to Mid-Size Employer Talent Outreach

In spite of their best outreach efforts, the ability to source military talent remains an elusive goal for many small to mid-sized businesses. They are often limited by staff bandwidth and resources to extend their outreach methods in contrast to corporate giants when sourcing military-affiliated talent. Though smaller than the Goliath's of the business world, there are a few simple free options employers of any size can utilize to prepare for hiring, share job openings, and source potential candidates.

(a) Leverage free online resources—For example, the Employer Roadmap, developed by USAA and Hiring Our Heroes, offers a host of free resources, including workbook pages, job description builders, and action plans based on company size.
(b) Foster relationships with veteran representatives or program coordinators at the following organizations to build a strategic talent pipeline for outreach success:

   (i) Local economic development, government, and community agencies. These include: DOL's American Job Centers, local VA Vet Center, universities, and non-profit organizations that serve veterans and their families;
   (ii) Military installations within the target hiring area—connect with the transition assistance program manager; and Onward to Opportunity (program managed by Syracuse University's Institute for Veteran and Military Families). Request inclusion on their list of local employers.

Non-profit Support: Veteran Service Organizations (VSOs), Military Family Service Organizations (MFSOs), and College Groups

Employers that reach out to program representatives in their communities and local universities can easily build a presence and connection, while creating shared value for the organization's current military-affiliated employees. Consider creating talent connection opportunities by offering these non-profits: meeting space; food and beverage service for their meetings or special events; volunteers; door prizes; free printing of event materials; and in-kind donations of products or special career or job coaching workshops through your military affinity group.

Partner with universities or community colleges that offer in-state tuition for veterans and/or military dependents, distance-learning, certificate programs, or other targeted military services. Confer with those contacts to create student veteran and military spouse internships, and new graduate rotational programs. Student veterans represent an especially valuable talent pool within the military hiring space. The college environment experience offers student veterans the benefit of easing their military to civilian transition, giving them a jump start to successfully assimilate into a civilian work culture. Through Student Veterans of America (SVA) chapters and student veteran resource centers across the country, employers may access veteran college students and graduates and begin to build their veteran talent pipeline by offering internships to student veterans, prior to their senior year, and fostering relationships with the student veteran resource centers on college campuses. For example, Comcast hires over 500 student veterans annually for summer seasonal positions. By featuring student veterans in their social media storytelling, Comcast attracts more potential talent to connect with and add to their veteran pipeline.

Be sure to include information about all educational opportunities and programs in the organization's new military hire welcome kit. Periodically, re-evaluate the changing nature of education programs receiving GI Bill eligibility. These steps will not only support the military-affiliated new hire to pursue education, it can be seen as a workforce development tool, increasing their value to the organization as they increase their specialized skills and education.

Spouses and children of service members offer opportunities to attract and retain workers who feel aligned with their employer's values, something that is very important, especially to Millennials, in today's workforce. Investing in the education of military families, even on a small scale, can make the difference between a future job versus a career or profession for a young adult or military spouse.

Keep Updated on Government Policy Changes that Incentivize and Facilitate Military Hiring

As government systems make tax incentives like the Work Opportunity Tax Credit (WOTC) easier to apply for and receive, more employers will leverage the financial opportunity to support hiring efforts. Tax incentives are just part of the ongoing dialogue, however.

Employers wanting to have the veteran talent advantage can successfully compete for this talent pool by offering benefits that fill support gaps for military family members. Be prepared to talk about employer benefits programs with military-affiliated hires, highlighting mandated and voluntary benefits with those most closely aligned with DoD-provided benefits, which typically cease when transitioning out of service. If offered in the civilian sector, they can add significant value to the veteran, or military spouse's employment experience. The by-product is that by supporting the military-affiliated employee's focus on their job, productivity may increase, adding to the bottom line.

Private sector employers should also become familiar with the employment opportunities offered through exchange, internship, and apprenticeship programs with different service branches. These programs have been underutilized because of historical lack of employer awareness about their existence; a difficult acceptance process resulting from confusion regarding qualifications; and program variations between branches. However, as coordination at the national level continues, there is great promise for an increased pipeline in the future.

Relocation Support

Organizations may readily apply a standard relocation program, typically offered to a transferring employee or new hire. However, for military families, consideration should be given to the potential frequency of relocations that increase stress for spouses as they attempt to find viable, meaningful employment, often without a support network in place within their new community. Specific types of support may range from guidance about relocation expectations; touring the new city/town; coordinating neighborhood searches with local real estate professionals; and providing information about schools and childcare options. Extend the assistance further with referrals to the local Department of Labor (DoL) Workforce Development representative to connect with the relocating military family member.

Welcome Kits

In addition to the usual benefits, payroll, and voluntary Equal Employment Opportunity Commission (EEOC) disclosure forms, customize new hire kits for military-affiliated hires to include a variety of relevant information and resources connecting the new hire with subject matter experts on military-related issues. Examples include: a personalized welcome letter; military affinity group leadership and military affairs team contacts; and local veteran service organization (VSOs) point of contact information. Consider including free resources from research organizations such as Purdue's Military Family Research Institute. Another example of an educational resource is the Institute for Veteran and Military Family's Veteran Certificate Transition Program (VCTP). The institute provides 36 different certificate programs to post-9/11 veterans and their families.

8.5.2   Post-hire Support

Leverage the potential to increase engagement, retention, and promotion rates of military-affiliated employees by proactively integrating their perspectives when creating policies, programs, or vetting third-party vendors. As with any other diversity and inclusion strategy, consider the impacts derived from offering services and benefits options that support military-affiliated families, such as:

Employee Assistance and Wellness Programs (EAPs)

When selecting a carrier, ensure vendors offer behavioral health professionals trained in identifying and navigating the effects from combat for the veteran, as well as the effects on the military family. They should be experienced with specialized knowledge regarding re-entry and have a track record of providing appropriate supports for the military community. Consider including program coverage for what are now more commonly offered, as well as emerging promising practices such as yoga, meditation, and equine therapy that support reduced stress (and address issues related to Post-Traumatic Stress (PTS) or Post-Traumatic Stress Disorder (PTSD) for military-affiliated talent).

National Veteran Service Organizations (VSOs)

Establish partnerships with the American Legion (AL), Disabled American Veterans (DAV), and others who have a long history of assisting veterans with processing their Veteran's Administration (VA) medical claims. The Military Child Education Coalition (MCEC) assists military families with educational issues for their children. These are just a few of the organizations that could be useful for your company. A local point of contact for VSO and MFSO organizations in veteran on-boarding welcome kits is a great way to proactively connect new hire veterans to local resources in the area, specific to their military needs.

Military Spouses and Caregivers

Throughout the job design and policy development processes, seek input and feedback from military spouses to ensure their perspective is considered. This input may be gleaned either from military spouses or caregivers within the organization, or through external employer partners and service providers.

An example of the need for flexible job design and transition assistance is when an employee who is military spouse must relocate, based on their active duty service member's Permanent Change of Station (PCS) military orders. In this circumstance, a variety of policy options adaptable to all sizes of employers can extend support during the transition:

(a) Determine whether business needs can be met if the current job function is performed in the military spouse's new location (i.e., remotely/virtually or if another office exists in the new location)
(b) Assess the potential to re-assign the employee to another job function, based on individual and organization needs
(c) Assist the employee with aligning skills to internal open positions for which he or she may apply and compete
(d) Tap into external employment opportunities with organizations in the new community, aligned with the commitment to support employment for military families

When possible, offer flexibility through job sharing, telecommuting, and work schedule options that increase the potential of military spouses or caregivers (of active duty, Guard or Reserve service members) entering or continuing in the workforce. Through thoughtful, well-planned job design, organizations will have the opportunity to hire military-affiliated talent, anywhere in the country, and/or retain that talent even when relocations occur.

Support of the National Guard and Reserve

To compete for Guard and Reservist talent, employers must be prepared to conduct periodic reviews of benefit programs to ensure they are keeping pace to support their employees who continue to serve. Organizations with the most competitive benefits package for Guard members and Reservists will be more likely to claim that talent pool by not making them choose between service and self. When conducting a cost-benefit analysis, utilize the ESGR as a resource to receive and compare the Guard and Reservist benefits, along with best practices of other state and national organizations.

Fill Talent Gaps

Small business owners should proactively plan to navigate potential talent gaps during periods of deployment, in order to minimize the impact to their business. Options include: job redesign, job sharing, and temporary replacement staffing. For large organizations with a handful of active duty service members, Guard members or Reservists, workflow during leaves of absence may be easily managed due to the size and scale of their operation. However, the impact on small to medium businesses may be much greater, as even the temporary absence of one employee can threaten the viability of that business.

Support Training and Deployments

A smooth reintegration begins with planning and coordinating with the service member and their manager prior to the activation. Establish a protocol that includes connecting with members of the National Guard and Reserve as they activate for deployment periods exceeding 30 days. Ensure that the manager, Human Resource partner, and employee are aware of their respective rights and responsibilities, and completed the ESGR offered training. Track activation periods from first notice through return to work status to facilitate the reservist's transition back into the workplace.

Utilize the Expertise of the Employer Support of the Guard and Reserve (ESGR)

This national, DoD-run program offers free guidance and training programs designed to educate employers, along with guard and reservists, on how to successfully navigate their respective rights and responsibilities. Ensure all human resource and payroll and leave management staff, along with managers responsible for guard and reservists, receive training on how to respond to, and manage active duty leaves of absence. Connect with the ESGR and establish open communications to learn about hiring events and demobilizations that may yield more talent for the organization's military pipeline.

Stay Connected During Active Duty Periods

A simple communication during times of separation ensures that the service member, military spouse, and family member(s) know there is a continuing employer commitment to their well-being. It is a great, no/low cost method, for maintaining a sense of continuity with co-workers for the deployed service member. This no cost/high impact action by Human Resources, the organization President, a direct manager, team, or military affinity group member, can foster employee loyalty, increase engagement, and improve retention.

8.6 Preparing for the Future

As each new chapter in the current war unfolds, there is a continuous need for collaborative efforts to deliver services, education and training to, and improve support and awareness among, a variety of stakeholders at both a national and local level. This requires authentic communication, purposeful programming, and a commitment to collaboration. Without these efforts we will continue to experience lack of match between employers, transitioning military, and their spouses seeking employment; myths and misperceptions in hiring/promotion practices affecting military-connected talent; stagnant or weakening employment opportunities for veterans and military spouses; increased economic insecurity within the military community, and, ultimately, incomplete solutions delivered in silos which, even at their best, will not achieve maximum impact. It therefore becomes increasingly important when looking at the "what and how" to consider "who" can contribute useful insights. Look for partners who can bridge knowledge gaps and assist with building viable, sustainable strategies—in all areas of the business. Consider the following:

8.6.1 Regularly Participate in Round Table Discussions, Strategy Planning Exercises, or Dialogues with Representatives Across All Sectors and Geographic Regions

The symposium that produced this book is a good example of a dialogue across all sectors specifically to stimulate ideas and transform them into measurable actions for the future conflicts. These types of events, when held on a regular basis, quickly establish the national dialogue and potential directions for the most pressing problems. For example, early in the conflict the focus was on employment. Now, with 5.5 M caregivers in the USA (Ramchand et al., 2014), the focus may shift from employment to supporting the needs of caregivers in employer benefits and work schedule flexibility. Or, collectively we could look to increasing program support for veterans interested in entrepreneurship. Research indicates 25% of transition service members would like to start their own businesses (Fairlie, Morelix, Reedy, & Russell, 2015). Monitoring trends for issues such as these that affect the workforce and impact military families will assist to proactively prepare for the next shift in focus.

Relationships with other stakeholders can be very helpful when creating effective programs. They also provide an essential feedback loop for federal agencies tasked with providing transition programming for veterans and their families. However, invest time and resources where they will have the most impact for the organization. Before joining coalitions learn about other member organizations, and clarify membership expectations. Prior to supporting a non-profit, research and examine their financials, ratings, and impact statements. Be a conscientious contributor, knowing that the organization's leadership will expect measurable, defined impact concurrent with enhanced business operations that deliver effective outcomes. Also consider who will serve as champion, and the role of strategist, both with responsibility for communicating the purpose and metrics associated with each partnership and budget item. When choosing national, state, and local coalitions to join in pursuit of supporting military families and your military-affiliated employees, consider several factors:

(a) What is this entity's purpose and does that purpose align with your organization's business goals in addition to your military-related programming? You will be better able to justify time and expense towards efforts that align with larger organizational goals than those outside your wheelhouse. For example, if you are a financial organization, joining a coalition around providing financial literacy services to military families or helping to get more military spouses into financial services is a more relevant investment than perhaps volunteering to build homes for veterans. Both are needed and worthwhile, however one has a more direct tie-in to your organization's expertise and business operations.

(b) Do you want to outsource or in-source any of the services and/or trainings that this group might provide? There are many models for how organizations choose to provide training, on-boarding, and mentorship experiences, as well as sourcing and recruiting functions. It depends on size, expertise, resources, and a host of other considerations. Go back to your leadership and discuss what your enterprise-wide strategy is (or what you want it to be) towards diversity recruiting, professional development opportunities, and in-house training and curriculum programming before deciding on outsourcing that function within the military realm.

(c) Does this group of organizations share best practices with each other regularly? Do they share their outcomes publicly and with transparency? Any expenditure of your resources and investment into the military community will continue to be scrutinized and judged against your own success metrics (increasing the percent of new hires who are military-affiliated, increasing retention of military-affiliated employees, company performance, etc.). Make sure you clearly understand the benefits of joining and investing your time and resources.

8.6.2 *Leverage Military-Affiliated Employee Data to Set Strategies and Allocate Resources*

Just as with designing relevant, cost-effective benefits and training programs, consider effective methods for incentivizing self-identification, data collection, and analytics to capture an accurate profile of an organization's military-connected talent. This is especially crucial for employers with federal contracts that must meet certain compliance criteria (i.e., The Vietnam Era Veterans' Readjustment Assistance Act of 1974—VEVRAA; and Uniformed Services Employment and Re-employment Rights Act—USERRA). Data collection combined with the ability to extrapolate meaningful reports for analysis, are integral components to the success of sourcing, recruiting, on-boarding, and retention functions. The concerns surrounding self-identification are often similar to those expressed by differently abled workers. One challenge is that many veterans and military spouses choose not to self-identify for fear they will not be hired, promoted, or given career-enriching assignments. However, over time and with corporate culture evolution, this challenge can dissipate as veterans, spouses, and reserve component members experience the commitment within their workplace to support military-affiliated employees.

Monitor the entire sourcing to on-boarding process and collect data so you can identify problem areas—know what lines of business, geographical areas, and levels of management are most populated by military talent, know your percentage of new hires and your total military-affiliated population. It is helpful to be able to know at which point in your talent acquisition and retention process organizations and veterans face the most challenges. The data will show you the exact points of difficulty within your operations—is it the jump from applicant to interview? Or perhaps interview to hire? Knowing the exact points of difficulty will help you know where you need to get better and hone your strategy.

Create tracking measures around career progression so you can also know the retention rates, performance, and satisfaction rates, of your military-affiliated employees, again by line of business, geographical area, and level of management or other categories that help you interpret data for your usage. Understand current and trending key issues and concerns such as health care, behavioral health care, education, career progression, and personal development. This will enhance opportunities to be proactive, rather than reactive to the prevalent topics as demographic shifts, life, and world issues affect the needs of veteran and military spouse retention and career progression issues. If your organization conducts a yearly employment engagement survey, consider creating or tagging-on a military-specific segment for military-affiliated employees. It is not enough to hire veterans. Businesses must strive to create an organizational culture where military-affiliated talent will choose to stay, contributing their experience and expertise to our bottom lines.

8.6.3 Expand Military-Friendly Efforts by Including Veteran Entrepreneurship

When looking at the holistic picture of how an organization engages with the military community, consider the role of entrepreneurship. According to the recent figures, 25% of veterans transitioning out of the service are interested in starting their own business (Fairlie et al., 2015). Veterans are overrepresented in the entrepreneur population; they employ nearly six million people; and generate annual receipts of approximately $2.1 trillion. Given that veterans hire veterans, this could be the next level of employer/veteran support sophistication.

Consider veteran-owned businesses in relationship to operations, sales, and third-party vendors. For example, in addition to military talent as part of a diversity staffing strategy, think of sourcing and procurement programs. Where do opportunities exist to expand the number of veteran and military spouse owned businesses in the vendor or Business to Business supply chain? Do vendor selection criteria include reference to contracts (possibly with a preference) for veteran-owned businesses? Does the organization sell products or services to small businesses, invest in entrepreneurs and small businesses, or have resources to promote business-to-business or business-to-consumer selling models? Is there a relationship with the Coalition for Veteran-Owned Business? Ultimately, organizations will select a vendor for optimum product quality, competitive pricing and service. Including "veteran-owned business" in the selection and vetting criteria keeps the dialogue up front and center, reinforcing the brand message "we support veterans and military-affiliated talent."

8.7 Expanding the National Dialogue

As employers and a nation, it is important to continue the dialogue about supporting military families; one that challenges us to think about what to consider beyond "of the moment issues" when preparing for the future and how to effectively deliver long-term solutions. For example, how will the changing demands and career paths within the military re-align with the private sector? This has become one of the biggest discussions for today's service members. Traditional career paths from the past are not necessarily going to work in the future. Where are the gaps, and how can the private sector address these trends?

Warfare has dramatically changed over the centuries. Technology plays a major role in those changes that affects incumbents assigned to new job functions. Employers should remain cognizant of support strategies and planning as part of the potential evolution for outsourcing certain jobs previously performed by military staff. An example where this shift could occur are job functions related to cyber information. Though the job function may be performed domestically, stress levels may be the same as if the incumbents were performing as overseas active duty staff. What choices might employers need to make with regard to providing benefits and support for them and their families?

It is important to maintain an ongoing dialogue on a community level to create community capacity. Yet it is also important to invite and foster solutions focused on relationships and scalability at the national level to address issues with second- and third-order effects that touch every community. For example, national convenings might have an agenda item such as: *What is the next iteration for the Veteran Jobs Mission? How can organizations share talent in instances of military relocation? What do successful retention and career mobility metrics look like?* Collectively, public, private, and non-profit stakeholders will decide who is best situated to create and curate a national resource or repository that transitioning service members, veterans, and military spouses could opt into and organizations can avail themselves of—or if one is even desired. Would the inability to identify a champion within the government lead employers to seek private sector alternatives with national coalitions or civilian talent locaters such as LinkedIn, Indeed, Monster, or Zip Recruiter?

While we continue to solve smaller pieces of the larger picture, we remember that as employers and business enterprises, we must use our first, best resources to find the best value. We must do what we can do best, enabling commerce, building communities through private enterprise, and hiring the best talent in the country.

How do we develop the next generation to create the optimum collective impact? Several national initiatives, including Joining Forces, have been extremely effective in galvanizing employers nationwide. No matter the form it may take with each new White House Administration or national convening, this type of national dialogue and concentrated effort spurred employers to collective, collaborative action. It created a cohesive national voice, while appealing to the private sector value of driving ingenuity and innovation. Leadership from the White House or the government will always be needed, but businesses are equally vital to create lasting impact and successful economic health for veterans and their families.

When reflecting on how human resource professionals, other business leaders, and organizations with a common core value can support military talent and their families, consider the potential of each choice and action. Choosing collaborative, proactive approaches as exemplified in this chapter, can collectively create opportunities that improve the economic security, and stability of military-affiliated talent, and their families. Those choices also create the space for optimized health and overall well-being for military families. As a result, the organizations also can thrive, financially and culturally. The resulting intrinsic value for all is beyond measure.

References

Bradbard, D. A., Maury, R., & Armstrong, N. A. (2016, November). *The force behind the force: Case profiles of successful military spouses balancing employment, service, and family (Employing Military Spouses, Paper No. 2).* Syracuse, NY: Institute for Veterans and Military Families, Syracuse University.

Fairlie, R. W., Morelix, A., Reedy, E. J., & Russell, J. (2015). *The Kauffman index. Startup activity: National trends.* Kansas City, MO: Ewing Marion Kauffman Foundation.

Institute for Veterans and Military Families. (2012). *Leading practices: Assimilation and employee assistance*. Syracuse: Syracuse University: Institute for Veterans and Military Families. Retrieved from: http://toolkit.vets.syr.edu/wp-content/uploads/2012/12/LP-Examples-Assimilation.pdf.

Maury, R., & Stone, B. (2014). *Military spouse employment report*. Syracuse, NY: Institute for Veterans and Military Families. Retrieved from: https://ivmf.syracuse.edu/article/military-spouse-employment-survey/.

Maurer, R. (2015, April 16). *Onboarding key to retaining, engaging talent*. Retrieved from https://www.shrm.org/resourcesandtools/hr-topics/talent-acquisition/pages/onboarding-key-retaining-engaging-talent.aspx

National Center for PTSD. (2016). *How deployment stress affects children and families: Research findings*. Department of Veterans Affairs; Revised February 23, 2016. Retrieved from https://www.ptsd.va.gov/professional/treatment/family/pro_deployment_stress_children.asp

National Center for Veterans Analysis and Statistics. (2017). *Women veterans report: The past, present, and future of women veterans*. Washington, DC: Department of Veterans Affairs. Retrieved from https://www.va.gov/vetdata/docs/SpecialReports/Women_Veterans_2015_Final.pdf.

Office of the Under Secretary of Defense, Personnel and Readiness. (2016). *Population representation in the military services: Fiscal year 2015 summary report*. Retrieved December 31, 2016, from http://www.cna.org/research/pop-rep

Ramchand, R., Tanielian, T., Fisher, M. P., Vaughan, C. A., Trail, T. E., Epley, C., Voorhies, P., Robbins, M. W., Robinson, E., & Ghosh-Dastidar, B. (2014). *Hidden heroes: America's military caregivers*. Santa Monica, CA: RAND.

Summerall, E. M. (2017). *Traumatic brain injury and PTSD*. National Center for PTSD, Department of Veterans Affairs. Retrieved March 2017, from https://www.ptsd.va.gov/professional/co-occurring/traumatic-brain-injury-ptsd.asp

Chapter 9
The Higher Education Community: Educating America's *Next* Great Generation

Kathryn McMurtry Snead and Lesley McBain

9.1 Background

One of the significant benefits the higher education community provides to the nation and our military families is educating the Next Great Generation of engaged citizens and leaders—service members, veterans, and their family members. As a marker of the significance of military and veterans' educational benefits, the *VA Annual Benefits Report 2000–2013* stated that approximately 400,000 beneficiaries enrolled in postsecondary education in 2000. The number of veterans and family members engaged in higher education increased threefold in the subsequent 14 years due to greater numbers of service members called up for Operation Iraq Freedom and Operation Enduring Freedom who were eligible for education benefits as well as more generous education benefits resulting from the Post-9/11 GI Bill and GI Bill transferability of benefits to family members.[1]

Additionally, 225,000–300,000 service members used military Tuition Assistance (TA) funding annually to enroll in postsecondary education courses and programs, thus reserving their Department of Veterans Affairs (VA) education benefits for educational programs after they separate from military service. Department of Defense

---

[1] GI Bill Transferability, VA website accessed in October 2015 (http://www.gibill.va.gov/post-911/post-911-gi-bill-summary/transfer-of-benefits.html).

K.M. Snead, Ed.D (✉)
Military and Veterans Partnerships, American Association of State Colleges and Universities, Washington, DC, USA
e-mail: sneadk@aascu.org

L. McBain, Ph.D.
National Association of College and University Business Officers (NACUBO), Washington, DC, USA
e-mail: lmcbain@nacubo.org

© Springer International Publishing AG 2018
L. Hughes-Kirchubel et al. (eds.), *A Battle Plan for Supporting Military Families*, Risk and Resilience in Military and Veteran Families,
https://doi.org/10.1007/978-3-319-68984-5_9

Voluntary Education Fact Sheets reported that service members successfully completed 10.5 million individual courses from fiscal years 2000 to 2014.[2]

Service members and family members benefited from changes in the Post-9/11 GI Bill and other actions taken by various parties. Data from the Military Compensation and Retirement Modernization Commission (MCRMC) indicated that

> [b]etween August 2009 and September 2014, there were 423,355 Servicemembers who transferred their Post-9/11 GI Bill benefit to 928,078 dependents. Of the Service members who transferred their benefits, 38.5 percent were officers and 61.5 percent were enlisted Service members, compared to a total force that is 16.4 percent officers and 83.6 percent enlisted. As of August 2014, 52 percent of children who received transferred benefits were younger than age 14 at the time of transfer (MCRMC, 2015, p. 167).

The estimated cost of these transferred benefits to military family members resulted in a $5.6 billion price tag for the VA Veterans Benefit Administration during the time period noted above. Given that less than half of those eligible for benefit transfer are college-aged, the cost estimates for this educational benefit remain in flux but could be staggering. The MCRMC Final Report noted "VA does not currently have a robust model for out-year cost projections for the Post-9/11 GI Bill or transferability. The Commission estimates the VA would pay an additional $76.5 billion between FY 2015 and FY 2024 for transferred benefits" (MCRMC, 2015, p. 167).

On the spousal front, the Department of Defense's (DoD) Career Advancement Account scholarship program for military spouses (MyCAA) was established in 2009 to help military spouses gain essential training for portable careers regardless of military duty assignments. Eligible spouses receive $4000 that can be used for approved training programs in high-demand employment fields. Funds can cover occupational license or credential examinations and associated courses leading directly to employment; they cannot be used for general studies or for pursuing a bachelor's or graduate degree. Program data provided by the Office of the Deputy Assistant Secretary of Defense for Military Community and Family Policy estimates that roughly 25,000 spouses completed an educational goal as a result of MyCAA funding between October 2010 (when the program was redesigned) and November 2013; many other military spouses enrolled in the program and were still in the career pipeline beyond the conclusion of the RAND Corporation study cited (Friedman, Miller, & Evans, 2015).

While the primary role the higher education community plays for military-connected populations is providing postsecondary education instructional programs, there are two other significant higher education intercepts that affect the broader community of military families—applied and scientific research and practitioner preparation and training.

---

[2] Data compiled from Voluntary Education Fact Sheets found at http://www.dantes.doded.mil/service-members/resourceslinks.html#sthash.KN7U8GpJ.dpbs.

9.2 Research

According to the National Center for Education Statistics, in 2014 postsecondary education institutions received more than $134 million dollars of federal obligations for research, development, and research and development plant funding. Obligated federal funds have remained fairly stable, ranging from $149 to 112 million dollars during the past decade (NCES, 2015). Research universities also solicit funds from nonprofit and philanthropic organizations on targeted research topics related to military-connected populations such as military-related injuries, post-traumatic stress, transition assistance, suicide, family relationships, educational attainment, and child and adolescent resiliency. Two institutions, Purdue University (IN) and Syracuse University (NY) have established research institutes that focus on issues affecting military-connected citizens—service members, veterans, and family members.

While data specifically related to the number and scope of scientific, sociological, and program evaluation assessments on topics related to the military family community conducted by higher education institutions have been difficult to capture, the potential impact on military-connected populations is significant. For instance, according to the National Science Foundation (NSF) Higher Education Research and Development (R&D) Survey (HERD), in FY 2013, the DoD funded over $56.8 million dollars in higher education R&D efforts related to psychology and over $94.5 million dollars in social science R&D in addition to its investments in engineering and scientific R&D conducted by higher education institutions (National Science Foundation, 2016, p. 3; National Center for Science and Engineering Statistics, 2015). In 2015, the DoD obligated over $11.2 billion dollars for applied and basic research conducted by colleges and universities (NSF, 2015). Granted, not all of those obligations were specific to military-connected populations, but the dollar amounts still indicate that researchers at higher education institutions are interconnected with the military community in ways that may not be immediately obvious to the outside observer. In addition, current grant projects open to higher education researchers and being solicited by Federal agencies include ones on military burn research, human performance sensing, and extremity regeneration (Grants.gov search October 25, 2015). These directly affect military-connected populations both during and after service.

9.3 Practitioner Preparation and Training

The higher education community also provides the instructional and training framework for K-12 teacher preparation and health care and behavioral science practitioners who work closely with military populations—including but not limited to teachers, nursing and health professionals, and social workers. All elementary and secondary teachers, health professionals (e.g., emergency medical technicians, clinical/medical lab scientists, registered and practical nurses), and social service workers (including social workers) obtain practical training and professional education from the higher education community.

It has become increasingly important within the last 10–15 years to embed knowledge of military populations into education, health care, and behavioral science curricula so that future healthcare practitioners and social service professionals understand their patient clientele in terms of the military mindset, unique characteristics, behaviors, and common medical and psychological challenges that military families face. The Association for Institutional Research (AIR) noted in the Freedom and Honor Warriors Transition Workshop program evaluation that

> An estimated 500,000 veterans serving in Iraq and Afghanistan will return home with post-traumatic stress disorder, or PTSD—a debilitating illness that is often marked with anger, depression, physical pain, disturbed sleep, social isolation, and thoughts of suicide. In addition to the personal devastation to a soldier's quality of life, the cost for treating PTSD creates a burden to the nation's health care system.[3]

Examples of collegiate programs seeking to develop culturally competent veterans service providers include Fayetteville State University, which offers bachelor's and master's degrees in social work that include courses on "Social Work Practice with Military Families (SWRK 375)," and "Social Work Practice and Traumatic Brain Injuries (SWRK 629)"; Mississippi State University's Veterans Certificate Program at the undergraduate and graduate levels;[4] and Texas State University's elective course (Helping Veterans Transition) offered both through classroom-based and online delivery for graduate students in their Master of Social Work (MSW) program.[5]

It is essential that K-12 teachers, particularly those in communities with a high density of military families, are trained to recognize, accept, and assist children of military families who may be dealing with family separations, deployments, and loss. According to the *U.S. Department of Defense 2011 Annual Report*, there are currently 2,000,000 military-connected students whose parents are members of the active-duty military, National Guard or Reserves, or veterans (U.S. Department of Defense, 2011). Approximately 60% of children of military service members are school-aged and a high proportion attend public schools. Incorporating teacher training modules to heighten awareness of social, emotional, and learning challenges specific to military-connected students, while building concepts of resiliency and coping mechanisms, helps both classroom situations and family relations.

It is worthy of note that a DoD program, Troops to Teachers, assists eligible military personnel to engage in classroom education in high-need public schools upon

---

[3] http://www.air.org/project/addressing-post-traumatic-stress-disorder-among-veterans-learning-what-works.

[4] http://iswd.msstate.edu/current-students/programs/veterans/.

[5] Fayetteville State University has partnered with the US Army and the US Navy to increase the number of Social Workers within the military. To learn more about the FSU-Army MSW Program at Fort Sam Houston, Texas, or the MSC Navy Social Work program, refer to http://www.uncfsu.edu/sw.

their separation from military service. More than 17,000 participants have acquired their teaching certification and are teaching in public classrooms since the program began in 1994 (U.S. Department of Defense n.d.).[6]

9.4 History: The Evolving "Problem"

Three key issues surfaced during the initial phases of Operation Iraqi Freedom (OIF) and Operation Enduring Freedom (OEF): institutional policies allowing service members and family members access to, withdrawal from, and readmission into the educational environment without educational or financial repercussions, financial support mechanisms and strategies to fill initial education benefit funding gaps, and transition programs and supports for military service as well as civilian support communities for veterans whose terms of enlistment were satisfied.

With the start of Operation Iraqi Freedom (OIF), significant numbers of service members were mobilized for deployment, often without advance notification to get personal affairs in order. Service members and family members' primary focus was on deployment planning and family action plans (wills, finances, child care arrangements), not academic procedures at the college where they were enrolled. For military family members enrolled in college courses, this often caused attendance absences and course withdrawals at times not in synch with academic calendars. Army National Guard (ARNG) mobilizations affected a significant number of states due to call-ups; thus National Guard members, reservists, and family members were forced to withdraw from college to meet unanticipated military and family obligations.

Many institutions across all sectors of higher education developed organic or grassroots responsiveness to deployment and mobilization issues, unique educational needs and supports for service members (active and reserve component, veterans, family members). In describing the higher education landscape for military populations during early years preceding 2001, McBain asserts that individual states:

> responded in different ways to the educational and other needs of veterans (both those currently deployed and those returning to civilian lives), as well as their spouses and dependents. At present, there is no centrally coordinated effort among states to work together to meet these needs given the combination of veterans and servicemembers' mobility and states' individual governance structures. However, there is increased attention and goodwill toward veterans' higher education efforts (2008, p. 5).

Proactive state college systems such as those in Arkansas, Minnesota, and Texas developed close relations with National Guard units engaged in mobilization events and Yellow Ribbon demobilization events. As military families went through pre- and post-mobilization preparations, educational institutions and advisors participated to apprise them of educational options. The Minnesota State College and

---

[6] http://troopstoteachers.net/AbouttheProgram/Overview.aspx.

University System (MNSCU) developed online courses that service members could complete while deployed overseas. East Carolina University (NC) offered distance learning courses in which a military spouse could enroll in the same course as the deployed service member at no additional cost as a way to support family communication and connections (on other than stressful topics such as finances and personal safety) during deployment.

With a growing numbers of service members and veterans who had completed their military obligations and set to engage in America's promise of access to obtaining a college degree in exchange for their military service, it became important for the higher education community to anticipate the transitional and educational needs of returning service members. One of the first national efforts to identify these occurred in May 2008 when the American Council on Education (ACE) convened a summit focused on "Serving Those Who Serve: Higher Education and America's Veterans." The chief education-related concerns student veterans presented were: financial challenges related to transitioning to veteran student status amid lagging processing of VA educational benefits; informational gaps about the college admission and enrollment process, cultural barriers between civilian student populations and the military culture from which they transitioned, and appropriate services and support for battlefield injuries and trauma-related challenges. Student veteran financial need and campus funding to expand programs and services remained key issues for service members, veterans, family members, and institutional leadership throughout the decade.

Later in 2008, higher education associations began to examine the national landscape to capture data on demographics, campus climates, and programs and services under development for military student populations. In a collaborative effort, four associations (the American Association of State Colleges and Universities [AASCU], American Council on Education [ACE], Student Affairs Administrators in Higher Education [NASPA], and National Association of Veteran Program Administrators [NAVPA] with financial support from the Lumina Foundation for Education produced a "first-of-its-kind national snapshot of the programs, services, and policies" (2009, p. iii) on college campuses serving veterans, military personnel, and family members. Results of two iterations of the national survey were published in *From Soldier to Student* to benchmark and measure institutional efforts to assist military-connected populations' transition to the college environment. *From Soldier to Student: Easing the Transition of Service Members to Campus* also included responses from focus groups of veterans and enlisted service members about potential challenges they anticipated and/or experienced related to pursuit of their educational goals. (Cook & Kim, 2009; McBain, Kim, Cook, & Snead, 2012).

While administrative policies and policies were under development and revision nationally and at many institutions, parallel initiatives on campuses initiated support services and programs for military-connected students. The common goal of the higher education community was to take care of and serve those who had served the nation. Examples of collaborative practices and organizations supporting military-connected students included the Military Family Research Institute's (MFRI) Operation Diploma, New Jersey State College and Universities' Operation College

Promise 3-day training for college personnel, University of Louisville Veterans Symposium, Cleveland State University's Supportive Education for the Returning Veteran (SERV) program, and Syracuse University's Entrepreneural Boot Camp.[7] New veteran advocacy and service organizations such as the Iraq and Afghanistan Veterans Association (IAVA) and the Student Veterans of America (SVA) were also formed. They actively engaged constituents nationwide in support of educational programs, legislation, and funding for military-affiliated populations. Grant funding by the Wal-Mart Foundation, MFRI, and Lumina Foundation aided the higher education community with campus support program start-ups and establish veteran one-stop centers.

9.5 Responses and Strategies

National responses to the key issues identified at the start of OIF/OEF took two primary forms: policy implementation—at national, state, and institutional levels—and/or program/service implementation. Brief summaries follow of key national policies and promising practices implemented by institutions of higher learning regarding military family educational needs and issues.

9.5.1 Policy Implementation (National and State Levels)

The higher education community supported the **Higher Education Relief Opportunities for Students Act of 2003 (HEROES Act)**, which gave the Department of Education broad authority to ensure that service members called to active duty are not worse off financially at the end of their service. Higher education associations supported and signed a HEROES Act community letter urging the extension of the Act until authorities could enact new legislation.

1. **Higher Education Opportunity Act, Readmission for Returning Service Members.**[8] To minimize the disruption to the lives of service members mobilized or called up to military service, Congress added requirements into HEOA that allowed them to return to an institution of higher education without penalty for service-related withdrawal. Under HEOA, a student who is called to active duty in the United States Armed Forces or the National Guard or Reserve for more than 30 days is entitled to reenroll in the same program, with the same enrollment status, number of credits, and academic standing. To qualify for readmission a service member is required to satisfy three conditions explicitly outlined in the legislation.

---

[7] http://vets.syr.edu/education/ebv/.

[8] http://www2.ed.gov/policy/highered/guid/readmission.html.

2. **In-State Tuition Rates for Armed Forces Members, Spouses, and Dependent Children. Section 114** of the HEOA enabled active-duty members of the Armed Forces and their family members to receive in-state tuition rates for attendance at public institutions of higher learning. As a further protection, if the family member is continuously enrolled at the institution, he/she must be allowed to enroll at in-state rates.

3. The legislative change with the most significant impact on military-connected populations was the **Post-9/11 GI Bill**. Prior to its enactment in June 2008, the Montgomery GI Bill (MGIB) was available to service members but had not kept pace with the cost of living, college tuition, nor cost of college attendance. The Post-9/11 GI Bill) is the most complex—and potentially most costly—version of the GI Bill in American history. Under the Post-9/11 GI Bill structure, institutions receive funds directly from the VA for tuition and fee payments, which has forced the VA and higher education stakeholders into a much closer working relationship. As noted earlier in the chapter, one of the provisions of the Post-9/11 GI Bill for family members was the inclusion of the Transfer of Benefit eligibility for selected service members. Incorporated in the legislation as a recruiting and retention incentive, the provision

allows service members (officer or enlisted, active duty, or Selected Reserve), to transfer unused education benefits to immediate family members (spouse and children). The service member must have at least six years of service, and commit to an additional four years of service in order to transfer benefits to a spouse or child.[9]

4. **The Post-9/11 Veterans Education Assistance Improvements Act of 2010**, also known as GI Bill 2.0, modified some more restrictive or narrowly defined aspects of the 2008 GI Bill after conversations among legislators. The new law expanded benefit eligibility for members of the National Guard to include time served on Title 32 orders or in the full-time Active Guard and Reserve (AGR) toward the 36-month service requirement. Two key changes were inclusion of a partial housing stipend for distance learners enrolled solely in online courses and replacement of the state-by-state tuition caps for veterans enrolled at public colleges and universities by a national in-state tuition threshold.

5. **The Presidential Executive Order 13607, "Establishing Principles of Excellence for Educational Institutions"** signed on April 27, 2012, directed agencies to implement Principles of Excellence for education institutions that interact with veterans, service members, and their families and to ensure beneficiaries have the information they need to make educated choices about VA education benefits and approved programs. It also directed federal agencies to provide meaningful cost and quality information on schools, prevent deceptive recruiting practices, and provide high-quality academic and student support services.

---

[9] Downloaded 11/16/15 from http://www.benefits.va.gov/gibill/handouts_forms.asp. *Education and Training. Post 9/11 GI Bill: Transferability* (U.S. Department of Veterans Affairs, 2015, p. 1).

Greater inter-agency collaboration between the Departments of Education, Defense and Veterans Affairs and the Consumer Financial Protection Bureau was one of the order's outcomes, though overlapping data collection and reporting efforts persist. Agencies examined data collected within the various organizations but because departmental program definitions and agency accountability requirements differ in prescribed outcomes and reporting metrics, multiple consumer information resources exist for military-connected students. The National Center for Education Statistics operates College Navigator, the Department of Education's website that compares colleges and universities in multiple ways including by price, region, and programs offered (NCES, 2014, n.d.). Veterans Affairs' Education Benefits Administration and the Department of Defense Voluntary Education division have developed military-affiliated search tools (GI Bill Comparison Tool and TA Decide) where military/veteran students can search for institutional data on colleges. To ensure student protection, the Executive Order called for the creation of a robust, centralized complaint process for students receiving federal military and veterans' education benefits. Collaboratively, the agencies established the Postsecondary Education Complaint System (PECS) that provides authorized personnel the ability to track, manage, and process formal complaints that have been submitted by, or on behalf of, uniformed service members, spouses, and other family members when educational institutions fail to follow the Principles of Excellence.

6. **Section 702 of the Veterans Access, Choice, and Accountability Act of 2014** enables veterans/military families (regardless of formal state of residence) who meet established criteria to receive in-state tuition rates for enrollment terms starting after July 1, 2015. Commonly known as the Choice Act Section 702, the legislation requires public institutions to charge in-state tuition rates to veterans and family members using GI Bill education benefits moving to a state in which a public institution of higher education is located and enrolling within 3 years of the beneficiary's military discharge.

9.5.2 State Policies/Implementation

Several state university systems were proactive in the recruitment of veterans well before implementation of the Choice Act in 2014. One such frontrunner was the Ohio Board of Regents who, through an Executive Order from the governor, established the Ohio GI Promise that "would allow qualified veterans, and their dependents, from anywhere in the country to skip the 12-month residency requirement and attend University System of Ohio schools at in-state tuition rates."[10] The Ohio Board of Regents and the University System also pressed for the evaluation and transfer of military credit as state priorities, establishing an Articulation and Transfer Advisory Council to support endeavors statewide.

---

[10] http://veterans.osu.edu/future-students/choosing-ohio-state/ohio-gi-promise/.

Other states taking a broad statewide approach in delivering educational opportunities for military families include California (specifically the California State University system), Minnesota, Iowa, and Texas. Although Minnesota has no military base within its state borders, the state has a sizeable National Guard presence. Many Guard units were mobilized shortly after September 11th, some mobilized overseas and others sent to military installations as rear detachments and/or backfilling assignments for those active-duty units deployed. As noted earlier in the chapter, the institutions that comprise the Minnesota State Colleges and Universities (MNSCU) were actively engaged in Yellow Ribbon Mobilization and Demobilization activities within the state and continued their involvement beyond early call-ups. One of the products of that collaboration was the development of VETS, Veteran Education Transfer System,[11] an educational planning tool to determine how evaluated credits for military training can count for college credit at various institutions within the MNSCU system. Funding for the system's multi-campus initiative linking military occupational specialties to campus programs was supported by Congressionally directed grant awards. The state of Iowa has developed a comprehensive Home Base Iowa initiative to welcome and entice veteran families to relocate to the state. Home Base Iowa offers financial incentives (e.g., property tax exemptions, home ownership assistance, Veterans Trust Fund), employment assistance, and educational opportunities to transitioning service members and veterans moving to Iowa.

Thirteen Midwestern states, supported by the Lumina Foundation, have collectively developed a Multi-state Collaborative for Military Credit (MCMC)[12] to aid course transfer and articulations of military training among participating state institutions. The Collaborative focuses on institutional practices in four areas (articulation of credit, licensure and certification, communications and information dissemination, and technology solutions) to help ease educational transitions and degree attainment of military-connected populations at colleges and universities.

9.5.3 Promising Practices at the Institutional Level

Since September 11, 2001, there has been significant development and implementation of promising campus practices in support of veteran and military families among educational associations and cooperating institutions. Early on, grassroots programs and initiatives surfaced on campuses about how best to address institutional barriers or military-affiliated student issues from a national perspective.

For instance, the American Council of Education partnered with the Walmart Foundation to engage the higher education community in promoting "awareness of innovation ideas and lessons learned, and disseminate insights and ideas to institutions of higher education" (ACE, 2011, p. 2). Walmart Foundation awarded Success for Veterans Award grants to 20 institutional recipients for a 3-year period beginning

---

[11] http://www.mnscu.edu/college-search/public/military.

[12] http://www.mhec.org/multi-state-collaborative-on-military-credit.

from June 2009. According to the final report of the *Promising Practices: Outcomes and Recommendations from the Success for Veterans Award Grants,* "[o]ne of the most critical effects of the grants has been the development of state and community partnerships on and off campus to support veterans programs." (ACE, 2011, p. 3). Additionally, the American Council on Education conducted a 3-day Veterans Success Jam[13] in May 2010 that engaged veterans, service members, and families as well as campus administrators, nonprofit organizations, and government officials in a national online conversation about the "challenges and opportunities facing veterans in higher education" (ACE, 2010, p.1).

Over the course of a decade, education associations and veteran service organizations have developed an evidence-based body of knowledge and practice centered on educational issues related to military-connected student populations. In essence, a specialized community of student personnel professionals has been established to assist veterans, service members, and their families effectively navigate higher education. Professional education associations such as the American Association of Collegiate Registrar and Admissions Officers (AACRAO), Council of College and Military Educators (CCME), Student Affairs Administrators in Higher Education (NASPA), National Association of Veteran Program Administrators (NAVPA), and Student Veterans of America have developed program tracks in their annual and regional meetings to present professional development and policy issues related to military and veteran student populations.

9.5.4 Future Scenarios

However, while these efforts are making headway in providing educational services and support for those who have served and their families, they only scratch the surface. Since the military-affiliated student population (i.e., active-duty and Guard/Reservists, veterans, and family members) is not monolithic, future scenarios for policy, practice, and research should be considered. A sampling of these follows:

- Consider when creating national or local policy that differences exist in military families encompassing not only branch of service and whether the service member is enlisted or officer, but in more traditional areas of demographic research such as race, gender, social class, and geographic region of origin. This also holds true for those in the Guard/Reserve and veterans. Higher education policy and research are just catching up to socioeconomic, gender, class, race, and other forms of overlapping diversity in the civilian nontraditional student population. The same attention must be paid to differences within the military family population—both on the national level and on campuses—in order to accurately craft policies that do not serve only one small segment of the whole and inaccurately present them as the totality of what it means to be a military family. For instance,

---

[13] http://www.acenet.edu/news-room/Pages/Veterans-Jam-2010.aspx.

the dependent child or spouse of a veteran using transferred Post-9/11 GI Bill benefits may not seek out the services being offered to veterans on campus because they do not feel entitled; the parent of a deployed service member who goes to school part-time and cares for that service member's minor child has different support needs from the student veteran who goes to school full-time and lives with a spouse and children. While national or institutional policies cannot account for every individual's life circumstances, they can be more inclusive and recognize that the "traditional" post-World War II model of a single or married white male veteran using GI Bill benefits has changed as the composition of the Armed Forces, and society as a whole, has changed.

- Focus on academic and empirical research that goes beyond the veteran or service member to address the family unit as a whole. While research is being done, as noted earlier in the chapter, on military dependents in the K-12 classroom, higher education researchers have not extended this research to what happens to military children's developmental trajectories in college and young adulthood.
- Focus on policy and research issues that are not solely deficit oriented. While it is vital to address problems such as physical, cognitive, or psychological disability suffered as the result of combat exposure and not gloss over the fact that many veterans and their families are facing tremendous lifelong challenges as a result of serving the nation, broadly depicting the service member, veteran, and military family as a traumatized population does not help them assimilate to civilian life and can set up negative stereotypes that higher education researchers and policymakers rightly decry when applied to students of color, women students, or other minority students. The same baseline respect should be afforded military families by civilian higher education researchers. Given the dearth of research on military-affiliated students, there is room to address the potential for demonstrating resiliency as well as overcoming deficit.

9.6   Lessons Learned

9.6.1   Collaboration Among Stakeholder Groups and Organizations Was a Lesson Learned Late by Many Organizations and Agencies

Colleges, veteran service organizations, and government agencies developed excellent programs and services but didn't work collaboratively or communicate strategically to inform potential clients/students/program participants. Better-publicized state or regional college collaborations might have reduced duplication of services that occurred and been cost-effective in sharing resources. Equally important is the potential synergy and national consciousness of broader social issues around military-connected populations: mental health support and services, homelessness, substance abuse, deployment- and healthcare-related financial stress, health care for military families, employment training, trauma-informed care, and sexual trauma. Characterizing particular issues experienced by veteran students such as "self-medication" as an "educational" challenge does not engage all potential problem-solvers and subject matter experts in the development of broader responses and/or support to post-traumatic stress exhibited in other societal sectors (e.g., employment, VA health care).

9.6.2 The Best Time to Evaluate Effective Policies and National Strategies for Our Military Personnel and Veterans Is During "Periods of Peace"

Perhaps the worst time is in the midst of military conflict when heightened demands for programs and services compete for limited financial resources and human capital under time and performance pressures. Whether as a consequence of the shift to the all-volunteer military force following the Vietnam War or due to competing pressure to help solve the country's economic crisis at the turn of the century, national policy leaders invested little time, effort, or resources for more than two decades (post-Vietnam War-pre September 11) in shaping policy that protected/safeguarded the educational rights and benefits of service members, veterans and family members. Education benefits had not kept up with cost of college attendance and therefore were no longer as attractive a motivator for joining the armed services. Policymakers were therefore caught off-guard when mobilizations, deployments, and readmission issues surfaced at the outset of OIF/OEF. Going forward, one lesson learned from the past conflicts is that legislative policies must be kept in place during peacetime hiatuses and periodically revisited to insure applicability. For instance, the Presidential Executive Order and the Readmission section of HEOA can remain in effect when the country is not engaged militarily so that should future conflicts arise, some protections and administrative relief are in place. While the policy and guidelines will likely need to be modified to address ongoing changes that occur in higher educational programs, at least the foundation for educational safeguards will be in place. Similarly, the greatest opportunity for conducting research on the effectiveness and impacts of education benefits and institutional policies—such as which institutional practices best worked for veteran retention or degree completion—is following a particular military conflict, during the drawdown period or in peacetime.

9.6.3 A Sea of Goodwill and Well-Intentioned Citizenry Should Never Displace or Replace Established Program Planning and Evaluation

During our most recent military conflicts many service providers, institutions, and nonprofit funding sources reacted quickly to implement new programs and services to fill perceived and "urgent" needs of military families. Helping veteran/military students and military families was the immediate priority—sometimes bypassing or overlooking procedural guidelines and needs assessment documentation to fill perceived program/service gaps. Government agency and philanthropic funding efforts to support military family programs and services contributed greatly in meeting the social, educational, and economic needs of military families. However, one of the lessons learned nationally was the importance of being proactive and developing formal program evaluations and need-based assessments prior to actual program implementation despite pressure for rapid action by advocates, military-affiliated populations, and media outlets. Responding quickly to implement service programs without such assessment, which were seen as unnecessary administrative delays, may have encouraged and exacerbated the proliferation of well-intentioned programs and services with no significant impact. Establishing outcome measures or building in program evaluations and assessments at the outset of a program—not reverse-engineering such things midway through when advocates and media outlets begin asking for data—is a crucial requirement to insure effective program results, responsible program implementation, and positively impact and resolve the identified military family need.

One case in point was the creation of My Career Advancement Accounts (MyCAA) scholarship program for military spouses by the DoD. It was broadly accepted by DoD and American citizens that supporting military spouse education in high-demand career fields was a sound idea, especially during the height of OIF. Initially established in 2009, the educational program had a short implementation timeline and insufficient program development planning. What resulted was a scholarship program for *all* military spouses without determination of individual financial need, and inadequate needs assessment and research on "high need" career fields. While highly popular among military spouses, the program was temporarily shut down when all annual allocated funds were depleted within months of implementation. According to Clifford Stanley, undersecretary of defense for personnel and readiness, "The MyCAA program popularity grew beyond our expectations and became too expensive to continue. Therefore, we are returning to the original intent of the program in a way that is attainable and fiscally responsible for the Defense Department…Military spouses will be guided along a more holistic approach to career planning."[14]

When MyCAA was relaunched in 2010, established eligibility criteria were in place and policy guidance carefully followed. According to analysis by RAND Corporation researchers (Friedman, Miller, & Evans, 2015), less than one-fifth of the military spouses who are eligible are taking advantage of the program; 54% of the respondents who indicated they were not using the educational benefit explained they lacked knowledge that the program existed. Despite heightened publicity and awareness campaigns on the part of DoD in 2013, significant numbers of military spouses remain unaware of the scholarship program.

---

[14] Press Release U.S. Department of Defense Office of the Assistant Secretary of Defense (Public Affairs), No. 632–10 July 20, 2010.

9.6.4 The Military-Connected Populations Across the Nation Could Benefit Tremendously from a National Marketing and Communication Strategy for Support Programs

Three phenomena warrant the need for a national communication effort for military families: consumer education in response to the growth in the number of products, services, and programs; shifting demographics of the military family unit; and mobile lifestyle. A plethora of excellent campus programs and local support services have been developed nationally, but greater communication and consumer information on existing programs needs to be shared widely.

According to the DoD *2014 Demographics: Profile of the Military Community*,[15] approximately 51% of service members are married; 42% of service members have at least one child. Annually the demographics of the total military force is in flux as xx number of enlistees join the military and 200,000 enlisted personnel and officers separated from military service (retirements, voluntary and involuntary separations). Young recruits entering military service may join as unmarried individuals and during their enlistment marry and/or have children. Military commands place great emphasis on Family Readiness Groups (FRGs) or support groups on installations, but new spouses and family members may not be informed of the readiness groups, may elect not to utilize base resources due to confidentiality issues, and/or seek to satisfy consumer education needs about programs and services through Internet access to electronic resources.

Mobile military families relocating across state and local boundaries need to be apprised of potential resources *before* they relocate, not during a personal or family crisis or after the fact. Establishing a national clearinghouse or central repository for information so military-connected individuals are empowered to research and access nationwide knowledge of existing supports, services, and resources would go far to build resiliency and interdependence among military families. National advisory groups may help coordinate and guide users to the most appropriate resources available. Program evaluations about anticipated outcomes, potential costs, and which programs have the best outcomes and positive impacts for military populations seeking assistance. Thus there is a need to develop a reliable communication strategy and dissemination plan to share effective resources, promising practices, and vetted consumer resources through a centralized and trusted source.

---

[15] http://www.militaryonesource.mil/footer?content_id=279104. Office of the Deputy Assistant Secretary of Defense (Military Community and Family Policy). (2016). *2014 Demographics: Profile of the Military Community*. ICF International.

9.6.5 The Higher Education Community, Government Agencies and the Legislative Branch Would Benefit Greatly from More Engagement and Information Exchange During Committee Discussions of Legislation

Proactively engaging in discussions with committee members and staff of various committees (HELP, House/Senate Committee on Veterans Affairs, Armed Services and sharing information on program outcomes, research findings, and viable solutions *before* draft legislation is developed may alleviate some of the defensiveness on both sides and heated hearings that have marked recently proposed legislation. Identifying (or building) communication channels to inform policymakers of institutional research in progress and/or potential findings that may afford viable solutions to national issues can remedy the current informational gap. The higher education community has subject matter expertise on all manner of public policies, economic development issues, education benefits, and research findings—including two national associations devoted to education research (the Association for the Study of Higher Education and the American Educational Research Association)—but frequently does not actively engage in national policy discourse specific to military-affiliated students and their families. The description of the university as an Ivory Tower removed from mundane or practical affairs of daily living, such as the well-being of military families and service members engaging in national service, is apt imagery for the separation of the higher education community from national policymaking in this sector. Simply stated, the university community mustn't wait to be asked to share potential solutions and knowledge—teaching and research faculty alike should engage in active policy development conversations and if need be, initiate those dialogues. A possible explanation for the reticence and lack of engagement may also be that researchers who are working on military-connected student issues within the university silo don't communicate in ways that committees understand.

Committee members and personnel at military- and veteran-serving agencies *also* have a responsibility to proactively engage with the higher education community to fulfill the shared goal of serving military-connected students. For example, when implementing the Post-9/11 GI Bill, VA administrators did not consult either the U.S. Department of Education or higher education associations until late in the implementation process. As a result, VA was unaware of standard higher education billing practices, specifically how institutions calculate tuition and fees, and proposed to implement a confusing and impractical redefinition of "tuition and fees" for the Post-9/11 GI Bill. While higher education researchers and associations do not expect committee members or government agencies to be experts on the nuances of higher education finance, it is reasonable for them to ask policymakers consult higher education experts on such matters *before* making decisions that can potentially harm student veterans and their families.

9.7 Recommendations

9.7.1 Establish an Alliance

Establishing a national Military Family Alliance would ensure that there are broad collaboration and communication channels created among stakeholder groups and organizations. Rather than supporting military families and addressing specific issues in topical or agency silos, cross-functional advantages may be created through cross-pollination, brainstorming on critical military family issues spanning multiple sectors, and the development of viable solutions resulting from collaboration.

The determination of what national organization or federal agency is "best" positioned to lead a national forum on Military Families should not be viewed as a turf battle but an opportunity for non-partisan collaboration. While the Joining Forces initiative,[16] launched by First Lady Michelle Obama and Dr. Jill Biden in 2011, has championed military family issues and heightened the national visibility of the challenges our military-connected populations experience, the Office of the First Lady does not have the authority, manpower, or resources to carry on the Military Family charge after the incumbent First Ladies leave office. The coordination of a Forum on Military Families might most effectively reside with a national advisory group or steering committee to insure that stakeholders from all key sectors are represented and engaged. Organizations such as Purdue University's Military Family Research Institute and/or Syracuse University's Institute for Veterans and Military Families that embody an interdisciplinary perspective on social, economic, and policy issues related to military-affiliated populations might be great agents for coordinating and galvanizing the myriad of stakeholders around the central issues of military families.

9.7.2 Establish a National Website

In conjunction with the proposed Military Family Alliance, establish a national Military Family Resource website to store and disseminate vetted and reliable consumer information about the various programs, services, and resources to assist and support military-connected individuals. The challenge for military-connected families (and service providers alike) is having a centralized and trusted source for accessing and/or disseminating information. There has been an explosion of service providers, support programs, and community agencies to assist military-connected citizens in a variety of areas including wellness and healthcare support, disability services, education transition programs, financial planning, and employment assistance. Unfortunately, some of these may be driven by a profit motive rather than focused on the best interests/needs of the military-connected individual. For optimal

---

[16] https://www.whitehouse.gov/joiningforces.

effectiveness of a centralized repository of program and service providers, the Military Family Resource concept must include a vetting process whereby program specialists and professionals within the subject area examine, review, and approve service providers for inclusion.

Access and availability of financial resource information is a key data need cutting across all service sectors supporting military-connected students. Whether focusing on college access and support for individual students, institutional student success initiatives, support service providers (by government, community or non-profit organizations, or evidence-based research that can contribute to future success, health, and well-being of military-connected populations), all pathways are challenged by the need for sufficient financial resources. Whatever form or structure the national repository takes, information on available financial resources—for individuals and program providers—must be incorporated. Military-affiliated populations interested in postsecondary education need accurate and timely information about financial resources for funding their educational goals. Education consumer information and financial funding options from the Departments of Education, Defense, and Veterans Affairs, Veterans Benefit Administration need to be centrally accessible. In the RAND analysis of MyCAA surveying spouses who desired to pursue postsecondary education options but were currently not doing so, 82% of respondents cited cost for not pursuing their educational goal (Friedman, Miller, & Evans, 2015).

This information should be outwardly facing for various user groups that include military-connected populations for personal information searches and resource exploration; college and university administrative stakeholders seeking to research promising practices or funding sources; academic and scientific researchers to acquire information on current trends and research findings and potential funding sources; state and national policymakers to understand the demographics and identified needs of military/veteran/military family populations.

One of the unique challenges in disseminating information to military family members is the place-based variations and availability of programs and services. Individual states, cities, and localities may offer widely diverse programs or services depending on the proximity of military installations, economic funding available, and the number of military-connected individuals residing within jurisdictions and boundaries. Families living in rural communities may have fewer support options or access to advisers and service providers than those military families living in urban areas or near military bases. State agencies currently have review processes for identifying community-based resources, so a national information resource might tap into state and community resources for disseminating information.

While a Web presence alone cannot address the full scope of the information challenge related to sharing programs and service information with military families, it is a positive start—particularly if the website is a centralized repository that contains vetted information and resources covering the full range of programs and services that military families may need over their lifetime. With the continuous flow of military personnel and family members joining the military services and transitioning as veterans, it behooves the nation to communicate with the military family audiences using a variety of methods as the circumstances and need for service information will vary over the audience's lifespan. Despite uneven access to the Internet within home environments, most cities offer access through public libraries, schools, and community centers.

9.7.3 Establish a Clearinghouse for Military-Connected Data

Just as military-affiliated populations have a need for a consolidated clearinghouse for relevant and timely information on health, education, and employment issues, so do researchers, educators, and policymakers need a national repository or clearinghouse for military-connected data. A data warehouse with search capacity and primary source data for topical issues (e.g., mental health, disability assistance, employment assistance, resiliency training, and educational research) and military subpopulations (veterans, enlisted personnel, military families, active or reserve components, and children of military personnel) would enhance ongoing research and policy decisions. Conceptually, the recommendation sounds like a simple solution but is in fact a complex challenge to execute. There has been a proliferation of knowledge, established practices, state and national policy, and demographic information generated about veteran and military populations over the past decade but no central repository or collection agency to help decision-makers access and utilize the collected data.

Creating a data warehouse and clearinghouse that has the capacity to serve the various stakeholders (users) with sufficient capacity to handle data queries and requests requires significant financial and government agency support. A current initiative under development by Veterans Affairs is *my*VA, a website that centers holistically on the broad array of veterans' programs, services, and benefits—health care, home loans, education, mental health, disability compensation, employment, and vocational rehabilitation. Efforts are underway to create relationship maps to help understand the Veteran's customer experience with all aspects of Veterans Affairs in order to help build trusted relationships. While still in the infancy stages of development, *my*VA could serve as the landing page or homepage for a Military-Connected Clearinghouse and data warehouse. Other government agencies and trusted partners of Veterans Affairs could serve as inter-agency affiliates and link their specific military family-related resources and programs through *my*VA.

Conceptually, military-connected individuals and the general public might access *my*VA for consumer information and resources for a specific need or topic of interest through a public-facing website. Other stakeholders (researchers, legislators, policymakers, university personnel) might access the data warehouse through a log-in procedure to investigate and utilize documents and shared data across governmental agencies. Having reputable military/veterans education-related data and research collected insofar as possible in one federal site location would assist interested parties in using said data/research to craft well-informed federal, state, and institutional policy; evaluate programs and services at the federal, state, and institutional level; monitor the treatment of military/veteran students and their families by higher education institutions; and evaluate Post-9/11 GI Bill expenditures.

The argument for developing a centralized repository and data warehouse is threefold: enabling a holistic approach to veteran and military-connected population issues, common access and data point connections across disciplines or service provision (e.g., impact of post-traumatic stressors on educational and employment outcomes) and reducing administrative and informational technology costs incurred by duplicative agency initiatives. While *my*VA might be the external entry point for consumer information and military-connected data, various government agencies might coordinate internal data sets. For potential military student education-related issues, the National Center for Education Statistics (NCES) might operate this website because of its role as the U.S. Department of Education's statistical agency within the Institute for Education Sciences (NCES, 2015). Since the research and data proposed to be collected and shared relates to military/veteran students and their dependents as a subset of students within postsecondary education, it is logical for the Department of Education to be the lead agency involved in this website and seek cooperation from other agencies as appropriate. Similarly, the repository must publicize and distribute academic and scientific research of military-connected populations; create a military-connected information center so that agencies, institutions, and citizens can access documented information sources on scientific research and best/promising practices with regard to the provision of support and service programs.

Reflecting upon the collective needs of future generations of military families and the national leaders who will inherit the roles of developing policy and program guidance for future military conflicts, the central theme and unifying must be collaboration—collaboration among intersecting stakeholders, including military family members themselves. The Military Family Research Institute's "Convening on Battle Plan for Military Families" held September 23–24, 2015 reinforced the myriad connections between the respective knowledge/service sectors that often go unnoticed and therefore are disjointed. The challenges and opportunities affecting military families cut across all sectors—federal government agencies, state and local governments and agencies, industry and employers, educational providers (K-12 and higher education), policy/program analysts and researchers, healthcare providers, service organizations, and philanthropic organizations. Pooling our collective knowledge and potential resources (programs services, funding sources, and expertise) on a regular (and frequent) basis helps "connect the dots" between stakeholders and reduce obstacles that impede the great human potential within our military-connected populations and communities where they reside. The proposed recommendations outlined above—establishing a national Military Family Alliance, developing Military Family Resource website, and creating a national repository or clearinghouse for military-connected data—would serve as solid foundation in supporting military families and building resiliency within military-connected populations in the wake of future military conflicts.

Additional Reader Resources

Educators and interested citizens may find the following resources and publications useful in understanding of the educational challenges, promising practices, innovative solutions, and potential development opportunities related to military-affiliated student populations.

- American Council on Education's Toolkit for veteran friendly institution. Retrieved from https://vetfriendlytoolkit.acenet.edu/Pages/default.aspx.
- Helping veterans succeed: A handbook for higher education administrators. American Association of Collegiate Registrars and Admissions Officers.
- From soldier to student: Easing the transition of service members on campus. Cook, B., and Kim, Y.
- From soldier to student II: Assessing institutional services for veterans. McBain, Kim, Cook, and Snead.
- Student Veterans of America's The Million Record Project. Retrieved from http://studentveterans.org/index.php/aboutus/what-we-do/million-records-project.

References

American Council on Education (ACE). (2008). *Serving those who serve: Higher education and America's veterans.* Retrieved from http://www.acenet.edu/news-room/Pages/Georgetown-Summit.aspx

American Council on Education (ACE). (2010). *Ensuring success for returning veterans.* Washington, DC: ACE.

American Council on Education (ACE). (2011). *Promising practices in veterans' education: Outcomes and recommendations from the success for veterans award grants.* Washington, DC: ACE.

Cook, B., & Kim, Y. (2009). *From soldier to student: Easing the transition of service members on campus.* Washington, DC: ACE, AASCU, NASPA, NAVPA.

Friedman, E., Miller, L., & Evans, S. (2015). *An assessment of education and employment goals and barriers facing military spouses eligible for MyCAA.* Santa Monica, CA: RAND Corporation. Retrieved from http://www.rand.org/pubs/research_reports/RR784.html.

Grants.gov. (2015, October 25). *Current grant solicitations.*

McBain, L., Kim, Y., Cook, B., & Snead, K. (2012). *From soldier to student II: Assessing campus programs for veterans and service members.* Washington, DC: ACE, AASCU, NASPA, NAVPA. Retrieved from www.acenet.edu/news…/From-Soldier-to-Student-II-Assessing-Campus-Programs.pdf.

Military Compensation and Retirement Modernization Commission. (2015, January). Final report of the Military Compensation and Retirement Modernization Commission. Arlington, VA: Military Compensation and Retirement Modernization Commission. Retrieved from https://www.ngaus.org/sites/default/files/MCRMC%202015_0.pdf

National Center for Educational Statistics. (2015). *Welcome to NCES.* Retrieved from https://nces.ed.gov/

National Center for Science and Engineering Statistics. (2015, February). Info brief: Higher education R&D expenditures resume slow growth in FY2013. Arlington, VA: National Science Foundation. Retrieved from http://www.nsf.gov/statistics/2015/nsf15314/nsf15314.pdf

National Science Foundation (NSF) (2015). *Higher Education Research and Development Survey, Fiscal Year 2014*. Retrieved from https://ncsesdata.nsf.gov/herd/2014/

National Science Foundation. (2016). *Higher Education Research and Development Survey Fiscal Year 2015*. Retrieved from https://ncsesdata.nsf.gov/herd/2015/index.html

U.S. Department of Defense (2011). *Annual report to Congress on plans for the Department of Defense for the support of military family readiness*. Retrieved from http://mldc.whs.mil/public/docs/library/qol/FY2011_Annual_DoD_Report_to_Congress_MilitaryFamilyReadinessPrograms_DoD.pdf

U.S. Department of Defense. (2016) *2014 demographics: Profile of the military community*. Retrieved from http://download.militaryonesource.mil/12038/MOS/Reports/2014-Demographics-Report.pdf

U.S. Department of Defense (n.d.). *Troops to Teachers: About the program*. Retrieved from http://troopstoteachers.net/AbouttheProgram/Overview.aspx

U.S. Department of Education, National Center for Education Statistics (NCES). (2014). *Digest of Educational Statistics*, Table 402.10. Retrieved from http://nces.ed.gov/programs/digest/d14/tables/dt14_402.10.asp?current=yes

U.S. Department of Veterans Affairs. (2015, August). *GI Bill transferability*. Retrieved from http://www.gibill.va.gov/post-911/post-911-gi-bill-summary/transfer-of-benefits.html

U.S. Department of Veterans Affairs, Veterans Benefits Administration. (2013a). *Annual benefits report*. Retrieved from http://benefits.va.gov/REPORTS/abr/

U.S. Department of Veterans Affairs, Veterans Benefits Administration. (2013b). *Education program beneficiaries: FY 2000 to FY 2013*. Retrieved from http://www.va.gov/vetdata/docs/Utilization/EducNation_2013.xls

U.S. Department of Veterans Affairs, Veterans Benefits Administration. (2014). *Annual benefits report*. Retrieved from http://benefits.va.gov/REPORTS/abr/

Westat. (2010). National survey of veterans, active duty service members, demobilized National Guard and reserve members, family members, and surviving spouses, Rockville, MD: Westat. Retrieved from http://www.va.gov/vetdata/docs/SurveysAndStudies/NVSSurveyFinalWeightedReport.pdf

Chapter 10
The Mental Health Response to Operation Enduring Freedom and Operation Iraqi Freedom: History and Recommendations for Change

Morgan T. Sammons and David S. Riggs

The US military has been on a continual war footing for more than 15 years, arguably the longest sustained period of conflict in this nation's history. Since the terrorist attacks of September 11, 2001, we have deployed combat units to theaters of operation in Afghanistan and Iraq, with numerous combat and support units deployed around the globe. While originally labelled the Global War on Terror, nomenclature has now accurately shifted to the "Long War." Beyond its mere duration, this period of war has been complicated by asymmetrical combat, ill-defined operational goals, and complex and shifting domestic and international alliances and policy considerations. The notion of a global battlefield with an elusive enemy targeting predominantly civilians also increases societal anxiety and inflects our response to the needs of returning service members, veterans, and their families.

In order to counter overwhelming force, enemy combatants rely on stealth and crude but effective improvised explosive devices (IEDs) rather than conventional ballistic weapons. No wonder, then, that blast-related injuries emerged as one of the most common forms of Long War wound. In spite of the duration of the current conflict, we have fortunately seen a relatively low number of battlefield fatalities. Almost three million American troops have been deployed to theaters of operation since 2001. Total casualties are, at this point, less than 51,000 with less than 7000 battlefield fatalities. As of February, 2016, 4411 US troops had been killed in Iraq (from both hostile and non-hostile causes) with most deaths occurring between 2004 and 2007 (Brookings Institution, 2010; Defense Manpower Data Center,

M.T. Sammons, Ph.D., A.B.P.P (✉)
National Register of Health Services Psychologists, Washington, DC, USA
e-mail: morgan@nationalregister.org

D.S. Riggs, Ph.D.
Department of Medical and Clinical Psychology, Uniformed Services University of the Health Sciences, Bethesda, MD, USA
e-mail: David.Riggs@USUHS.edu

© Springer International Publishing AG 2018
L. Hughes-Kirchubel et al. (eds.), *A Battle Plan for Supporting Military Families*, Risk and Resilience in Military and Veteran Families,
https://doi.org/10.1007/978-3-319-68984-5_10

2016). The largest single group of fatalities, during the most intense period of conflict 1742 (39.3%), resulted from improvised explosive devices (Brookings Institution, 2010). Between 2001 and 2016, there were 31,951 non-fatal casualties in Iraq (Defense Manpower Data Center, 2016), with most occurring between 2004 and 2007. In Afghanistan, 2345 US service members have died of both hostile and non-hostile causes during Operation Enduring Freedom, and 20,071 have been wounded (Defense Manpower Data Center, 2016).

After 2007, a precipitous decline in all reported casualties occurred. This decline was principally due to a reduction in the intensity of conflict, but improved personnel protection against blast (e.g., vehicle design and armoring), enhanced personal protective gear, and advances in battlefield medicine also were responsible. Battlefield medicine has, along with trauma medicine in general, made significant strides, to the point that injured combatants who survive until they reach a field level care facility have a 90% chance of survival—unprecedented in the history of combat medicine (Defense Health Board, 2015).

In the context of asymmetrical combat, improved survival rates, and anxiety and frustration driven by uncertainty, it is little wonder that psychological injuries rather than physical injury were identified as the "signature wounds" (Tanielian & Jaycox, 2008) of this drawn-out conflict. It is not surprising, then, that we now are focusing more intently on psychological injuries, and that we are expending considerable effort to prevent and treat psychological injuries incurred in combat. Just as we continually seek improvements in personal protective equipment to minimize physical injury, we also continually seek mechanisms to strengthen resilience or otherwise lessen the impact of psychological injuries.

Considerable progress has been made in assessment and treatment strategies since psychological distress (in particular, post-traumatic stress) and the neuropsychological sequelae of traumatic brain injury were identified as "signature injuries." Hoge et al. (2015) provided an excellent summary of advances in military mental health treatment over the past 15 years. They correctly noted that pre-deployment screening was essentially nonexistent before 2003, that mental health services in theater were largely lacking, and that treatment initiatives in US military hospitals and the Department of Veterans Affairs (VA), while aspirational, were largely disjointed and generally service- and status- (e.g., veteran versus actively serving personnel) specific. This meant that despite common injuries, returning combatants were treated in highly compartmentalized environments. To an even greater extent than exists today, there was little crossover between military treatment facilities and similar VA programs (the public-private Intrepid Centers of Excellence and the five VA polytrauma centers were notable exceptions).

Those who did seek treatment early in the war were hobbled by access issues, ongoing stigma, and perhaps most significantly a lack of consensus about diagnostic strategies and effective treatments. By 2008, over half of US combatants who had suffered a blast-related injury had not been evaluated for treatment, and only around half of individuals with presumptive PTSD had sought treatment (Tanielian & Jaycox, 2008). The situation is improving. Now, diagnostic capabilities, including mental health assessments, are available at all but the most far-forward, field medic level (Level 1 or direct battlefield care; Defense Health Board, 2015), and intensive efforts at educating combatants, caregivers, and families regarding symptoms of traumatic stress and brain injuries have dramatically increased awareness of these conditions and helped to reduce the stigma associated with them.

In 2007, there was increasing notice in the press about the mental health needs of combatants and an exposé that severely criticized treatment efforts at the Army's Walter Reed Army Medical Center in Washington, DC (Priest & Hull, 2007). In response, Congress appropriated over $500 M to military medicine and the VA specifically to address the issues of mental health and traumatic brain injury. Like many large appropriations, this funding was both a blessing and a curse. The military services and the VA were charged with coordinating care and treatment efforts, challenging the historical separation between the two agencies (until then, it was in fact illegal for active duty service members to receive anything other than very limited care at VA facilities). Because these allocated funds came from annual congressional appropriations, most of the funds needed to be spent quickly, leaving little time for effective planning. The first author, along with representatives from each service branch, was appointed by the Assistant Secretary of Defense for Health Affairs to a work group directed to develop and coordinate with the VA a plan for expenditure of these funds. This group, the so-called Red Cell, attempted to provide a framework for integrating service delivery among the military services and the VA, coordinate care for veterans and family members, and provide for an education and training structure that would be able to produce accurate, timely information for clinicians, veterans, and the public regarding the physical and psychological consequences of combat. The desired outcome of the Red Cell was to provide veterans and service members with lifelong standardized and comprehensive screening, diagnosis, and care for all levels of TBI and psychological health conditions, in conjunction with education for patient and family members. The charter of the Red Cell was to build an integrated, comprehensive Department of Defense (DoD)/DVA program to identify, treat, document, and follow-up those who have suffered TBI or psychological health conditions while either deployed or in garrison. Then as now one of the major difficulties encountered by veterans and family members seeking to access services was the plethora of often poorly vetted sources purporting to provide information or service members to often-vulnerable veterans and families. The establishment of the DoD's Defense Centers of Excellence for Psychological Health and Traumatic Brain Injury and the Center for Deployment Psychology provides two concrete examples of positive initiatives coming out of the work of the Red Cell.

Despite these efforts, we are still confronted with the fact that there remain myriad private and public entities that seek to provide veteran-related services. Negotiating these entities and their bona fides still represents a considerable challenge for stressed or grieving veterans and families. Reports of suspect or fraudulent activities by the so-called charitable agencies suggest that veterans' services have become a target of opportunity for fraudulent activity. As a charity monitoring group, Charity Watch, reported in 2014, what is believed to be the largest government settlement (over $24M) against a charity fundraising group suspected of fraud was obtained against the Disabled Veteran's National Foundation (https://www.charitywatch.org/charitywatch-feature/146). In response to concerns of widespread fraud among such charities, an oversight body, the National Association of Veteran Serving Organizations (www.navso.org), was established in 2015.

In sum, then, we have been remarkably fortunate in terms of the number of fatalities resulting from 15 years of combat operations. Further, peculiar features of the Long War have led to a focus on psychological health issues that providers and veterans groups remain not entirely prepared to address. As previously noted, advances in battlefield medicine and personal protective gear have contributed to lower mortality, and a focus on the long-term sequelae of battlefield injuries is therefore to be expected. This alone, however, cannot account for the extremely large number of cases of post-traumatic stress disorder and other psychological injuries among our combat veterans (Sayer et al., 2011), nor can it entirely account for the large number of poorly described post-blast neurocognitive deficits we now focus on the treatment of combatants. We must contextualize both individual symptom expression and collective response in terms of prevailing societal attitudes to lengthy, relatively unpopular conflicts that have uncertain end points. The first author has argued elsewhere (Sammons & Batten, 2008) that we cannot completely understand the epidemiology of OIF/OEF mental health concerns unless we recognize that we have never in any previous conflict paid as much attention to the psychological effects of engaging in warfare than we are doing now. Further, our current emphasis on the psychological sequelae of combat is related, in part, to their relative predominance vis-à-vis physical injuries but also reflects, as Wessely (2005) observed, a societal discomfort with acceptance of risk. These caveats in no way should be taken to invalidate the fact that psychological trauma is an acknowledged consequence of participation in combat. However, they do add context to the discussion and may serve to explain some of the confusing array of conditions and symptoms which are our obligation to treat. It is within this context that we review the history of our response to psychological and blast-related injuries during the current conflict and seek to provide several suggestions to improve future care delivery.

In this brief review, we focus only on the activities of organized mental health delivery systems within the DoD and VA. There are numerous civilian groups comprising mental health professionals and others that continue to provide highly valuable services to veterans and families with mental health needs. In terms of community reintegration and sustained recovery, such services may in the long run be as or more beneficial than those provided by mental health professionals, but they are outside the purview of the current discussion.

10.1   Blast-Related Mild Traumatic Brain Injury (mTBI)

It is increasingly clear that mTBI and PTSD are often comorbid conditions sharing common etiological mechanisms (Howlett & Stein, 2016). Although mTBI is widely acknowledged as the signature physical injury of the ongoing conflict, exact numbers of those who have been exposed to blast or suffer the sequelae are elusive. In part, this is due to absent screening initiatives early in the conflict. Definitional terms, such as distance from a blast, minimum threshold for symptoms requiring evaluation, and latency between exposure to blast and definitive evaluation and treatment further complicate accurate tallying of blast-related injury. By some estimates, at least 32,000 combatants have been treated for moderate to severe traumatic brain injury since 2000 (Fang et al., 2015). This number refers only to those receiving emergent treatment in theater, so the percentage of those with mTBI who go without assessment or treatment is considerably higher.

As noted above, less than 32,000 non-fatal battlefield casualties were reported in Iraq during the most intensive combat years. But these numbers reflect only casualties reported in theater. The numbers seen subsequent to return from deployment tell a different story. Between 2002 and 2012, approximately 250,000 OIF/OEF veterans were reported by DoD to be suffering from blast-related TBI, with the overwhelming majority of these (approximately 212,000) being mild TBI (dePalma, 2015). Over 70% of these also had comorbid diagnoses of PTSD. dePalma (2015) reported that this diagnostic comorbidity resulted in the highest treatment costs per veteran of any diagnostic grouping in the Veteran's Administration. That is, over five times the number of veterans wounded in OIF/OEF conflicts are now either seeking care for long-term sequelae of blast or psychological injury or deemed in need of such care. The disparity between reported rates of injury and health-seeking behavior of veterans is striking.

Efforts at accurate screening of TBI are becoming increasingly sophisticated as are research rubrics related to blast-related TBI, now recognized as being etiologically and symptomatically distinct from other mild TBI, such as sport-related concussions (Nelson, Davenport, Sponheim, & Anderson, 2015). As those authors pointed out, DoD has developed new diagnostic and research tools (or adapted existing ones) in response to an unprecedented number of blast-related TBI, but more precision is needed, particularly in the area of acute assessment of TBI—as acute stage assessment is critical in determining longer term sequelae of blast.

It is not surprising that societal influences evidently play a significant role in the expression of mTBI symptoms, and in particular their linkage with post-traumatic stress type symptoms. Such differences are indirectly illustrated by a recent investigation of Canadian combatants returning from OIF/OEF activities (Garber, Rusu, & Zamorski, 2014). Not only did a much lower percentage of returning combatants report exposure to a blast (5.2% of those surveyed), but in this survey, most respondents reporting mTBI did not express long-term post-concussive symptoms. There was, however, a much stronger association between report of post-concussive symptoms and those servicemembers with mental health symptoms. Other authors also report that in cases of minor brain injury, cognitive function at 1 year does not differ from uninjured controls, and that factors other than concussion, including premorbid psychological symptoms, are more predictive of longer term sequelae (Nelson et al., 2015). While still developing, increasingly accurate neuropsychological assessments that better differentiate symptoms of TBI from PTSD are now available.

10.2   Expanding the Provider Base: The Mental Health Professional Workforce

At the beginning of 2003, when the United States invaded Iraq, military mental health services existed in a constellation that had remained unchanged for several decades. Most mental health services were facility based and concentrated in large medical centers that were in large part separated from fleet or troop concentration areas. A few psychologists and psychiatrists were attached to deployable units, such as special forces units or aboard aircraft carriers, but the concept of an embedded mental health provider had no real currency. After the invasion of Iraq, this changed rapidly. Behavioral health providers were a part of the initial battle plan, and psychologists and psychiatrists accompanied Army and Marine Corps combatants on their march into Baghdad. By 2005, the armed forces had initiated a screening program, one goal of which was to assess deploying combatants for a history of mental health difficulties that might indicate heightened vulnerability to combat stress. This was the well-known Pre-Deployment Health Assessment, which later was accompanied by a second screener, the Post-Deployment Health Re-Assessment, designed to be offered in theater to alert providers to the existence of deployment-related health issues. In addition, the Army initiated a large-scale screening effort for deployed personnel, the Military Health Assessment Team, which was deployed in successive iterations from 2006 onwards. Psychologists and psychiatrists, along with social workers, were deployed to operational sites in Iraq and Afghanistan, where they provided direct services to combat units and consultation to medical and command units regarding the psychological health of troops. Domestically, a major push to increase the number of mental health providers was undertaken.

There has been a remarkable expansion of mental health providers in the military healthcare system (MHS). Between 2007 and 2013, the Army and Navy significantly expanded the number of positions for clinical psychologists and to a lesser extent those for psychiatrists. In the direct care system (i.e., those healthcare facilities operated by military medicine), the number of mental health providers has grown significantly. Using Navy clinical psychology as an example, the community has grown from approximately 125 at the beginning of the war to 200 active duty psychologists today. Ranks of clinical psychologists in the VA also expanded significantly. In 2004, the Veteran's Administration (VA) employed approximately 1500 psychologists, that number now exceeds 4000.

Military mental health assets are increasingly deployed with troops assigned to combat missions, by some estimates the number of the so-called operational mental health providers has more than doubled. Clinical psychologists are now attached to all aircraft carriers in the fleet. The Army has embedded providers with a growing number of deploying units. Increasingly, psychologists and psychiatrists are deployed in clinical roles on operational platforms such as USMC expeditionary strike groups. In general, there has been at least a 50% increase in the number of mental health personnel assigned to operational units.

It cannot be gainsaid that much has been done to improve service provision to combatants, veterans, and their families. Hoge et al. (2015) rightfully point out advances in numerous areas, including expanded services in theater, systematic implementation of evidence-based treatment interventions for PTSD, better care coordination, and better programmatic outcome evaluation.

Some of these developments are truly ground-breaking. Indeed, it is justifiable to say that the current conflict has marked the beginning of a new epoch in military mental health treatment. The use of embedded mental health providers in combat units has never been as extensive as it is today. The US military has engaged in multiple and substantial efforts to destigmatize battle-derived psychological distress. In addition, we have included the ability, at least putatively, to withstand such stress as an element of pre-deployment assessment and training. Combatants now must not only be prepared to withstand the physical rigors of war, we are increasingly concerned if they can withstand the attendant psychological risks. Pre-deployment screening, enhanced education and training, immediate battlefield access to mental health services, and a sustained effort to destigmatize psychological injuries truly mark a new era in the history of the US military. It is almost certain that historians of the future will look back upon this period as the first in which psychological injuries were formally incorporated into the battle plan.

Given that systematic planning for widespread prevention and treatment efforts for mental distress is only around a decade old and has perforce developed within the rigid hierarchical confines of the US military, it is not surprising that there have been significant challenges to many of these efforts. To illustrate some of these challenges, we will use the example of treating PTSD. Effective treatments for PTSD and related disorders have been developed and tested over the last 25 years, but most of these efforts have been completed with survivors of civilian traumas (e.g., automobile accidents, sexual assaults, physical abuse). Questions remain as to how effective these treatments are with symptoms that incurred on the battlefield. Replicating civilian studies on samples of military personnel are expensive, time-consuming, and have delayed the delivery of potentially useful treatments to military personnel struggling with PTSD. Although the use of these treatments has proven somewhat helpful for military personnel, we still do not fully understand the limits (if any) of treatments developed and tested on civilian populations when they are applied to the emotional distress associated with combat deployments, particularly when those deployments continue. Further, many questions remain as to how to most efficiently and effectively disseminate new or underused treatments to providers throughout the large, widely dispersed care system that is the MHS.

In the case of many mental disorders, the delivery of effective treatment is further complicated by diagnostic conundrums and questions of individual vulnerability and resilience. For example, it is entirely normative for persons to be emotionally distressed by the experience of combat, such strong emotional responses have been convincingly described since the time of the *Iliad*. It is extraordinarily difficult to predict, however, when and under what conditions these normative responses become pathological, persistent, and severe and associated with formal diagnoses of PTSD or related disorders. For PTSD and indeed many mental disorders, we are lacking clear lines of delineation that permit differentiation in both form and severity between normative (non-diagnosable) reactions that resolve with no intervention, diagnosable disorders in need of treatment, and long-term disabling responses that prove resistant to treatment. Even limiting the discussion to a single disorder such as PTSD does not remove all these challenges, as no two individuals manifest the disorder in the same way and, beyond a few common indicators, the symptoms and problems associated with PTSD tend to change over time. Although strides have been made in identifying effective treatments for individual psychological disorders, it has proven extremely difficult to identify which available treatments (pharmacological or psychological) will prove most effective in any one patient. The importance of the therapeutic relationship is central to all therapies (Lambert & Barley, 2001). It is also the case, though largely unexamined, that different treatments will be differentially effective at various points in the deployment cycle (e.g., while deployed, following deployment, in anticipation of a subsequent deployment). In sum, symptoms of disorders common among servicemembers and veterans are frustratingly difficult to predict, the severity of an initial psychological injury does not necessarily predict severity of expressed symptoms, and responses cannot be reliably tied *a priori* to any particular intervention.

We add to this complexity another factor that is frequently overlooked but which deserves comment—that is the system of perverse incentives that we have constructed in our efforts to validate and treat those who suffer unseen injuries of war—the VA Disability Rating system. For many veterans and servicemembers, access to treatment in VA facilities is determined by the identification and disability rating of a disorder. Only by receiving a formal diagnosis and a rating of a compensable disability will access be granted. Thus, with all good intentions, we have created a system that perforce focuses on pathology and that reinforces pathology rather than recovery and wellness. Ironically, the contingencies within the VA disability system may function in direct opposition to those among active duty personnel, particularly when deployed, where symptoms are often minimized so as to "remain with the team" or in response to continued stigma associated with mental health symptoms. How much this factor complicates epidemiology and treatment outcome is unknown, but it is indubitably present.

10.3   PTSD

Diagnosis and treatment of PTSD in returning veterans is a complex and evolving problem. As outlined above, tensions arise from diagnostic imprecision, the disability determination system, stigma, and a need to provide effective treatment for veterans with bona fide psychological injuries. Added to this well-meaning advocacy efforts and political pressure to respond rapidly to any identified shortcoming, we have managed to create a system that is poorly equipped to provide consistent and effective services to those identified with PTSD.

Treatment of PTSD is further complicated by the presence of significant comorbidities. For example, there appear to be clear comorbidities between mTBI and PTSD symptoms, with several studies demonstrating a strong epidemiological link between mTBI and PTSD symptoms. Some data suggest this may be mediated by the severity of the brain injury, with combatants who experienced a blast-related loss of consciousness reporting much higher rates of PTSD versus those who did not experience loss of consciousness or other altered mental status (Howlett & Stein, 2015). The ability to differentiate between symptoms mediated by organic blast-related causes and psychological effects of blast exposure, both clearly pertinent to understanding the veteran's range of symptoms, remains unresolved. Adding to this complexity, we must also recognize that other disorders and experiences, such as alcohol abuse (Blanco et al., 2013), depression, sexual abuse, and other traumatic life experiences also share a high degree of comorbidity with PTSD.

Making even simple estimates of the number of servicemembers suffering from combat-related psychological distress is frustratingly difficult. Estimates vary considerably based on when (relative to deployment), how, and in what setting the assessments are made. In 2012, over 20% of all veterans treated in a VA healthcare facility had a diagnosis of PTSD (Institute of Medicine, 2014). Even though this number represented only the percentage of those seeking VA treatment who had a diagnosis of PTSD, it is higher than most estimates of OIF/OEF servicemembers who suffer from PTSD. This number also reflects the fact that many of those seeking care in the VA are veterans of earlier conflicts, particularly Vietnam. Still, between 2003 and 2012, the number of OIF/OEF veterans with a diagnosis of PTSD trebled, from approximately 200,000 to over 600,000. Almost all of these veterans have a disability rating of 30% or greater, with over 450,000 being given a rating of over 50% disabled (Institute of Medicine, 2014). The VA disability rating system, then, indicates that approximately 20% of servicemembers from OIF/OEF have received a moderate to severe disability rating on the basis of a PTSD diagnosis, an astonishingly high number. These numbers stand in contrast to other epidemiological findings. For example, Wisco et al. (2014) found point and lifetime prevalence in a sample of veterans to be 4.8% and 8%, respectively, lower numbers than have been reported elsewhere. These numbers are not remarkably different than lifetime prevalence estimates of PTSD in the general population, estimated by Kessler et al. (2002) to be around 8%. These and other large discrepancies between epidemiological findings and diagnoses in particular settings make estimating the true incidence of PTSD in veterans challenging.

Marmar et al. (2015) reported a lifetime prevalence of 26.2% for both PTSD and sub-threshold PTSD in a sample of Vietnam era veterans. Thus, by at least some measures, the diagnoses of PTSD are more common in OIF/OEF veterans than among veterans of earlier conflicts. This doubtlessly reflects a variety of influences, including expanded definitions of the disorder, increased awareness of the stress-related consequences of combat, successful initiatives to reduce stigma associated with mental illness, and VA compensation policies. Whichever of these factors is most explanatory is in certain respects immaterial, as it is clear that both DoD and the VA must meet increased demands for PTSD-related services for some time to come.

In response to this massive influx of patients, the VA has developed a robust network of services aimed at veterans with PTSD; these include specialized outpatient and inpatient options aimed solely at veterans with PTSD. The DoD, on the other hand, was criticized in the 2014 IOM report for offering relatively disjoint treatment options for PTSD, largely branch-of-service and location-dependent, and for which standardized treatment outcomes were lacking.

10.4 Stigma

Stigma remains a barrier to careseeking, particularly among active duty service-members. A recent survey of over 1000 veterans found that not only did an astonishingly high percentage (72%) report symptoms consistent with PTSD, but that veterans who had greater concern about public perception of mental illness were less likely to seek mental healthcare (Kulesza, Pedersen, Corrigan, & Marshall, 2015). Not surprisingly, these researchers also found that veterans were less likely to negatively judge fellow veterans who sought mental health treatment.

Efforts at stigma reduction have had mixed results. A review of the topic concluded that there were some indications of a reduction in stigma within the military, but that strong conclusions were precluded by methodological differences among studies (Acosta et al., 2014). In contrast, Hurtado, Simon-Arndt, McAnany, and Crain (2015) reported that after a brief intervention with enlisted and commissioned Marine Corps officers, negative perceptions of stigma actually increased slightly on several key variables, including risk to careers and perceptions of malingering. Unlike commissioned officers, enlisted leaders did not report improvement in stigma awareness after this intervention, suggesting that those immediately aware of most Marine's stress-related symptoms may continue to harbor negative perceptions of mental disorders. Other recent studies also confirm that anxiety over possible negative career repercussions continues to deter help-seeking behavior, despite numerous attempts by military and civilian leaders to destigmatize psychological injuries (Brown & Bruce, 2016).

10.5 Suicide

Suicide, among other forms of violent behavior, is the most feared outcome of combat-related stress, and a clear focus for DoD and VA clinicians and healthcare planners (Ursano et al., 2014). Rates of suicide have increased significantly across all branches of the US armed forces since 2001. Although diagnoses such as PTSD, depression, and TBI have been related to suicide risk, factors other than a primary psychological diagnosis may be more strongly predictive of suicidal behavior (Haller, Angkaw, Hendricks, & Norman, 2015). These researchers found that in a sample of 252 predominantly male veterans with histories of suicidal ideation, both reintegration stress and substance abuse had far more associated with suicidal ideation than PTSD or depression. Similarly, in a very large cohort study of OIF/OEF veterans ($n = 45,741$) who were screened for suicidal ideation and depression, Maguen et al. (2015) found that European-American ethnicity, a prolonged time between redeployment and initial screening, and substance abuse problems were predictive factors most associated with complaints of suicidal ideation. Patton, McNally, and Fremouw (2015) found that increased age, health problems, and marital status were more predictive of murder-suicide in military veterans. Findings like these make it essential that preventive strategies are not confined to diagnoses of PTSD, and instead take into consideration the significant adjustment issues faced by combatants returning from deployment. Indeed, it can legitimately be argued that an exclusive focus on PTSD is inherently risky, as it tends to downplay or ignore more predictive factors like substance abuse and reintegration issues in both domestic an occupational environments.

10.6   Access

Another factor of importance to planners, particularly those working with members of the Guard, Reserve, and their beneficiaries, is that access to behavioral healthcare drops rather precipitously for those in non-urban areas. When using a liberal definition of "remoteness" (i.e., being located more than 30 min away from an authorized behavioral healthcare provider), a recent RAND study found over 1.3 million eligible veterans and dependents living in remote areas (Brown et al., 2015). These individuals received significantly less behavioral healthcare than those living in more urban environments. Also of importance is the fact that more of those living in remote areas were more likely to be prescribed psychotropics, perhaps a reflection of the fact that most behavioral healthcare in such environments is provided by generalists in primary care clinics.

10.7   Societal Changes as Drivers of Military Health Service Demands

It is not surprising that over the 15-year span since the United States has been engaged in Afghanistan and Iraq, societal changes have affected perceptions of veterans and the type of treatment they receive. Not only have we seen far greater emphasis on the psychological needs of servicemembers and their families; tectonic shifts in healthcare, the view of the military, and how society at large interacts with the military have occurred during this period of time. Each of these issues carries long-range consequences for how we provide services to military members, veterans, and their families. For example, the passage of the Affordable Care Act extended provisions for mental health coverage under the Mental Health Parity Act and other legislation. Putting the treatment of emotional disorders on the same reimbursement footing as physical disorders has expanded treatment options for many, and in its own way has assisted in reducing stigma associated with seeking mental health treatment.

More importantly, the very definition of military families has fundamentally changed, as most recently demonstrated in the 2015 US Supreme Court decision *Obergefell v. Hodges*, which established the right of same-sex couples, including same-sex military couples, to marry. When the military's "Don't Ask, Don't Tell" policy was overturned in 2011, spousal healthcare benefits could be extended to servicemembers who resided in states that had legalized same-sex marriage. *Obergefell v. Hodges*, by overturning remaining prohibitions on same-sex marriage will make a larger population of spouses eligible for care in the direct care and purchased care systems. Estimates of the number of lesbian and gay servicemembers vary, but in general can be assumed to roughly approximate those in the public at large, or approximately 5% of the total active duty force. Currently, nearly one million veterans are estimated to have same-sex partner. The number of gay and lesbian servicemembers and their spouses and families, and the potentially unique healthcare needs of this population, is therefore likely to become a significant issue for healthcare planners, as it is probable that the VA will become the largest mental health provider for lesbian, gay, bisexual, and transgendered veterans (Averill, Eubanks Fleming, Holens, & Larsen, 2015). Demands for population-specific policies and interventions will undoubtedly increase although it is difficult to predict how this might impact the overall demand for services (Blosnik, Gordon, & Fine, 2015). On the one hand, mental health utilization rates for LGB servicemembers and veterans will probably not differ from those of other veterans. A recent online survey of a small number ($n = 356$) of lesbian and gay veterans (Simpson, Balsam, Cochran, Lehavot, & Gold, 2013) suggested utilization rates similar to those for heterosexual veterans although women with sexual trauma were likely to be higher utilizers of mental health services. Of this group, however, only 33% reported open communication regarding sexual orientation with provider, and 25% reported avoiding services due to perceived stigma. As LGB servicemembers, veterans and their families become increasingly comfortable in disclosing their sexual identity, and if the DoD adopts policies allowing transgendered individuals to serve, the need for population-specific treatment strategies will grow.

10.8 Recommendations

Almost 10 years ago, when the military services and the VA were struggling to devise unified, effective responses to the large number of psychological casualties from OIF/OEF, it was proposed that a combined service center called the "Center of Excellence for PTSD and TBI" be established. The first author argued that this title would place too much emphasis on pathology, and that our initiatives should be less focused on diagnostic entities than on instilling a sense of recovery and well-being. In the end, the Defense Centers of Excellence for Psychological Health and TBI was established. This subtle change in nomenclature, unfortunately, does not seem to have had the desired effect. We continue to be preoccupied with the diagnosis of PTSD and specific treatments for this disorder and pay relatively short shrift to those factors that assist servicemembers in the natural course of recovery from trauma-related symptoms. Likewise, in mTBI, we have made little progress in our ability to distinguish physiological from psychological effects of blast, determine a natural course of recovery from blast-related mTBI, or identify interventions to promote recovery. Below we outline several ways in which directed efforts may help servicemembers, veterans, and their families to address the psychological and interpersonal challenges of military service and combat deployments. In our view, if the United States is to adopt "lessons learned" from our experience to date with the psychological effects of combat, we will need to focus on the following broad areas to ensure optimum readiness in the future:

(a) Research and development into a number of areas such as techniques to differentially diagnose the often overlapping, functional disorders (including mTBI) as well as effective treatments for the various psychological reactions (diagnosable and not) related to combat exposure

(b) Appropriate staffing of the current military and VA mental health workforce to include steps in anticipation of having to upsize the mental health workforce in response to future military operations, with flexibility to determine (and delay if necessary for the sake of developing and promoting the therapeutic alliance), exactly when the patient is ready to begin evidence-based treatment

(c) Expanded provision of evidence-based training to military, VA, and civilian mental health providers delivered by culturally competent providers with provisions for the rapid deployment of new treatment developments throughout the MHS

(d) Complete integration of the electronic health record interface between VA and DoD

(e) Overhaul of disability-based eligibility criteria for VA services and the compensation strategies for mental health disorders

(f) Development of specific evidence-based interventions for common psychological responses to combat stress that can be implemented by both providers and the community. An expanded discussion of these items follows

Enhanced diagnostic specificity for PTSD and other possible psychological sequelae of combat exposure is essential. Furthermore, it is increasingly apparent that the field would benefit from the identification or development of markers for individuals at risk for persistent problems in the aftermath of psychological trauma. A parallel need is the development of effective means for reducing the consequences of trauma either prior to (resilience) or soon after (early intervention) exposure to the traumatic event.

At present, no effective interventions for enhancing the somewhat amorphous construct of "resilience" exist although it is not dissimilar from long-demonstrated personality constructs like hardiness. Recently in the popular press, a great deal of attention has been paid to the concept of "grit," which purportedly measures determination and the willingness to overcome adversity (Duckworth, Peterson, Matthews, & Kelly, 2007). These concepts are interesting, and they clearly define essential human characteristics. But we have no evidence to suggest that they can be altered via the application of any standardized intervention. Accordingly, we believe that large-scale programmatic development of such interventions has a low probability of success. We point out that components of military training that are aimed at enhancing leadership, unit cohesion, and the warrior ethos address hardiness, "grit," and determination. Whether these programs effectively enhance these characteristics is unknown, but the development of additional programs outside the command structure seems unwise.

Similarly, the data are unclear whether harm-reduction interventions used in the immediate aftermath of a potentially traumatizing event are of value. Prophylactic pharmacology has not been shown to be useful (Burbiel, 2015). At the moment, it seems safe to say that cognitive behavioral therapy or other related therapies like Cognitive Processing Therapy offered in the immediate aftermath of trauma help certain individuals in the short-term, but long-term effectiveness is uncertain. Unlike interventions designed to alter core personality constructs like "grit" or hardiness, however, it is feasible to investigate whether post-trauma psychological prevention is generally effective, and what type of therapy yields optimal results. Additional research specific to military personnel, particularly in the context of repeated combat deployments, will clarify this question and should be performed.

Improved diagnostic understanding for TBI, particularly mTBI, is required. The effects of repetitive mild head trauma are demonstrable, whether such injuries are occurred in combat or on the playing field. All current evidence indicates that neuropathology stemming from blast-related mTBI is qualitatively different from mTBI arising from blows to the head. Whether this observation extends to the neurocognitive and emotional sequelae of blast-related mTBI is unknown. Recently, some TBI researchers have reported on a structured diagnostic interview that appears to have promise in detecting a history of mTBI as much as 2 years post-incident (Walker et al., 2015). While this small study of approximately 100 veterans needs further replication, it may assist in determining a standard. Regardless of the eventual approach, it is important to develop a low-technology methodology for detecting a history of mTBI.

We must also improve our understanding of the natural course of recovery from these injuries and develop effective interventions to remedy the consequences of mTBI. Biomarkers for mTBI are being actively investigated, as are neuroimaging techniques that might better elucidate subtle structural damage that might accompany mTBI. This research, while in relative infancy, may assist us in understanding symptoms that are specific to mTBI vice psychological disorders. How this information, if attainable, will assist us in devising effective interventions is a murkier issue. The development of pharmacological treatments to address inflammatory responses and neuronal or glial damage associated with mTBI might be prioritized by the National Institutes of Mental Health under their new strategic plan. Here, however, preventive strategies are likely to yield better results in the short term, so the refinement of effective armoring with blast resistance should be a priority for military research and development. More precise neurophysiological and psychological assessment of mTBI, then, will assist in differentiating its effects from symptoms of PTSD and other stress reactions. It should be understood, however, that victims of blast or other physical assault are at higher risk to develop psychological sequelae and, as noted above, investigation of specific psychological and pharmacological interventions for such responses should be a priority.

As important as it is to better understand PTSD and mTBI, data are clear that neither of these disorders have the strongest associations with suicidal ideation or behavior, indeed, deployment status has not been found to be an independent predictor of veteran's suicidal behavior (Reger et al., 2015). Although efforts to identify and develop evidence-based interventions for PTSD and TBI must continue, it is equally important that we devote more resources towards understanding reintegration problems at home and at work, ongoing substance abuse issues, and other factors that affect the ability of veterans to make successful transitions home from combat. The effect of pre-existing psychological trauma, such as a history of childhood abuse (which some have found to be higher in military samples than in the population at large; Afifi et al., 2016) on long-term recovery from psychological and physical wounds in military personnel is also deserving of further study. We caveat that given the relative absence of sensitivity and specificity of large-scale pre-deployment screening as demonstrated by the PDHA/PDHRA as well as by unsuccessful mass screening efforts undertaken in prior conflicts, we do not believe that large-scale screening for servicemembers without a prior diagnosis is likely to be effective.

We must take full advantage of advances in the assessment and treatment of the psychological consequences of combat deployments. Furthermore, during periods when we are deploying significant numbers of personnel into combat, it is imperative that new advances in care be moved into clinical practice rapidly and effectively. To this end, it is recommended that systems for disseminating and implementing new advances in understanding and treatment of combat-related psychological disorders throughout the military and VA healthcare systems be jointly developed and maintained. Models for such dissemination efforts have been developed in both the VA and DoD, such as those resources currently offered by DoD's Center for Deployment Psychology, which aims to enhance training of both civilian and military mental health providers. With the exception of skills specific to operational mental health providers, there is no rationale for separating training of military and VA providers, nor is there a rationale for separating evaluative strategies aimed at measuring efficacy of interventions. Civilian academic and training programs would be wise to incorporate specific training on military-specific needs; some training institutions, like the University of Southern California's School of Social Work, have already done so. Further consolidation of the VA/DoD electronic health record will allow for such comparisons and provide more seamless care.

The demand for behavioral healthcare within the MHS and VA care systems continues to increase, even as the wars in Iraq and Afghanistan reduce in intensity. The cause of this is probably multiply determined. Claims for PTSD are on a per-servicemember basis dramatically higher than in previous conflicts (Sayer et al., 2011). Positively, effective efforts at stigma reduction, education of military planners, servicemembers and their families, and expanded access to evidence-based care have all contributed to reduce barriers to treatment for this bona fide battle injury. Clearly, changes are needed to address the increased demand for care. This will likely require increasing the capacity and efficiency of the existing care systems.

In anticipation of behavioral healthcare needs associated with future conflicts, it is recommended that efforts be made to leverage existing civilian care providers. This will likely require establishing networks of care in civilian communities that can be accessed by military servicemembers, veterans, and their families as well as preparing civilian providers to work effectively with these populations. The recent development of the Veterans Choice program in which veterans may receive care from civilian providers suggests one model for such a program. Programs such as "Give An Hour," where psychologists and other licensed therapists donate clinical hours to treat servicemembers and their families, can assist in extending clinical availability, particularly in the case of family members who are ineligible for services in the VA or who cannot access treatment in military facilities. Such programs have demonstrated the ability to provide treatment to reasonably large numbers of veterans and their families. These services, however, are not predicated on any particular expertise of the therapist in working with military trauma, simply a willingness to volunteer. Moreover, the majority of sessions delivered to a given patient are significantly fewer than required to complete a course of evidence-based therapy. In the end, while these programs are laudable, they cannot substitute for a workforce that is specifically schooled in working with military members and their families.

Regardless of the service delivery locale, the current conflict has taught us that we lack appropriately trained mental health professionals in both the DoD and VA healthcare systems. In the past, reductions in force (RIF) algorithms used by military planners have linked reductions in medical and mental health military personnel end-strength to relatively inflexible "ratios"—e.g., we need one physician for every x number of troops. While exceptions to these ratios have existed for certain medical specialties, mental health has rarely been included as an exception. This leads, as we have seen in the civilian setting, to mental health provider shortage areas that are so common as to be the norm (Health Resources and Services Administration, 2016). We suggest that the mental health workforce be protected from algorithmic reductions that accompany reductions in force. Instead, we recommend an epidemiological algorithm that incorporates:

(a) Estimations of current mental health morbidity
(b) Projections based on extrapolated utilization data associated with prior conflicts and current levels of demand in the MHA's direct and purchased care system and the VHA
(c) Projections based on potential increased utilization that may occur if more effective stigma reduction initiatives are implemented

We also note significant gaps in training both military and civilian psychologists, psychiatrists, and other mental health providers. At both the pre-and-post doctoral level, psychologists and psychiatrists who have not received training in the military medicine system often lack sufficient exposure to the investigation, differential diagnosis, and treatment of military-specific trauma and related disorders (Tanielian et al., 2014). This leads to a potential overreliance on diagnoses of PTSD, currently the most commonly recognized pathological stress response, rather than more nuanced understanding of normative and non-normative responses to severe stressors. Without specific training in effective interventional strategies, military personnel are likely to be misdiagnosed, with attendant ramifications for effective treatment.

Coordination between branches of the service and the VA, while demonstrably improved in recent years, requires continued attention. The recent suggestion by retired Chairman of the Joint Chiefs of Staff ADM Mike Mullen that all veterans be granted access to VA care regardless of disability rating (ADM Mike Mullen, personal communication, September, 2015) has profound implications for both better access to care and as a potential solution to the perverse incentives inherent in a lifelong disability rating system. The true costs of expanding VA services to all veterans regardless of disability rating should be carefully explored. They are likely to be far lower than those incurred by present inequities of healthcare provision, and they have the distinct advantage of exposing veterans to mental health providers who have specific training in military trauma.

Just as DoD is now exploring alternatives to the current length-of-service retirement system (i.e., the requirement of 20 years of active service before becoming retirement-eligible), VA accessibility for non-combatant military members with shorter terms of service might be considered. Likewise, it is essential that the VA expand currently limited programs to offer services to families of veterans. Effective treatment for many psychological disorders involves systemic involvement of family members. TRICARE insurance has expanded health service provision to military members and their families and is now seen as a major recruitment and retention tool in the military. Making the VA a TRICARE provider is imminently accomplishable and would serve to reduce fragmentation of care and cost burden to military families. While this is both politically and bureaucratically challenging, extending TRICARE eligibility to the VA system is perhaps the most transformative change short of complete integration of the DoD and VA healthcare systems that can be accomplished in the current generation. Not only would it provide for more seamless care for active duty and veteran populations and their families, it would force integration of currently fragmented healthcare informatics systems. The Veteran's Health Administration (VHA) and the Defense Health System (DHS) utilize two separate informatics systems that, if combined, would improve patient care but also could provide powerful disease management and disease modeling capability. Unfortunately, interoperability is limited. Clinical information in the electronic health record in each system can only be accessed via a read-only "legacy bridge" system. Current disease modeling projects, such as the VHA's "Reach Vet" program that provides predictive analytics for suicide risk (Aaron Eagan, personal communication, 15 November, 2016) would be vastly enhanced if data in the VHA's CPRS system were combined with the DHS's M2 data repository. Making the VHA a component of the DHS's purchased care system would also enhance our capability to understand and predict health-seeking behaviors of eligible military and veteran's populations—potentially a significant cost-saving mechanism.

Most difficult to accomplish will be the development of an alternative system to the current disability-based VA compensation scheme. Inherent tensions in a rating system that reinforces and indeed compensates differentially for disability associated with PTSD has led to a system that artificially perpetuates otherwise recoverable symptoms of a disorder that, in most individuals, is neither life-long nor incapacitating. Altering this system will be a long-term initiative and one that will be inherently controversial. Veterans' advocacy groups will rightfully argue that it is the responsibility of the nation to care for those wounded in its defense. While this obligation must never be shirked, it is equally important that we develop alternative schemes that reinforce adaptation and wellness and engender the expectation of a return to normalcy. The consequences of PTSD and TBI are real, but they need not be life-long, and often are not.

The perverse incentives associated with providing lifelong disability for recoverable psychological injuries must be addressed compassionately and in a manner that does not disenfranchise those who are truly incapacitated by the symptoms of PTSD. Available evidence suggests that higher levels of compensation are associated with disincentives to employment (Tsai & Rosenheck, 2013); and unemployment is likely to worsen the burden associated with a mental health diagnosis. Evaluation systems that require the endorsement of ongoing symptoms in order to receive compensation have the effect of iatrogenically perpetuating a disability, to the detriment of the veteran's long-term psychological and often physical health. The problems this system creates are as substantial as those created by ignoring the physical and emotional wounds of combatants, and we do veterans a great disservice by not devising intelligent and caring solutions.

Revising the Veteran's Administration disability rating system is, as noted, complex and sure to be fraught with controversy. Such difficulties will be magnified if attempts are made so in the midst of a future conflict. It would behoove planners to initiate this task now, independent of demand occasioned by future large-scale military actions. Two essential elements will require examination: eligibility for VA care and the disability compensation system. The disability compensation system is currently based on percentage-based estimates of total disability, as is the current system for determining compensation for those medically discharged from active duty. A percentage disability is associated with not only eligibility for healthcare and other VA benefits but also monthly pension amounts, almost unavoidably creating an adversarial system between the servicemember claiming disability and disability examiners. Restructuring this system in a way that preserves equity for veterans is a task of enormous dimensions, but to ignore it perpetuates a system that does not serve veterans and their families well. The "moral hazard" argument does not seem to have led to the misuse of healthcare resources its proponents feared (Barry, Goldman, & Huskamp, 2016). We should, instead, give more weight to the moral imperative of providing care to those who have sacrificed much in defense of our country.

Finally, in our zeal to provide effective treatments for psychological wounds arising from participation in combat and to care for those who have given much in the service of their country, we have oftentimes ignored the healing power of the community. However well validated, psychological and medical treatments for mental and physical disorders play a necessary but limited role in long-term recovery. We pay scant attention to those adaptive processes that assist combatants in adjusting to civilian life. Resilience and recovery are lifelong endeavors, and we need to better understand community mechanisms that assist veterans in the often prolonged path to effective reintegration. We also need to devise metrics that assist us in better understanding the effectiveness of the numerous civilian organizations that provide professional services to veterans and their families, including programs like "Give an Hour" that coordinates the donation of services to veterans and their families by mental health professionals. While admirable in their intent and mission, we currently lack mechanisms for understanding their contribution to the well-being of servicemembers and veterans.

As mental health providers, our chief aim should not be simply limited to the eradication of symptoms. The consequences of participation in combat and other traumatic activities outside the normal range of human experience cannot be denied. There is no medical or psychological solution that can possibly expunge the fundamental human response to the horrors of war, and it would be both dangerous and foolish to try and devise such a solution. Our task instead must be to assist combatants in adapting to their experiences and to assist them in leading lives that, while irrevocably changed, are no less fulfilling than before.

References

Acosta, J., Becker, A., Cerully, J. L., Fisher, M. P., Martin, L. T., Vardavas, R., et al. (2014). *Mental health stigma in the military.* Santa Monica, CA: RAND. http://www.rand.org/pubs/research_reports/RR426.html.

Afifi, T. O., Taillieu, T., Zamorski, M. A., Turner, S., Chung, K., & Sareen, J. (2016). Association of child abuse exposure with suicidal ideation, suicide plans, and suicide attempts in military personnel and the general population in Canada. *JAMA Psychiatry.* https://doi.org/10.1001/jamapsychiatry.2015.2732. published online 27 January 2016.

Averill, L. A., Eubanks Fleming, C. J., Holens, P. L., & Larsen, S. E. (2015). Research on PTSD prevalence in OEF/OIF veterans: Expanding definition of demographic variables. *European Journal of Psychotraumatology, 12.* https://doi.org/10.3402/ejpt.v6.27322. eCollection 2015.

Barry, C. L., Goldman, H. H., & Huskamp, H. A. (2016). Federal parity in the evolving mental health and addiction care landscape. *Health Affairs, 35,* 1009–1016.

Blanco, C., Xu, Y., Brady, K., Pérez-Fuentes, G., Okuda, M., & Wang, S. (2013). Comorbidity of posttraumatic stress disorder with alcohol dependence among US adults: Results from National Epidemiological Survey on alcohol and related conditions. *Drug and Alcohol Dependence, 132,* 630–638. https://doi.org/10.1016/j.drugalcdep.2013.04.016. Epub 2013 May 20.

Blosnik, J. R., Gordon, A. J., & Fine, M. J. (2015). Associations of sexual and gender minority status with health indicators…. *Annals of Epidemiology.* https://doi.org/10.1016/j.annepidem.2015.06.001. Jun 19. pii: S1047-2797(15)00222-7.

Brookings Institution, Saban Center for Mideast Studies (2010). *Iraq Index.* Retrieved February 3, 2015, from http://www.brookings.edu/iraqindex

Brown, N. B., & Bruce, S. E. (2016). Stigma, career worry, and mental illness symptomatology: Factors influencing treatment-seeking for operation enduring freedom and operation Iraqi freedom soldiers and veterans. *Psychological Trauma, 8*, 276–283. https://doi.org/10.1037/tra0000082.

Brown, R. A., Marshall, G. N., Breslau, J., Farris, C., Osilla, K. C., Pincus, H. A., et al. (2015). *Access to behavioral healthcare for geographically remote service members and dependents in the US*. Santa Monica, CA: RAND Corporation.

Burbiel, J. C. (2015). Primary prevention of posttraumatic stress disorder: Drugs and implications. *Military Medical Research, 2*, 24. https://doi.org/10.1186/240779-0053-2.

Charity Watch. (2014). *Huge amounts of donations squandered by "F" rated charity before settlement is reached*. Retrieved September 24, 2014, from https://www.charitywatch.org/charitywatch-feature/146.

Defense Health Board. (2015). *Combat trauma lessons learned from military operations of 2001–2013*. Falls Church, VA: Office of the Assistant Secretary of Defense for Health Affairs. Retrieved from http://www.dtic.mil/get-tr-doc/pdf?AD=AD1027320.

Defense Manpower Data Center (2016). *Defense Casualty Analysis System updated as of 6 February 2016*. Retrieved February 8, 2016, from https://www.dmdc.osd.mil/dcas/pages/casualties_oif.xhtml

dePalma, R. G. (2015). Combat TBI: History, epidemiology, and injury modes. In F. H. Kobeissy (Ed.), *Brain Neurotrauma: Molecular, neuropsychological, and rehabilitation aspects* (pp. 5–14). Boca Raton (FL): Taylor & Francis.

Duckworth, A. L., Peterson, C., Matthews, M. D., & Kelly, D. R. (2007). Grit: Perseverance and passion for long-term goals. *Journal of Personality and Social Psychology, 92*, 1087–1101. https://doi.org/10.1037/0022-3514.92.6.1087.

Fang, R., Markandaya, M., DuBose, J. J., Cancio, L. C., Shackelford, S., & Blackbourne, L. H. (2015). Early in-theatre management of combat related traumatic brain injury: A prospective, observational study to identify opportunities for performance improvement. *Journal of Trauma and Acute Care Surgery, 79*(4 Suppl. 2), S181–S187.

Garber, B. G., Rusu, C., & Zamorski, M. A. (2014). Deployment-related mild traumatic brain injury, mental health problems, and post-concussive symptoms in Canadian Armed Forces personnel. *BMC Psychiatry, 14*, 325. https://doi.org/10.1186/s12888-014-0325-5.

Haller M., Angkaw, A.C., Hendricks, B. A., & Norman, S. B. (2015). Does reintegration stress contribute to suicidal ideation among returning veterans seeking PTSD treatment? *Journal of Suicidology and Life Threatening Behavior*. doi: 10/1111/sltb.12181, published online 3 Aug 2015.

Health Resources and Services Administration (2016). *County and county-equivalent listing— mental health*. Retrieved January 19, 2017, from https://datawarehouse.hrsa.gov/tools/analyzers/hpsafind.aspx

Hoge, C. W., Ivany, C. G., Brusher, E. A., Brown, M. D., Shero, J. C. Adler AB, et al. (2015). Transformation of mental health care for US soldiers and families during the Iraq and Afghanistan wars: Where science and politics intersect. *American Journal of Psychiatry in Advance*. doi: 10/1176/appi.ajp2015.15040553.

Howlett, J. R., & Stein, M. B. (2016). Post-traumatic stress disorder. In D. Laskowitz & G. Grant (Eds.), *Translational research in traumatic brain injury* (pp. 339–352). Boca Raton (FL): Taylor & Francis. Retrieved from https://www.ncbi.nlm.nih.gov/books/NBK326723/?report=printable.

Hurtado, S., Simon-Arndt, C. M., McAnany, J., & Crain, J. A. (2015). Acceptability of mental health stigma-reduction training and initial effects on awareness among military personnel. *SpringerPlus, 4*, 606. https://doi.org/10.1186/s40064-015-1402-z.

Institute of Medicine. (2014). *Treatment for posttraumatic stress disorder in military and veteran populations: Final assessment*. Washington, DC: The National Academies Press.

Kessler, R., Andrews, G., Colpe, L., Hiripi, E., Mroczek, D. K., SLT, N., et al. (2002). Short screening scales to monitor population prevalences and trends in non-specific psychological distress. *Psychological Medicine, 32*, 959–976.

Kulesza, M., Pedersen, E., Corrigan, P., & Marshall, G. (2015). Help-seeking stigma and mental health treatment seeking among young adult veterans. *Military Behavioral Health, 3*, 230–239.

Lambert, M. J., & Barley, D. E. (2001). Research summary on the therapeutic relationship and psychotherapy outcome. *Psychotherapy: Theory, Research, Practice, Training, 38*, 357–361.

Maguen, S., Madden, E., Cohen, B. E., Bertenthal, D., Neylan, T. C., & Seal, K. H. (2015). Suicide risk in Iraq and Afghanistan veterans with mental health problems in VA care. *Journal of Psychiatric Research, 68*, 120–124. https://doi.org/10.1016/j.psychres.2015.06.013.

Marmar, C. R., Schlenger, W., Henn-Haase, C., Qian, M., Purchia, E., Li, M., et al. (2015). Course of posttraumatic stress disorder 40 years after the Vietnam war. *JAMA Psychiatry, 72*, 875–881.

Nelson, N. W., Davenport, N. D., Sponheim, S. R., & Anderson, C. R. (2015). Blast-related mild traumatic brain injury: Neuropsychological evaluation and findings. In F. H. Kobeissy (Ed.), *Brain Neurotrauma: Molecular, neuropsychological, and rehabilitation aspects* (pp. 451–470). Boca Raton (FL): Taylor & Francis.

Patton, C. L., McNally, M. R., & Fremouw, W. J. (2015). Military versus civilian murder-suicide. *Journal of Interpersonal Violence*. https://doi.org/10.1177/0886260515593299.

Priest, D. & Hull, A. (2007). Soldiers face neglect, frustration at Army's top medical facility. Washington Post, Sunday, February 18, 2007.

Reger, M. A., Smolenski, D. J., Skopp, N. A., Metzger-Abamukang, M. J., Kang, H. K., Bullman, T. A., et al. (2015). Risk of suicide among US military service members following operation enduring freedom or operation Iraqi freedom deployment and separation from the US military. *JAMA Psychiatry., 72*, 561–569. https://doi.org/10.1001/jamapsychiatry.2014.3195.

Sammons, M. T., & Batten, S. V. (2008). Psychological services for returning veterans and their families: Evolving conceptualizations of the sequelae of warzone experiences. *Journal of Clinical Psychology: In Session, 64*, 921–928.

Sayer, N. A., Spoont, M., Murdock, M., Parker, L. E., Hintz, S., & Rosenheck, R. (2011). A qualitative study of U.S. veterans' reasons for seeking Department of Veterans Affairs disability benefits for posttraumatic stress disorder. *Journal of Traumatic Stress, 24*, 699–707. https://doi.org/10.1002/jts.20693.

Simpson, T. L., Balsam, K. F., Cochran, B. N., Lehavot, K., & Gold, S. D. (2013). VA healthcare utilization among sexual minority veterans. *Psychological Services, 10*, 223–232.

Tanielian, T., Farris, C., Epley, C., Farmer, C. M., Robinson, E., Engel, C. C., et al. (2014). *Ready to serve: Community-based provider capacity to deliver culturally competent, quality mental health care to veterans and their families*. Santa Monica: RAND Corporation.

Tanielian, T. L., & Jaycox, L. (Eds.). (2008). *Invisible wounds of war: Psychological and cognitive injuries, their consequences, and services to assist recovery* (Vol. 720). RAND Corporation. Retrieved from http://books.google.com/books?hl=en&lr=&id=DHfiWi2AcdAC&oi=fnd&pg=PP1&dq=Tanielian+Invisible+Wounds+of+War+Psychological+and+Cognitive+Injuries,+Their+Consequences,+and+Services+to+Assist+Recovery&ots=QGc6R8Q64g&sig=g6OH4HZswOvNapFVez9EtIlohQA.

Tsai, J., & Rosenheck, R. A. (2013). Examination of veterans affairs disability compensation as a disincentive for employment in a population-based sample of veterans under age 65. *Journal of Occupational Rehabilitation, 23*, 504–512. https://doi.org/10.1007/s10926-013-9419-z.

Ursano, R. J., Colpe, L. J., Heeringa, S. G., Kessler, R. C., Schoenbaum, M., Stein, M. B., et al. (2014). The Army study to assess risk and resilience in servicemembers (Army STARRS). *Psychiatry, 77*, 107–119.

Walker, W. C., Cifu, D. X., Hudak, A. M., Goldberg, G., Kunz, R. D., & Sima, A. P. (2015). Structured interview for mild traumatic braing injury after military blast: Inter-rater agreement and development of diagnostic algorithm. *Journal of Neurotrauma, 32*, 464–473.

Wessely, S. (2005). Risk, psychiatry, and the military. *British Journal of Psychiatry, 186*, 459–466.

Wisco, B. E., Marx, B. P., Wolf, E. J., Miller, M. W., Southwick, S. M., & Pietrzak, R. H. (2014). Posttraumatic stress disorder in the US veteran population: Results from the National Health and Resilience in Veterans Study. *Journal of Clinical Psychiatry, 75*, 1338–1346. https://doi.org/10.4088/JCP.14m09328.

Chapter 11
The Unique Role of Professional Associations in Assisting Military Families: A Case Study

Jason T. Vail

11.1 Introduction

The landscape of assistance and support for military families is a vast one, with involvement from all manner of players and participants, all bringing their own individualized strengths to bear on the tremendous growth in the needs of military families over the course of the last decade-and-a-half. While many of these participants bring money, staff, or programs to the effort, the community of professional associations brings something unique: Despite sometimes relatively small budgets and staffs, they are composed of large groups of dedicated members who have great depth of experience and knowledge in their areas of expertise, with impressive credentials and broad—often nationwide—reach. When engaged, these professional association members can be extremely effective forces for action and change.

The following is a case study of one such professional association: The American Bar Association, and how it has been able to build upon its position as the voice of the legal profession to play an active role in connecting the national legal community to work addressing the civil legal needs of military families. From this case study may be derived examples, lessons, and recommendations that may guide any professional association, whether national, state, or local, in doing the same.

J.T. Vail (✉)
American Bar Association, Chicago, IL, USA
e-mail: jason.vail@americanbar.org

© Springer International Publishing AG 2018
L. Hughes-Kirchubel et al. (eds.), *A Battle Plan for Supporting Military Families*, Risk and Resilience in Military and Veteran Families,
https://doi.org/10.1007/978-3-319-68984-5_11

11.2 Professional Associations and the American Bar Association

A professional association is generally a type of nonprofit organization with the purpose of furthering the interests of a particular profession and members who are engaged in that profession. Interests may also extend to those of the public interest generally. It is also common for professional associations to play a role in the education and training of members of a profession, including ongoing updating of skills and provision of specialized certification.

Given the above definition, the American Bar Association is typical of a professional association. The ABA is one of the world's largest voluntary professional organizations, with nearly 400,000 individual members and more than 3500 internally affiliated entities. It is committed to doing what only a national association of attorneys can do: Serving its members, improving the legal profession, eliminating bias and enhancing diversity, and advancing the rule of law throughout the United States and around the world. Founded in 1878, the ABA is committed to supporting the legal profession with practical resources for legal professionals while improving the administration of justice, accrediting law schools, establishing model ethical codes, and more. Membership is open to lawyers, law students, and others interested in the law and the legal profession. Its national headquarters are in Chicago, and it maintains a significant office in Washington D.C.

11.2.1 The ABA's Involvement in Military Legal Assistance

The work of the ABA in the area of legal assistance for military families is conducted through its Standing Committee on Legal Assistance for Military Personnel, otherwise known as the LAMP Committee. The LAMP Committee is the successor to the American Bar Association Special Committee on War Work, which was created in 1941. The original jurisdiction of that committee during World War II included legal problems of the members and veterans of the armed forces and their dependents (American Bar Association).

In 1943, when the War Department established legal assistance offices at all Army stations, the committee fostered working relationships between state bar association military committees and the legal assistance offices in their areas. Then, at the end of World War II, the committee focused its attention on the delivery of legal assistance to veterans, their dependents, and their widows. Special emphasis was placed on enforcing reemployment rights of discharged service members and the liquidation of obligations that had been deferred by the Soldier's and Sailor's Civil Relief Act (American Bar Association). In 1953, the name of the Committee was changed to "The Standing Committee on Legal Assistance for Servicemen," and in 1976 the committee was renamed "The Standing Committee on Legal Assistance for Military Personnel." (American Bar Association)

Committee Structure

The ten members of the LAMP Committee are appointed from the membership of the American Bar Association by the President-elect to serve staggered 3 year terms. The Committee members receive guidance and counsel from active-duty military advisors and maintain contact and coordination with other ABA entities and interested persons through designated liaisons. The LAMP committee is advised by a Military Liaison Advisory Committee, composed of advisory personnel from each of the services who are appointed by and serve at the discretion of the Judge Advocates General of the Army, Navy, Air Force, and Coast Guard, and the Staff Judge Advocate to the Commandant, Headquarters Marine Corps. The Commandants of the Army and the Air Force JAG Schools and the Commanding Officer of the Naval Justice School also serve as members of the Liaison Advisory Committee. The Department of Defense (DoD), other ABA committees involved with military law and the Board of Governors of the Association appoint liaisons as well. The committee is served by staff of the American Bar Association who provide logistical and administrative services to the committee (American Bar Association, 2016b).

The scope of the committee's jurisdiction is defined by its charter under the ABA Constitution and Bylaws at Article 31, § 31.7, which reads:

> The Standing Committee on Legal Assistance for Military Personnel has jurisdiction over matters relating to legal assistance for military personnel and their dependents. This includes all civil legal matters related to military service, whether directly or incidentally, and whether arising during periods of active-duty service or following transition to civilian status. It shall foster the continued growth of the military legal assistance programs and promote the delivery of legal services to military personnel and their dependents and to persons accompanying the armed forces outside the United States, for their personal legal affairs (except those involving proceedings under the Uniform Code of Military Justice). It shall advocate for policies improving access to legal services and civil legal protections for military personnel and their dependents. It shall maintain close liaison with the Department of Defense, the Department of Homeland Security with respect to the U.S. Coast Guard, the Department of Veterans Affairs, the military services, bar associations, and appropriate committees of the Association to enhance the scope, quality and delivery of free or affordable legal services to eligible legal assistance clients. (American Bar Association, 2016a)

11.2.2   Evolving Programs of the Committee: 2001–2007

Traditionally, the committee's involvement in the delivery of legal assistance services to military personnel and their families has been indirect: The committee provided direct support military legal assistance attorneys, thereby translating into the delivery of high-quality legal services to military personnel and their dependents. The committee historically played this "background" role in three key ways: First, by supporting the education and professional development of military attorneys through the provision of free continuing legal education courses developed and sponsored by the committee, delivered on-base at rotating locations during the year, as well as by webinars. Second, the committee published supportive legal books and reference resources on a variety of military law and legal assistance topics through ABA's publishing division. Finally, the committee engaged with the ABA's governmental affairs office to promote federal and state laws and policies that strengthen civil protections and rights afforded to military families under the law.

Following the September 11, 2001, terrorist attacks and subsequent activation and deployment of service personnel, it became apparent to the ABA and the members of the committee that continuing to simply support existing military legal assistance resources was an insufficient response to an explosion in demand for legal services as a result of dramatically increased operational tempo. Because of the committee's longstanding, close connection with the military services and the involvement of the service branches' legal assistance leadership, as well as the fact that the committee's membership has historically been made up of highly experienced, retired military personnel, the implications for the growth in legal assistance demands at that time were quite clear. In response, the ABA, through the Standing Committee, undertook two key steps to address the growing challenge to meet servicemembers' civil legal needs: First, by pulling together a consortium of state-based bar association programs to meet the demand for legal services, called Operation Enduring LAMP, and second, assembling a working group of experts to comprehensively assess the anticipated legal needs of military families in the coming decade. Both of these initiatives were instrumental in laying the groundwork for a much greater activist role that the ABA would play in legal service delivery in the future.

Operation Enduring LAMP

In November 2001, ABA President Robert E. Hirshon, with input and counsel from the Standing Committee, urged the civilian bar to prepare itself and stand ready to assist their fellow Americans who were mobilized for military service, as well as the families who were left behind. In that inaugural announcement, he committed the ABA, through the Standing Committee, to a sustained effort in support of the armed forces, and called it Operation Enduring LAMP (Podgers, 2007).

Originally established to augment the uniformed services' existing legal assistance effort by providing supplementary attorney resources through state bar associations in the face of the rapid, large-scale mobilization of reservists, Operation Enduring LAMP grew to 56 programs in 42 states. Creation of this type of network was the Standing Committee's first significant effort to directly connect military legal assistance attorneys with members of the civilian bar, which acted as a type of reserve force: While the servicemember was away from home, his or her family members could call upon these civilian lawyers when they needed someone to turn to for free legal counsel. Likewise, the program contemplated that when the reservists returned to civilian life, many of them would confront reemployment and other legal issues that could be dealt with through the assistance of the Operation Enduring LAMP volunteers.

Ultimately, the legal support delivered through the program was provided by volunteers with the various participating bar associations rather than by the ABA itself, which instead acted as a coordinating entity, encouraging involvement and providing a central clearinghouse of resources. It became apparent, however, that this type of loosely affiliated network created a patchwork of services and resources that varied from state to state, depending on the level of the state bar's recruitment and activity. Furthermore, with regular turnover of leadership within the bars, often annually, the commitment to the effort by changing leadership would vary as well. Thus, the shortcomings of the state-by-state approach were soon realized, inspiring a stronger, more direct response as detailed later.

The Working Group on Protecting the Rights of Servicemembers

Though the ABA was encouraging state bar associations to play an active role in providing supplementary legal services to military families through Operation Enduring LAMP, the expansive mobilizations of reservists and National Guard members beginning in 2003 was unprecedented, and the scope and extent of the legal assistance needs of the servicemembers and the families they left behind were difficult to predict. As the exclusive center of expertise within the ABA on issues of legal assistance delivery in the military, the Standing Committee had been working consistently to elevate these issues and concerns up through the ABA's internal and political channels to reach those in leadership positions. As a result, the ABA President in 2003, Dennis W. Archer, announced the formation of a new Working Group on Protecting the Rights of Servicemembers, with the objective of examining the legal needs of servicemembers in light of the quickly changing role and composition of the country's active military forces (American Bar Association, 2004). The Working Group was constituted to take the lead in analyzing and recommending protections and programs that may be needed to ease the legal burdens that the men and women in uniform bear as they are deployed around the globe, with particular attention paid to the broad areas of consumer law and family law that can present special concerns to military personnel.

The Working Group focused on four central policy initiatives, which are summarized as follows:

- Servicemembers Civil Relief Act and consumer law: A number of issues under the law at that time were identified for possible amendment, including lack of coverage for National Guard members when on state duty, unclear application of lease termination protections for military family members, and confusing taxation liability for servicemembers not actually residing in a particular jurisdiction. It was also clear that much needed to be done to educate the judiciary about the specific rights and protections available to servicemembers and dependents in civil proceedings (American Bar Association, 2004).
- Family law: Many issues were addressed in this area, particularly with regard to child custody and visitation, as well as child support. Specifically, the Working

Group proposed solutions to the then-inability for military parents to present telephonic testimony in court while stationed elsewhere, the need for expedited hearings for those servicemembers who may be unavailable due to military duties, and the lack of ability by the courts to order substitute visitation for children with relatives of deployed servicemember parents (American Bar Association, 2004).

The Uniformed Services Employment and Reemployment Rights Act/employment law: For those serving in the Guard and Reserves, this law provides many protections, but additional areas of need were identified, including the loss of performance bonuses and promotional ability in civilian employment due to extended absence due to military duties, the lack of coverage for those veterans whose service-connected disabilities do not manifest until a period after returning to civilian employment, and gaps in enforcement and advocacy on behalf of veterans within various governmental entities (American Bar Association, 2004).

The Expanded Legal Assistance Program: This program allows special accommodations to military attorneys to represent clients in state courts where the attorneys were otherwise not admitted. The Working Group determined that few states had adopted rules allowing for military attorney admission under this program, and thus a great deal needed to be done to advocate for states to create such rules (American Bar Association, 2004).

Other areas that the Working Group examined were the special legal needs of survivors of deceased servicemembers, access to voting, in-state tuition assistance to servicemembers and their families, and loan forgiveness or loan repayment assistance. Because of the vast array of expertise spanning all areas of legal practice within the ABA (with over 3500 internally affiliated entities, as noted above), as a result, the Working Group comprised representatives from a number of ABA entities, including the ABA Sections of Family Law; Real Property, Probate, and Trust Law; Labor and Employment Law; Taxation; Government and Public Sector Lawyers; State and Local Government Law; Tort Trial and Insurance Practice and the Young Lawyers Division; and the Military Lawyers Committee of the General Practice, Solo and Small Firm Section (American Bar Association, 2004).

At the ABA Annual Meeting in August 2004, the Working Group released its comprehensive report. This wide-ranging analysis of the legal needs of military families and where gaps existed in protections and services would serve as a roadmap for the work of the ABA and the LAMP Committee in the next decade on.

11.2.3 Evolving Programs of the Committee: 2007 to Present

From its work with Operation Enduring LAMP and the findings of the Working Group Report, the committee reached two important conclusions: First, that the scope of civil legal problems was broad and expanding, and second, that a distributed patchwork of services delivered by bar associations in only some states and with varying levels of service would be insufficient to provide a uniform, consistent, and predictable response to growing need. The LAMP Committee concluded that a more aggressive response would be necessary to overcome a clearly growing gap in access to justice for military families. In so doing, however, the committee was extremely mindful of the fact that the ABA, as a national entity, has certain strengths by virtue of such a position, but at the same time lacks the deep, local penetration, and relationships that are the hallmark of state and local bar associations. Thus, the committee embarked over the next several years to implement initiatives that involved it directly in the delivery of legal services to military families, building on the unique strengths of an association like the ABA (the ability to create resources and educate and mobilize volunteers on a nationwide basis) while building connections with state and local organizations and entities and deferring to the strengths of these groups to deliver "on the ground" legal services. Four key initiatives would emerge during this time: ABA Military Pro Bono Project, Operation Standby, ABA Home Front, and the ABA Veterans' Claims Assistance Network.

ABA Military Pro Bono Project

Where Operation Enduring LAMP was an effort to get state bar associations to recruit and support civilian volunteer attorneys to provide civil legal services that would supplement those delivered by military legal assistance, the results were inconsistent: Not all state bars participated, and the range of services provided varied from state to state. Often, the level of commitment, resources, and range of services devoted by any one state bar would relate directly to whether that state bar had a dedicated entity (like the Standing Committee) focused on military and/or veterans' issues; fewer than half of the states have such entities. A significant further shortcoming of the program was driven by frequent relocations of military personnel to different locations around the country, which often resulted in legal problems arising in states where the servicemember was no longer stationed. Thus, for example, a soldier who completed a Permanent Change of Station (PCS) from Virginia to California might subsequently be subject to a lawsuit by a former landlord in Virginia. In that instance, a California bar volunteer attorney would be unable to assist with responding to the Virginia lawsuit, and the loose affiliation of bar programs under the Operation Enduring LAMP brand was insufficient to provide strong, cross-jurisdictional collaboration among the states to address these types of issues.

In addition to these cross-jurisdictional problems, a further difficulty with the Operation Enduring LAMP concept became evident as more and more servicemembers were being deployed overseas: Once in a combat zone, a servicemember would not be in a position to connect with a state bar program to resolve a legal problem that the servicemember—and, in many instances, the family left behind—was encountering. Of utmost importance, especially in a combat zone, is service readiness, which can be significantly impacted by distraction due to a legal problem on the other side of the world.

Separate from these issues, however, is a longstanding limitation on delivery of legal assistance services by military attorneys: As a general rule, military attorneys cannot represent servicemembers and/or dependents in state civil court, which means these attorneys are limited to providing only legal advice and, sometimes, limited scope services that fall short of in-court representation. There are a number of reasons for this: Military attorneys are often stationed in states where they are not licensed to practice; there aren't enough military attorneys available to devote the kind of time commitment necessary to conduct in-court litigation while also serving a high caseload of clients; military regulations generally prohibit state court appearances; and technically, the client of the military attorney is the service branch, not the individual servicemember. So with the exception of very limited circumstances where a state court appearance is authorized and available under an Expanded Legal Assistance Program (noted above) court rule, in most cases where a military attorney meets with a client who requires representation in court, the client will have to seek such representation elsewhere.

In response to all of these issues, the LAMP Committee collaborated closely with its DoD partners on a new model, called the ABA Military Pro Bono Project, where the LAMP Committee would develop a nationwide roster of volunteer attorneys to handle all manner of civil legal problems for servicemembers, and would also connect those servicemembers referred to the ABA directly from military legal assistance attorneys to the volunteer attorneys to provide representation, including in state courts (Zack, 2011). By operating on a national, as opposed to statewide basis, the ABA could easily connect a military family in one state with a volunteer attorney in the state where the legal problem resided. And by using a model that funneled all cases through military legal assistance attorneys, a deployed servicemember needed only to initially meet with his or her JAG, after which the ABA would take the JAG's referral and do the work to secure an attorney to assist with resolution of the problem, which would free the servicemember from concern about having to obtain legal counsel on his or her own.

Also of great importance in developing this new initiative was the recognition that the high cost involved in securing civilian legal counsel placed such representation out of reach for many junior-enlisted military personnel and their families. Earning too much income to qualify for traditional civilian legal aid assistance but not enough to afford a private attorney, and not able to be represented in court by military attorneys, these military families fell into an access-to-justice gap that often left them without the critically important legal help necessary to resolve their legal problems.

Conceptualized in 2007 and officially launched in September 2008, the ABA Military Pro Bono Project continues to operate with great success. As of October 2016, the Project has secured pro bono assistance in 49 states and D.C. for a total of 1438 military members and families, though the cases have originated from every corner of the world—from the United States to ships at sea, Iraq, and Afghanistan, and from bases located in all manner of foreign lands. The types of cases referred to the Project have remained consistent throughout, as a significant proportion of the cases are family law matters. Approximately 72% of the cases referred to the Project involve family law issues, most often involving issues of divorce, child custody, and visitation; about 10% involve consumer and creditor matters, such as debt collection, bankruptcy; and the other cases involve landlord–tenant disputes, guardianship, trusts and estates matters, and other legal issues. In breaking down the cases referred to the Project by service branch, 31% are Army, 31% are Navy, 22% are Air Force, 14% are Marine Corps, and 2% are Coast Guard. As of October 2016, of the 1438 cases placed with pro bono attorneys, many are still active and work by the volunteers is ongoing. Volunteer attorneys have reported that 1260 of these cases have been completed and closed. These attorneys have reported their hours and typical billing rates as a way to quantify the value of the rendered services. From their responses, a total of 25,095 donated billable hours valued at $7,257,692 were provided for the 1260 closed cases. Relying on this representative sample, the 1438 placed cases represent about $8.3 million in donated billable hours. Based on these numbers, each servicemember who is connected with a volunteer attorney receives an average of over $5700 worth of donated legal services. And because the Project limits its services to junior-enlisted servicemembers (at an E-6 paygrade and below) who likely are otherwise unable to afford to hire an attorney outright, these donated hours of work by the volunteer attorneys make all the difference between the servicemember having competent legal counsel to resolve the matter at hand and trying to navigate the legal system completely unassisted.

Operation Standby

Though civilian legal counsel is often necessary to resolve a legal problem where a military attorney cannot due to the limitations on in-court appearances noted above, in many instances, the advice and assistance of a military attorney is sufficient. This is again, however, an area where cross-jurisdictional issues create challenges identified by the LAMP Committee: Military legal assistance attorneys are typically stationed in locations where they are not admitted to practice, and they have clients who have legal problems that may arise in any state, so these military attorneys typically cannot advise about the particular state law involved in their clients' legal issues. This significantly limits what a military attorney can do for a client and may result in an easily resolvable legal issue going unaddressed because the military attorney does not have knowledge of a specific state's law or local procedures.

In order to address this problem, in 2011 the LAMP Committee launched an initiative called Operation Standby. The LAMP Committee recruited volunteer attorneys across the country practicing in all of the substantive legal areas covered by military legal assistance, and these attorneys specifically volunteered to be available for consultations with military attorneys on their areas of expertise in their states. State-by-state directories were created with contact information for volunteer attorneys separated out by their areas of expertise, and these were made available behind a secured website login available to only military attorneys on the Military Pro Bono Project website. So, for example, if a military attorney stationed in Nebraska wanted to assist a client having a family law problem in North Carolina, the attorney could log in and pull up the North Carolina Operation Standby list, locate a family attorney's contact information, and then reach out to that attorney for guidance on how to advise his or her client.

Operation Standby has proven to be a tremendous resource for military attorneys, which greatly enhances the level of service they can provide to their clients. As of October 1, 2015, 704 attorneys in 48 states and D.C. are registered with Operation Standby, and of these, 276 attorneys (39%) specify family law as an area of expertise. Annual surveys of Operation Standby volunteers and the military attorney users reveal that the highest need and utilization of Operation Standby is for family law questions.

ABA Home Front

In developing its programs to support military legal assistance services through consultation and referral resources, it was important to ensure that those military families encountering a legal problem would seek out assistance through their military legal assistance offices so that they could get connected with counsel to resolve the problem, whether by a military attorney or a civilian volunteer. In its survey of informational legal resources available online to military families, the LAMP Committee determined that there was not a credible, reliable, and accessible place where military-connected individuals could go and both receive information as well as be directed to available legal services; without such a resource, many military families might not seek out assistance and not get connected with help, thereby making an existing legal problem even worse.

In order to help military families understand the legal rights and protections available to them, as well as direct them to appropriate legal assistance resources, in 2011 the LAMP Committee launched a website developed with the ABA Division for Public Education called ABA Home Front (Ward, 2011). Recognizing that there are many websites with resources for military families, a great deal of thought was put into how to create an educational portal that would be a unique and useful resource instead of "yet another website" that duplicated already ongoing efforts. Research on existing legal-focused sites for military families revealed very little in the way of comprehensive, user-friendly websites dedicated to legal education and referral. The design of the site, therefore, was driven by both an intent to improve upon what little was already available while also creating resources where none existed.

The ABA Home Front website includes numerous articles and "FAQ" content that addresses many of the common legal questions and situations encountered by military families. Written in a style accessible to non-lawyers, these educational materials both inform about legal rights as well as provide direction on where to obtain direct legal services, whether through a nearby military legal assistance office if available, or other resources run by legal aid, pro bono, lawyer referral, or bar association programs. The website routinely receives about 7000 unique visitors monthly, the majority of whom come to the site as the result of using Google to search for information on their issues. ABA Home Front continues to be an important "front line" of assistance to make sure that all who are in need of legal help understand their rights and seek assistance.

ABA Veterans' Claims Assistance Network

In recent years, the focus of the LAMP Committee has begun to shift from the shrinking numbers of service personnel deployed overseas to the steadily growing population of those who are now transitioning off of active duty. The committee anticipates that in the near term the legal needs of this group will continue to grow because even though they may no longer be serving in the armed forces, they and their families will continue to experience the effects—both legal and nonlegal—of their service. An area of the most significant growth is in the need for legal assistance with VA disability compensation benefits.

In order to receive VA disability benefits, a veteran's application must include all of the necessary medical and other documentation that clearly meets the eligibility criteria established by law and regulation. Failure to prepare a fully developed claim package can result in delays of months—or even years—in receiving an initial decision from the VA. And if the decision is a denial, navigating the appellate process can take even more months or years before a final award may be granted.

Many service personnel transitioning to civilian status have applied, or will be applying, for VA disability benefits, and while there are many legal resources available to assist with appeals of denials, the LAMP Committee sees an important role to play in connecting veterans with attorneys to assist, pro bono, with preparation of the initial claim package. In so doing, the veteran's chances of success at the VA's first determination is greatly enhanced, and even if not successful, the attorney-prepared record will be a much stronger basis for an appeal than if the veteran is left to prepare the package unrepresented.

Thus, in 2013, the ABA began negotiating with the VA on an agreement to govern a pilot project that would test the feasibility of using pro bono attorneys to assist unrepresented veterans with the preparation and completion of their disability claim packages. The significance of this negotiation cannot be understated; there had not been any prior direct collaboration between the VA and the legal community of this nature ever before. On the contrary, the VA and the legal community had a generally adversarial relationship, so a commitment to work together toward the shared goal of assisting veterans was groundbreaking in this context. It is possible that such an agreement would not have come about at all had it not been for the White House General Counsel's Office serving to convene the parties and assist in brokering the agreement. But after several months of lengthy, and sometimes contentious, discussions, the agreement governing a pilot project was finalized by the VA and ABA.

The pilot project, operated by the LAMP Committee and called the ABA Veterans' Claims Assistance Network (VCAN), launched in three VA Regional Office areas (Chicago, IL, St. Petersburg, FL, and Roanoke, VA) in September 2014, and intakes were conducted through April 2015 (McMillion, 2014). Of those that were eligible for representation through the pilot, 140 veterans were connected with pro bono volunteer attorneys for assistance with their claims, and case closing data from these cases indicate that the represented veterans were successful at about a 2:1 rate, with each case receiving an average of about 35 h of donated billable hours valued by the volunteers at just under $10,000.

Though both the creation, and sometimes the operation, of the pilot presented many difficulties and challenges that needed to be worked through, in the end, both the ABA and VA viewed the collaboration and the pilot project itself a successful means of providing representation and assistance to veterans in the claims process who might otherwise go without. Throughout the operation of the pilot, it was frequently apparent that VA systems and processes were quite incompatible with the traditional means of attorneys working with clients, and these incompatibilities created many unanticipated bottlenecks and delays during the pilot. The parties are now in the process of finalizing a new agreement, which makes a number of improvements throughout the entire process of outreach, intake, referral, and case closure that will eliminate many of the systemic problems that arose during the pilot and will result in an effective and efficient program serving the legal needs of veterans.

11.3   Lessons Learned and Recommendations for the Future

The dramatic expansion of the work of the ABA in the area of legal assistance for military families over the past 15 years has resulted in three key lessons learned that may be applicable to any national association similar to the ABA that might be working to support military families. These all draw upon the unique strengths and capacities of national associations and the resources they can bring to bear in helping military families.

11.3.1   A Comprehensive Review of Needs is Critical at the Outset

As noted above, the civil legal assistance needs of military families shifted dramatically in the early 2000s. Prior to that time, the LAMP Committee had been mainly concerned about civil legal assistance for members of the active-duty services during periods of peacetime. The mobilization of thousands of reservists and National Guard members from around the country for deployment into combat presented a new and unknown challenge in legal service delivery. Many of those being deployed came from areas of the country where there were no military installations (and military legal assistance offices), and many were leaving behind civilian lives and employment to go overseas for extended, and sometimes multiple, tours. Their legal needs would be quite different, both during and after activation, and it was absolutely necessary to immediately convene a large and diverse group of experts to make predictions for how legal needs would evolve, and to develop a roadmap for addressing these needs. By convening the Working Group to swiftly develop its Report on Protecting the Rights of Servicemembers, the LAMP Committee had a foundation upon which it could design appropriate responses to anticipated needs—and indeed, the Report revealed that its initial effort through Operation Enduring LAMP would be inadequate to meet expected demands, and a more active approach would be necessary.

One of the great strengths of professional associations is that they are populated by the best and the brightest in their respective fields. More than that, however, these often are also practitioners who engage with their respective issue areas in a direct way, including through client interaction, and therefore have a clear understanding of both current and foreseeable future issues and trends that is rooted in practical experience. Thus, when looking to respond to military families' emergent needs, the first step must be to bring together these experts to carefully analyze the current state of affairs, predict what might occur in the future, and make recommendations for effective action. Professional associations can make a significant contribution to the wider community of military family service providers in this way, as their expert analysis can not only provide a structure for the professional association's responsive efforts, but it can also provide needed guidance to many other organizations and providers who also work in the field, but lack the same depth and breadth of expertise. With regard to the LAMP Committee's Working Group Report, many states have looked to its recommendations to implement their own laws protecting servicemembers' rights; for example, many have expanded their own state-based versions of the Servicemembers Civil Relief Act, and some have also enacted child custody protections for deployed custodial parents, which was one area where the Report correctly anticipated a substantial increase in need.

11.3.2 National Associations Should Leverage their Unique Nationwide Scope

As became apparent during the recent conflicts, the legal issues faced by military families are often compounded by the itinerant nature of military life, particularly when overseas deployments are involved. This presents complications when attempting to resolve a military family's legal problem by a local organization, as the problem may have its roots well outside of the locality or even the state. In many other nonlegal fields, there is often the need to go outside the jurisdiction in order to effectively assist a military family, and where there is not strong coordination among similar local organizations nationwide, these needs can be a barrier to providing needed help.

From its initial efforts with Operation Enduring LAMP, the ABA learned that reliance upon a loose affiliation of state-based programs that lacked both nation-wide coverage as well as uniform standards and services resulted in a system where only some might receive the help they needed, while others would fall into gaps where no help was available. Undoubtedly, the state-based programs—many of which grew and developed, and continue to operate today—were extremely important to ensuring access to justice for many military families, but the LAMP initiative revealed that a strong, nationwide "hub" that could not only assist in coordinating the states' service delivery, but also to engage its own resources to fill areas of need where no resources exist or are inadequate, was a necessary component of a program to assist military families nationwide.

When undertaking a comprehensive examination of the current and future state of military families' needs, as recommended above, it is important that national associations survey what state and local programs and resources exist to meet that need, and then explore how the national association can act in a way that helps coordinate these disparate efforts as well as address substantive and geographic areas where local efforts are not present or sufficient. By their very nature, national professional associations are uniquely positioned to fill this role, and thus they play a critical role in ensuring a safety net that will capture all military families in need nationwide.

11.3.3   Collaborations are Vital to Ensure Successful, Non-duplicative Efforts

While professional associations have many strengths, these can also be liabilities about which associations should be mindful. When looking to take a strong leadership role in its area of expertise, such as the LAMP Committee did in establishing its national programs, the association should be careful not to supplant or duplicate activities already occurring a local levels. While professional associations have advantages in their ability to engage high-level experts to develop strategies, or to serve in coordinating roles on a national basis, or to employ resources where none exist, it should be recognized that more localized efforts often have a much better understanding of the particular resources and needs "on the ground" in their areas, and they can be understandably resentful if they perceive non-local entities as actively encroaching in these areas. Thus, it is extremely important that any approach taken by a professional association be first and foremost one of a collaborative spirit, and with due deference to those already working in the area on a more localized level.

The LAMP Committee took this approach when designing its two national pro bono initiatives, the Military Pro Bono Project and VCAN. With the Military Pro Bono Project, the LAMP Committee, in collaboration with partners in the DoD, carefully assessed the pro bono resources already being secured by the military services' legal assistance offices, and it became apparent that prevailing income eligibility guidelines employed by local legal aid and pro bono programs rendered most military families ineligible to receive their services. Thus, the LAMP Committee designed financial eligibility requirements for the Project that would capture and assist all those junior-enlisted military families that could not otherwise obtain legal aid or pro bono help through local programs, and thereby become not a competitor for the same clients, but rather a complimentary resource when a military legal assistance attorney could not make a local pro bono or legal aid referral due to the family's income. As a result, the legal aid and pro bono community—as well as the military community—views the ABA as an important partner in providing access to justice for a wide range of low- and moderate-income military families who cannot afford full-fee legal representation.

Similarly, when designing VCAN to provide help with VA disability claim preparation, the LAMP Committee was well aware of similar assistance provided by veterans service organizations (VSOs). Though not staffed by attorneys, these organizations have been the traditional backbone of VA claims assistance delivery, and it could be easily anticipated that they would view the systematic involvement of attorneys in this area—which had never before been attempted—with suspicion. That said, however, the dramatic growth in VA disability claims filings and the associated VA backlog demonstrated that the VSOs alone were insufficient to meet demand and that there was an important role for the nation's lawyers to serve as a supplementary "force multiplier" in delivering claims assistance services in conjunction with the VSOs. Additionally, attorneys, by their nature, bring additional skillsets to claims development work that may not otherwise be available with VSOs. So it was important to the LAMP Committee, when working with its partners in the VA Office of General Counsel, to design a program that would work in tandem, rather than in competition, with the VSOs, by ensuring that all veterans contacted about legal resources available through the VCAN pilot project were equally advised about the availability of help through VSOs. Additionally, all of the special treatment and accommodations made by the VA in its processes under the agreement between the VA and ABA were made equally available to the VSOs as well. As a result, of those veterans who responded to the initial notices about the program, the data show that they opted for VSO assistance about as often as they chose the ABA option, thereby benefitting both entities equally. This result went a long way to ensuring that the VCAN pilot program was viewed by all participants—the VA, ABA, and VSOs—as a very successful collaboration to provide help to veterans who would have otherwise gone through the VA system unrepresented.

Clearly a national organization of the ABA's stature had unique opportunities to engage directly with the DoD and the VA at high levels, and it is recognized that many professional associations may not have the same manner of access. Nonetheless, any work done in the military family/veterans space by any association is likely to involve collaboration opportunities and potentials for duplication of efforts, so the lessons learned here remain the same: Fully understand the players in the space, the work they do and the resources they bring, and work together to find ways of developing complimentary programming that, in combination, delivers the most good while avoiding concerns about who gets to "take credit" for positive outcomes.

11.4   Conclusion

All manner of professional associations can and should be encouraged to examine how their own unique positions, cultures, and compositions may be engaged in supporting the needs that military families have today. The experience of the American Bar Association demonstrates that through the application of expertise, the advantages of its position as a national organization, and the prioritization of collaboration can help any professional association become a leader in supporting our nation's military families.

References

American Bar Association. (2004). *Report of the Working Group on Protecting the Rights of Service Members*. Chicago: American Bar Association.

American Bar Association. (2016a). *Constitution and Bylaws*. Chicago: American Bar Association.

American Bar Association. (2016b). *Standing Committee on Legal Assistance for Military Personnel*. Chicago: American Bar Association.

American Bar Association. (n.d.). *History & organization*. Chicago: American Bar Association.

McMillion, R. (2014, September 1). Program will mobilize lawyers to help reduce VA claims processing backlog. *ABA Journal*.

Podgers, J. (2007, September 1). Engaged from the start. *ABA Journal*.

Ward, S. F. (2011, May 17). ABA launches website to help military families. *ABA Journal*.

Zack, S. N. (2011, June 1). ABA military Pro Bono project offers civil legal assistance to US service members. *ABA Journal*.

Part III
States and Communities

Chapter 12
Nonprofit Contributions: Reflections and Looking Forward

Michael L. Gravens and Mary M. Keller

12.1 Background—Combining Challenge and Opportunity

During the past 15 years of armed conflict, nonprofit organizations have not only been supportive of military members and veterans but have also proven vital to the well-being of their families and the communities in which they reside. The responsiveness, timeliness, and dedicated commitment of nonprofits have been instrumental in addressing and meeting the needs of all. Given the extensive wartime requirements, both in the numbers of those affected and the depth of issues experienced by family members, our nation and those who serve have greatly benefited by this collective group known as nonprofits.

The nonprofit environment comprises mostly smaller organizations. The National Council on Nonprofits states that 82.5% of all reporting public charities had annual revenue of under 1 million dollars. Today, over 45,000 nonprofit organizations self-identify as serving military families or veterans. Most of these nonprofits are small and/or local. The vast majority (over 43,000) focus on serving veterans with a far smaller number (over 1600) serving military families (Bush Institute, 2014). Whether serving military families, veterans, or both, these organizations come in various identified categories, diverse roles, and business models with different means of delivery in programs and services.

Notably, a few nonprofits have nationwide name brand recognition and have been serving for many years. A selected few of these nonprofits achieved national recognition as they originated to fill evident gaps in the years following 9/11. Other organizations are niche providers, yet have become nationally known within their spheres of influence. By far, the most prevalent are the many nonprofits that exist today because a local service gap was identified, and an organization was created to meet community

M.L. Gravens, CSM (USA, Ret.) • M.M. Keller, Ed.D. (✉)
Military Child Education Coalition, Harker Heights, TX, USA
e-mail: mary.keller@militarychild.org

© Springer International Publishing AG 2018
L. Hughes-Kirchubel et al. (eds.), *A Battle Plan for Supporting Military Families*, Risk and Resilience in Military and Veteran Families,
https://doi.org/10.1007/978-3-319-68984-5_12

needs in the post-9/11 environment. Regardless of their recognition factor, longevity, size, or capacity, nonprofit organizations are a crucial complement to the family programs and services currently provided to our military members, veterans, and their families by the local, state, or federal government.

12.2   History and Key Events

For most military families, multiple and extended deployments have been a routine part of life since 2001. This holds true for active duty, National Guard, and Reserve Component families. The high mobility, continued family separations, complex transition issues, as well as the too frequent traumas of injury, illness, or loss of a loved one highlighted the need for additional support beyond that routinely provided by the Departments of Defense (DoD) or Veterans Affairs (VA) (Kudler & Porter, 2013; Military Child Education Coalition, 2012).

Throughout the history of our nation, support services for military and veteran family members have been secondary in focus as compared to the resources directed towards the military member and veteran. Understandably, first and foremost was the need to ensure the military member was equipped and prepared to perform his or her duties and that the veteran was adequately cared for as appropriate. Since the inception of the volunteer force in the 1970s, and most certainly since 9/11, there has been a growing recognition that the military member and family or veteran and family need to be treated as one unit (Bush Institute, 2014). The Afghanistan and Iraq wars heightened the recognition that in order to maintain a volunteer force while our military fights in extended conflicts, it is imperative that service members know that their families' needs are met and their families are well cared for during multiple deployments (MacDermid Wadsworth, 2016).

After the terrorist attacts of 9/11, the American public proclaimed support of our military and sought to respond accordingly. While the DoD and VA stepped up their efforts to identify and better support the needs of families through expanded programs and services, they also, albeit slowly, embraced the resources and capabilities offered by communities and the private sector, to include nonprofit organizations. Unfortunately, still today, many barriers to access and pertinent data continue to exist though some small strides have been made (Blue Star Families, 2014).

As the conflicts continued from 2008 through 2014, military members were returning home from war only to find their local communities locked in recession. The consequences of sequestration and shrinking of available federal dollars continued to have negative impacts on services and programs provided by DoD and the VA. Budget challenges also affected the capability of nonprofits as the competition for resources becomes more challenging. Communities and organizations of care and support continued to be instrumental in helping to fill the gaps but are showing signs of fatigue. In addition to budget challenges, military members face obstacles when transitioning from the DoD as active service members to the VA upon separation from the military.

The DoD and VA are massive bureaucratic systems, and despite continued efforts to make the transition process smoother, obstacles still remain. Once a military member attains veteran status, he or she may face long wait times for processing and accessing benefits. Veteran-focused nonprofits not only must identify gaps in service experienced by veterans but also must consider relevant areas that can maintain donor appeal. As a result, operation problems within the nonprofits tend to manifest. For example, nonprofits Nonprofit organizations budget challenges must figure out how to deliver on both donor intent and, most importantly, how to reach identified recipients in ways that have clearly measurable outcomes. Fortunately, positive movement is taking place in senior leader-led progress towards DoD and VA collaboration with the government agencies and nonprofits providing services and advocacy, with the encouragement of public–private partnerships. Local frustrations continue with access and communication, especially with the practical realities associated with access to and outreach to those who need support. The mixture of good to great NGOs with those who are either not capable or are potentially harmful or exploitive is another challenge facing the public–private partnerships. While a good to great nonprofit can result in practices and systems worthy of attention, an ineffective or harmful nonprofit can add to a cycle of distrust within the veteran community.

An excellent example of how a senior leader influenced and shaped the non-governmental environment was demonstrated by Admiral Michael Mullen. While serving as the Chairman of the Joint Chiefs of Staff (2007–2011), he began publicly speaking of a "sea of goodwill" of American support. In 2010, the Office of the Chairman of the Joint Chiefs of Staff published a white paper titled, *A Sea of Goodwill: Matching the Donor to the Need* which called for community-level action teams to address what Admiral Mullen referred to as the "reintegration trinity" of education, employment, and access to healthcare (USG DoD, 2010).

Mullen's focus on public engagement in supporting military and veteran families brought their needs to national attention while also highlighting that no single agency or organization can do it all. His *Sea of Goodwill* emphasized the need for building key partnerships between national and local community efforts. He recognized that governmental agencies, non-governmental organizations, institutions of higher learning, and community-based organizations and local businesses all have a collaborative role to play. Tying together these many efforts is, in effect, the concept of the *Sea of Goodwill*.

From the onset of the conflicts that arose following 9/11, nonprofit organizations have played a pivotal role in supporting military and veteran families. Whether augmenting or supplementing programs and services as requested by DoD or the VA or providing new and innovative endeavors, nonprofits have continuously sought to fill the gaps and meet the needs. Few envisioned that the needs would be so great and those needs would continue, simply evolving as our military and their families serve in today's ever changing global, social, and economic environment. Now, more than ever, nonprofit organizations are crucial in helping provide training, education, advocacy, and direct support services to military and veteran families.

12.3   Responses and Strategies

At the national level, First Lady Michelle Obama and Dr. Jill Biden formally launched the White House Joining Forces Initiative in 2011, highlighting the needs of military members, veterans, and their families in the areas of employment, education, and wellness. They called upon not only nonprofits but every sector of society to include businesses, colleges, and other educational programs, philanthropic organizations, religious institutions, communities, and government to provide opportunities, resources, and support needed for those who have served (Kudler & Porter, 2013). While it is difficult to determine the long-term outcomes, this initiative helped put the issues onto the public stage. Many nonprofits within those broad areas responded to this high profile call for action within their domains and means to do so. Having a national voice on these topics empowered the engaged nonprofits to secure attention and clarity for the need of public support.

Recognizing the positive influence and impact that nonprofit organizations have in advocacy and providing programs and services, other key leaders at the senior cabinet member level of the federal government have sought to hear the collective voices of the nonprofits and most certainly, that of the veteran service organizations. In recent years, both the Office of the Secretary of Defense and the Office of the Secretary of Veterans Affairs have periodically joined in roundtable sessions with nonprofit organizations whose collective expertise, advocacy, and service interest span the full spectrum of needs. The selected organizations meet with the respective secretaries and their key staffs for briefings and discussions on vital matters pertaining to military members, veterans, and their families. Topics routinely range from current and future policy decisions and impacts, sequestration, benefits, wellness, and family program issues (Blue Star Families, 2012).

As our nation, our national leaders, and the DoD responded and progressed in supporting our military during the time of war, it became evident that the need was great and more had to be done to support military spouses and their children. The well-being of military families, both spouse and child, was crucial to the service member, and therefore, ultimately of critical importance to DoD and its quest for mission accomplishment. In response, in the early war years, DoD developed and funded numerous programs and services to help military families adapt to the military community and assist them with the challenges that come with a military lifestyle (MacDermid Wadsworth, 2016).

While DoD initiated and staffed many of the programs and services, often they recognized the gaps they could not fill and turned to nonprofit organizations to fulfill DoD requirements and provide staff for programs and services. Beyond outsourcing by DoD, many nonprofits, both pre-9/11 (legacy) and post-9/11, through their own initiatives, have developed and continue to execute programs and services that seek to enable spouses and children to survive the multiple deployments of their military member to become resilient and thrive during prolonged periods of adversity and challenge. Since September 2001, nonprofit organizations of many specialties have come into being. While some focus on overall military family well-being, others specifically support the spouse. Other nonprofits have made their mission to support the children and youth of those who serve.

Identified in Admiral Mullen's *Sea of Goodwill*, two other distinctive areas of focus and growth in the number of nonprofit organizations are based on addressing wellness issues affecting our military and their families and on supporting veterans. The need for support in these areas is nationally recognized by the American public. The needs are commonly identified with those returning from combat with specific physical wounds or injuries. They are also associated with deployment-related post-traumatic stress disorder (PTSD) or other reintegration issues, whether with family or society (Springle & Wilmer, 2014). Growth in veteran supporting organizations is appropriately based on the wide range of needs spanning wellness and healthcare, employment opportunities, housing, and education.

Admiral Mullen expressed the importance of providing a lifetime continuum of care to our warriors, veterans, and families. He also recognized that no single agency or organization has the resources or capacity to provide that lifetime of care and support (USG DoD, 2010). Hence, a team effort by government agencies, private sector groups, communities, and nonprofit organizations who have committed themselves to supporting our military, veterans, and their families is essential.

One of the prevalent independent strategies of the post-9/11 era continuing strong today is that of nonprofit organizations collaborating with others to achieve shared goals. "Collaboration" is an often-expressed term among nonprofits and usually indicates a sharing of work load, information, and resources for mutually benefitting reasons. The agreements on collaboration are normally informal and nonbinding, often based on nothing more than mutual verbal consent, though at times followed by memorandums of agreement or understanding.

Collaboration efforts may be between nonprofits or in public–private sector partnerships. They vary in scope, from local to state to national capacity, but are usually specific in agreed upon collaborative efforts in specific functions. It is not uncommon for like-minded organizations to be habitual collaborators with trusted informal partners. The challenge is that more often than not these collaborative efforts happen by chance, rather than by intent. This is pointed out in "Driving Community Impact: The Case for Local, Evidence-based Coordination in Veteran and Military Family Services and the AmericaServes Initiative" (IVMF, 2015).

> A clear gap in services for veterans and military families persists across America. Contrary to what most might expect, however, this gap is far from lack of public concern…Rather, the gap lives between the public, private and nonprofit organizations that service them…. [because of] a lack of collaboration, coordination and collective purpose. (p. 3)

On a larger scale, some key collaborations have been sustaining and impactful in creating a collective voice with specific findings and recommendations regarding the way forward in supporting military members, veterans, and their family members. Through by-invitation convenings, retreats, and other gatherings, leading nonprofit organizations bring together not only peers whose missions span various sectors, such as employment, wellness, and education but also include key senior leaders from government agencies and influential non-governmental organizations.

Recurring strategies within these brainstorming sessions may include identifying current barriers to forward progress in service with proposed solutions, creating strategies to bridge the gaps of needs not yet met, and achieving consensus to identify big ideas for future implementation (Blue Star Families, 2015).

In today's post-9/11 environment, one successful collaboration model currently in practice possesses a more refined and deliberate effort and is known as the *collective impact* concept. Though the term is often expressed in many conversations and forums, stand-alone collective impact initiatives normally require a centralized infrastructure, a dedicated staff to serve as the backbone of the team and coordinate activities, and a more structured process so as to empower the accomplishment of the initiative. Successful efforts normally include an agreed upon common agenda, shared measurement of progress, continuous communication while working towards goals, and mutually reinforcing activities among the participating members of the initiative (Kania & Kramer, 2011). Collective impact initiatives require significant investment of effort and resources by the nonprofit organizations and may sometimes compete with a nonprofit's specific mission as charged by their board of directors. Having a centralized infrastructure with dedicated staff helps remove some of the workload for all involved and provides clarity of focus. However, this infrastructure requires significant financial investment and funders who see their role as contributors towards a larger goal rather than short-term goals with immediate impact and ensuing recognition.

The within-sector strategic partnerships formed may or may not be based on noted strengths of a fellow nonprofit they wish to incorporate into their own business model, or the partnership may possibly form to offset an identified weakness within its own structure or business model (Bush Institute, 2015). While there are obvious benefits for nonprofits to be on the receiving side of work efforts, information, or resources, a mutual trust and willingness to cooperate with a similarly purposed nonprofit must rise above competitive tendencies for such collaborations to reach full potential (USG DoD, 2014).

12.4 Scenarios: Nonprofits in Action

Sesame Workshop is an excellent example of a "civilian" nonprofit expressing its care by responding to the needs of military families—both the parents and their children. Through its Talk, Listen, Connect programs, Sesame Workshop developed the resources to provide military parents with a means to effectively communicate and help their young children cope with military lifestyle issues such as deployments and parental injury. (MacDermid Wadsworth, 2016).

America Joins Forces with Military Families: White Oak is a descriptor used by a collaborative group of leaders and organizations in the nonprofit, government, and private sectors who have met every other year since 2010. Gathering in a retreat environment, this convening connects leaders from many major military-related nonprofits with various government branches and agencies, including the White House, DoD,

VA, and influential non-governmental organizations. The purpose is to facilitate solutions that raise both awareness and means to accomplish identified objectives that well support the military and veteran community (Blue Star Families, 2015).

The Military Child Education Coalition (MCEC) program known as *Living in the New Normal Public Engagement* (LINN PE) convened caring community leaders who are committed to the well-being of military-connected children. Conducted over a 7-year period (2007–2013), these engagements typically involved key state and community leaders and those from business, education, healthcare, service clubs and others, as well as active duty, National Guard and Reserve component military leaders. Goals included creating short- and long-term action plans and establishing ongoing local committees. Funded through grants and with the national support of DoD, MCEC public engagements (LINN PE) spanned 34 states and four major military communities. The outcomes continue to impact local and state efforts on behalf of military and veteran-connected children. For example, school districts needed better data about military-connected students as part of their standard pupil management systems. As a result, 14 states have adopted a military student identifier (MSI). Five other states, through administrative action, are also participating in identifying their military-connected school-aged youth. At the national level, for the first time, the military-connected student is recognized as a discrete cohort through the reauthorization language of the Elementary and Secondary Education Act (ESEA). This act, now termed *The Every Student Succeeds Act (ESSA),* was signed into law by the president in December 2015. Though this is significant progress, the ESSA language limits the requirement for the states to direct the local school districts (LEAs) to report the data about the children with parents who have indicated that they are serving active duty. The Military Child Education Coalition, with the support of committed partners, is continuing to work for the children of the National Guard and Reserves also to be recognized and reported via the LEAs to the states to the National Center for Educational Statistics.

Hiring our Heroes, a program of the U.S. Chamber of Commerce Foundation, is a successful nationwide initiative designed to provide employment opportunities for transitioning service members, veterans, and military spouses. The program has two overriding strategies: (1) grassroots engagement and (2) public–private partnerships. By using the U.S. Chamber of Commerce's huge network of state and local chambers as well as strategic partners from the public, private, and nonprofit sectors, this endeavor provides hundreds of thousands of hiring opportunities for transitioning service members, veterans, and military spouses.

Got Your 6 (GY6) demonstrates a collective impact group in action. The small staff of GY6 provides focused leadership and generated generous donor support for over 30 nonprofit organizations. Collectively, the nonprofits sought to reach noteworthy agreed upon goals with measured outcomes across the six pillars of Education, Family, Health, Housing, Jobs, and Leadership. Examples of outcomes during the period of 2011–2014 include over 6 million h of volunteer service given by veterans and military family members in their local communities; over 120,000 health care students and professionals trained in addressing health care needs of returning troops; and over 110,000 educators trained in meeting the needs of military and veteran-connected students.

The Points of Light *Community Blueprint* provides a framework for action by communities across the United States and is currently in place in over 20 states. By implementing the Blueprint, communities are able to engage and demonstrate visible support for military members, veterans, and their families. Dedicated to volunteer service, Points of Light is able to mobilize those who seek to support our military and veterans through acts of community service. By implementing locally created community solutions, local leaders, businesses, and nonprofits seek to help in areas such as employment opportunities, behavioral health, and veteran homelessness. Simultaneously, the Blueprint also provides opportunities and engagements for military members, veterans, and family members who wish to make a positive impact within their local communities.

12.5 Results/Evaluation

The good ideas that have worked well for nonprofit organizations, regardless of whether a legacy or start-up operation, have wide reach, relevance, are evidence-based, and impact both the military and non-military communities.—Patricia "Patty" Shinseki, Military Child Education Coalition, Board of Directors, Emeritus

In 2014, the George W. Bush Institute commissioned the Institute for Veterans and Military Families (IVMF) at Syracuse University to conduct a study of leading practices among successful nonprofit organizations. Study results note that of 25 participating nonprofit organizations, there exists a strong pattern of reliance upon strategic relationships with private and philanthropic sectors as well as with each other. The reasons and purposes for partnership were numerous and varied—from financial support and consultation to sharing of complimentary services. The most effective organizations created partnerships with fellow providers and collaborated in efforts and resources.

The IVMF study also highlights private sector partnerships that offer a wide range of pro bono services supporting nonprofit operations and service delivery in fulfilling their mission requirements. The generous application of expertise and manpower provides a windfall of talent for the receiving nonprofits and enhances the capabilities of their staff, supports the end-user of the organizational offerings, and often enables the delivery of services that would otherwise not be available.

The partnership and pro bono contributions often include a generous application of volunteers to serve with the nonprofit. While the volunteer service may be a huge benefit for the nonprofit, the pro bono organization can also fulfill its internal goals and objectives by providing meaningful community service projects for its employees. Challenges sometimes arise because many times nonprofits require consistent volunteers with specific, dedicated skills. Best results come from good relationship management as well as being thoughtful and caring stewards of the volunteer force with the nonprofit. The need for a volunteer management strategy is crucial for a successful long-term relationship in this endeavor (Bush, 2014).

The IVMF study also highlights one well-identified area that still needs focus and solutions: bridging the civilian–military divide. The divide has become a common term of reference for both the military and private sector when describing the challenges that military members face as they transition back into the civilian sector. This challenge continues for many veterans who struggle with readapting to a civilian culture, while some veterans may never have experienced life as an adult in the civilian workforce. Likewise, with less than 1% of the American population having served in the military, civilian employers and their workforce are often challenged with building relationships with those who have served in the military (Bush, 2015).

Many dedicated nonprofits (along with private sector businesses and government organizations) have worked tirelessly in providing job opportunities, educating employers, and preparing both transitioning military members and veterans in the nuances of civilian employment. Though not garnering nearly as much public attention, military spouses also struggle with employment, professional credentialing, and licensing issues as they, along with their military member, experience frequent moves, and transitions. Numerous nonprofit organizations recognize this added hurdle for military and veteran families and strive to provide opportunities. Still, as with other military member and veteran issues, much remains to be done including the education of service members and their spouses about available opportunities, legitimate support, and proven ways to navigate systems.

Nonprofit organizations that are employment-centric keep tallies on the numbers of veterans who receive job opportunities or meaningful employment and use those as an outcome; however, what seems to be missing is a solid metric of the true impact of their efforts. Likewise, organizations that the IVMF research team labeled as "deliberate relationship builders" that seek to integrate veterans into society as a whole find it challenging to truly measure meaningful engagement between veterans and non-veterans of civilian society (Bush, 2014).

Nonprofits who serve in a "voice" or advocacy capacity for military and veteran families have become purposely engaged in recrafting the portrayal of military and veteran families. Too often, in all forms of media, marketing, and public dialogue, the military member, the veteran, the spouse, and the child have each been depicted as a victim and at times dysfunctional, needing sympathy.

At best, the norm has been to cast the military and veteran community as either heroes or victims—one size fits all. While this image may be an effective tool used by a few organizations for fundraising purposes, it is neither accurate nor beneficial to the overall military and veteran community.

The call to action for nonprofits that serve military and veteran families is to turn the message from negative to positive. The military spouse and child, while experiencing challenges and adversity that their peers may not encounter, are generally strong and resilient and have much to contribute to their community. Many nonprofits who operate within the military and veteran family space are striving to change the current portrayal and hardily embrace the positive message of military and veteran families, but much work is still needed.

The 2015 America Joins Forces with Military Families White Oak Retreat IV also identified bridging the civilian–military divide as one of three critical areas for focused attention, stressing the importance of positively framed messaging designed to encourage and elevate the dialogue. The second critical area identified at the Retreat was the need for bridging barriers to collaboration at all levels in order to identify the best opportunities for needed direct support services, impactful information, and referral services. Bridging the gaps in existing services to targeted sub-communities (such as military children, caregivers, and the wounded) was the final critical area discussed. The intent is to leverage local, scalable programs and thereby strengthen the bond between the stakeholders and the constituents both in the present conflict environment and into the future (Blue Star Families, 2014).

12.6   What about the Children?

There is a significant need for more developmental research to better understand and respond to the needs of children and youth, both when their parents are in the military and during the transitions to civilian life. Michelle D. Sherman points out that this appeal is true for both military- and veteran-connected children. The VA estimates that from 2011 to 2016, more than 1 million personnel will exit the military. Fifty-eight percent of post-9/11 veterans are married (and if they got married while serving, there is an almost 12% chance that is a dual military couple). As Sherman stated, "there is another growing population of children whose needs are generally overlooked, namely the children of veterans. When service members leave the military, they transition to a veteran status; this change involves not only the service member, but his/her entire family as well….and the civilian community often has fewer structural supports and may be less attuned and responsive to the military family culture" (2014).

12.7   Staying the Course

Though the senior leaders of our country frequently expressed in 2001 and afterwards that our nation would be in the current fight for a long time, many among us never expected the conflict(s) would go on for this long and with no end in sight. Additionally, we now know that the second- and third-order effects of war will be with the military and veteran families for years, if not for life. The possibilities for future conflicts loom large as well. What is on the minds of many, both in the nonprofit arena and elsewhere, is how do we sustain the current level of support in both the public and the private sectors? How do we generate the necessary revenue for the nonprofits to continue their mission and not roll back programs and services? All indications show that the federal government will presumably reduce funding for military and veteran family programs. The American public also shows signs of war fatigue and may reduce giving to those nonprofit organizations that support our military and veteran families so well.

Themes of concern among nonprofit organizations are of military downsizing, plunging budgets, and evaporating interest by the public sector for military and veteran families and those who support them. Concurrently, as government resources decrease, it is natural for tension and conflict to build among nonprofits as they compete for funds for their programs and services from the same funding sources (Blue Star, 2014). In similar fashion, the IVMF study stated that, "in the nonprofit world, competition for funding can be just as fierce as competition for customers between for-profit enterprises..." (Bush Institute, 2014).

Despite the challenges of funding deficits, acknowledging the need for continued collaboration at all levels remains prevalent among nonprofit organizations. Whether a nonprofit is a nationally recognized name brand or a new organization, many in the nonprofit sector see the need for connection with other like-minded nonprofits or cross-sector affiliations. As identified by Kania and Kramer, nonprofits consider the alternative to collective impact to be isolated impact. That image is of countless nonprofits pursuing their own solutions and often at odds with others. The collaboration can improve capacity and ability to reach goals (Kania & Kramer, 2011).

Nonprofit organizations face inherent challenges in distributing their services as widely as possible yet not overreaching their own resources, personnel, and infrastructure. Finding that balance is tricky. As always, nonprofit organizations need to constantly stay focused on fiscal development so they can sustain the programs and initiatives they provide. It is a never-ending battle to ensure that money is available to launch and support all the good work that nonprofit organizations are poised to do. Leanne Knobloch, Department of Communication, University of Illinois

12.8 Lessons Learned

Draw from the past, frame the present, share for the future...

The lessons learned over the past 15 years concerning the operations, impacts, and perhaps missed opportunities of nonprofit organizations are innumerable. Thinking about "what more might have been done" while also being mindful of shaping the future efforts of nonprofits in an ever-changing environment, we offer a few considerations gathered from select people and sources within the military and veteran family community. While certainly not all encompassing, we believe these are pertinent points worthy of review:

- There is an imperative need for continuous collaboration and the sharing of information among nonprofits, the public sector, and government agencies such as the DoD and Veterans Affairs. Since 2001, much time and effort has been and continues to be expended in seeking current and relevant data, defining gaps, overcoming barriers, and finding resources to provide the necessary programs and services. While everyone involved, regardless of their respective responsibilities, has truly sought how to best serve and support military and veteran families, a common view is that collectively, we were too slow in coming together and still today are not where we need to be in the process.

Having said that, beyond the communicating and sharing, engaged partners need to agree on and carry out specific action plans (Blue Star Families, 2015).

- Though nonprofits have been diligently providing resources, support, and advocacy since 9/11, "new faces" enter the military and veteran family arena every day. Relentlessly, nonprofits must continue to engage, educate, and motivate those within the public and private sector on the needs and challenges associated with those who serve. The nonprofits must diligently inform or train health care professionals, educators, government program and service personnel, potential donors, military and community leaders, and the general public on the current environment regarding the military and veteran family community. Military-connected children illustrate the need for continued efforts. When there is focused support with leaders, professionals, and influencers ensuring that processes, programs, and policies are in place and well implemented, these children will not only survive the challenges associated with a military lifestyle, they will thrive (Military Child Education Coalition, 2015).
- Nonprofit organizations must remain relevant in supporting military and veteran families and continually have a vision of where they, as an organization, are going in the future.
- What is the next need and how will the nonprofits meet that need within their area of responsibility? What worked in the pre-9/11 era and the early years of the post-9/11 era may not be effective today or in the future. Program and service offerings must be current and effective, worthy of funding during a time of constrained resources. The individual nonprofit organizational structure as well as staff training must precisely fit the mission. The military and veteran community continues to evolve as does the operating environment. Should a nonprofit simply wish to maintain the status quo with both the military and veteran families as well as with funding sources, they may be hardly pressed to remain a vital contributor (Bush Institute, 2014).
- Nonprofit engagement in helping to build local communities of care for military and veteran families is essential for not only the well-being of the those who are either serving or have served, but also empowers and boosts the efforts and reputation of the nonprofit organization within the community. Becoming established and known as an organization that is making a difference with programs and services is key. Reputation is everything. Being a trusted agent who both well serves and well represents as a selfless voice for the military and veteran community gets things done with all engaged local players within the community.

12.9 Recommendations

1. Identify Innovative "Big Ideas"

Whether at the federal, state, or community level, fresh, innovative thinking is still in great demand as we continue in efforts to provide first-class support for military and veteran families in an ever-changing world. What may have been a great idea with an ensuing program in the early days of post-9/11 may no longer be relevant. Likewise, within the nonprofit sector, if for nothing more than the survival of the organization, there is an imperative to continually reinvigorate the way daily business is done. Programs and services may become stale and must evolve as long as the need for the program exists. However, more importantly, not only identifying what the long-standing gaps are, but also envisioning what the new gaps will be and determining how our organization might meet those needs is crucial, both for those whom we serve and for the nonprofit. While innovative thinking is the genesis for great change, creating evidence-based solutions and programs is the second equation in the formula for success. Admittedly, acquiring the necessary evidence-based data in a timely fashion may be as challenging as capturing the initial vision. Regardless of whether operating in small-town USA or at a national level, nonprofits must have an accurate vision and an actionable plan with the resources available to execute the plan.

2. **Treat the Military and Veteran Family as One Unit**

   As with many elements of the Departments of Defense and Veterans Affairs, unless a niche-provider, nonprofits have a natural tendency to focus solely on the military member or the veteran and omit integration of the family—spouse and child—into whatever particular service they provide (Bush Institute, 2014). Some nonprofits make the case that family inclusion is neither mandated in their mission statement nor funded by sponsors or donors. By default, they may be leaving out an integral component impacting the success of their efforts with the military member or veteran. Research indicates a strong correlation between the well-being of the family of military members and the military members choosing to remain in military service (Lerner, Zaff, & Lerner, 2009). Of the active duty military members, 55.3% are married with 42.2% of those having children (DoD, 2014). Engaging in the needs and considerations of the family not only well serves our nation, but also invites a natural affinity between the nonprofit organization the military and veteran member and their family. While only the military member volunteers to wear the uniform, the entire family plays a vital role in that service to our nation.

3. **Research is Needed to Better Understand Implications for Children and Youth**

   I often find myself telling those in the military and veteran communities that children are left out of our conversations. There is little data on the achievements of military children and a lack of community support. And lately I've noticed when we are included, it's a negative narrative. (Margaret Clevenger, 2015)

   Nonprofits can contribute in important ways to the translation to practice and the local context. They provide the field experience and help contribute to the balance. This is only strengthened into strategies and solutions that are sustainable if there is a solid research framework to build upon; otherwise, there is a continued risk of adding programs that are neither informed by the research nor practice.

The paucity of research about military children and their families is significant. Cozza, Lerner, and Haskins in both the Future of Children: Policy Brief (2013) and the Society of Research in Child Development: Social Policy Report (2014) emphasize strongly "the need for future rigorous developmental research about military-connected children and families that could more definitively inform future programs and policies" (SRCD, 2014, p. 1). Michelle Sherman extends this urgency by pointing to the sorely needed focus on a life-course perspective by including the veteran child in research agendas: "The course of the transition from a military child to a veteran child is unknown; our ability to extrapolate from the current knowledge and promising programs for military children to the experiences and needs of the veteran children is uncertain." (2014, p. 16).

When capturing practices worthy of attention and those worthy of replication, one must consider the array of demographic, developmental, and social contexts for military- and veteran-connected youth as well as their families. Considering that there are many normative settings where most military- and veteran-connected children and their families live, there are special opportunities for nonprofits to partner with local organizations and institutions. Spotlighting the Los Angeles Public Schools and their collaboration with local nonprofits as well as the University of Southern California (USC), Ron Astor wrote in a blog for the Huffington Post:

> This type of partnership aimed at the reintegration of veteran families into public schools and civilian communities should serve as an example and a challenge to mayors, school superintendents, veteran organizations and universities across this country. Large civilian institutions in big cities can work together to improve supports for students who might be facing battles due to the war, long after their parents return home. (2015)

The question is, can nonprofits be nimble enough to respond to the complex and dynamic conditions and experiences of military and veteran-connected children and their families. It is a dynamic complexity for nonprofits to pay attention to these multifaceted variables when studying and unpacking what has worked; what can potentially work; under what conditions; and, with what populations—especially when trying to address resilience and respond to risk in youth. *Awareness of the effects of contexts has implications for including context variables both in the conceptualization and the measurement in research…one example is the attention to national, regional and historical contexts as explaining variability.* (Benbenishty & Astor, 2014)

4. **Prepare for the Future**

After these many years of war, some nonprofit organizations may find themselves feeling uncomfortable as the environment evolves into something new. As the expression goes, "the only guarantee we have is change." Many post-9/11 organizations operating in the military and veteran community since 2001 have simply grown and expanded without thought to structure or effectiveness; it has long been simply about meeting the mission need. Those same organizations are now witnessing military downsizing and budget constraints with reduced services, programs, and benefits yet see a high probability of continuously engaged military forces operating in an era of persistent conflict. Clearly, the nonprofit world is changing, yet there appears to be a continued need for selfless nonprofits who fill critical gaps in support, particularly at the state and community level.

Regardless of where the nonprofit operates, whether in employment, wellness, family, housing, education, or other areas, there is a constant oversaturation and redundancy of nonprofits. Whether a government agency is looking for contractual support of a vital program, or a military or veteran family is looking for help, there is difficulty sorting through the "noise and clutter" of countless, often competing nonprofit organizations. Looking forward, in order to survive and flourish while continuing to provide vital programs and services, nonprofits will not only need to originate their own *big ideas*, but will also need to truly apply strategic planning and organizational effectiveness towards the execution of their current and perhaps *next* mission statement.

Greatness is not a function of circumstance. Greatness, it turns out, is largely a matter of conscious choice, and discipline. Jim Collins

Acknowledgments We would like to express our thanks and appreciation to the following people for generously sharing their perspectives and insights:

Geoffrey J. Deutsch, President & CEO, Armed Forces Services Corporation & Military Child Education Coalition National Advisory Committee

Leanne Knobloch, PhD, Department of Communication, University of Illinois & Military Child Education Coalition Science Advisory Board

Chris Marvin, Principal, Marvin Strategies Consulting Services

Michelle D. Sherman, PhD, University of Minnesota & Military Child Education Coalition Science Advisory Board

Patricia "Patty" Shinseki, Military Child Education Coalition, Board of Directors, Emeritus

David W. Sutherland, COL (USA, Ret.), Chairman, Easter Seals Dixon Center

References

Armstrong, N., McDonough, J., & Savage, D. (2015). *Driving Community impact: The case for local, evidence-based coordination in veteran and military family services and the America-Serves initiative.* Syracuse University- Institute for Veterans and Military Families.

Astor, R. (2015). L.A.'s challenge to all large U.S. Metropolitan cities: Support Veterans' and Service Members' children in civilian public schools. *Huffington Post*, Blog post: November 30, 2015. Retrieved from http://www.huffingtonpost.com/ron-avi-astor/las-challenge-to-all-larg_b_8486408.html

Benbenishty, R., & Astor, R. (2014). Expanding the scope of research on military children: Studying adversity, resilience and promotion in normative social settings. *Commentary for Military and Veteran Families and Children: Policies and programs for Health Maintenance and Positive Development. Society for Research in Child Development, 28*(3), 17.

Blue Star Families. (2012). Blue Star Families blog: Roundtable with secretary of Defense Hagel. Retrieved from http://www.bluestarfam.org/blog/roundtable-secretary-defense-hagel

Blue Star Families. (2014). *America joins forces with military families: White Oak III summary report.* Retrieved from http://www.bluestarfam.org/resources/research-and-policy-1/white-oak

Blue Star Families. (2015). *America joins forces with military families: White Oak IV summary report.* Retrieved from http://www.bluestarfam.org/resources/research-and-policy-1/white-oak

Clevenger, M. (2015). We're having the wrong conversation about Military Brats. *Task & Purpose*, Blog post: August 24, 2015. Retrieved from http://taskandpurpose.com/author/margaret-clevenger/

Collins, J. (2005). *Good to great and the social sectors. A monograph to accompany good to great.* Retrieved from http://www.jimcollins.com/books/g2g-ss.html

Got Your 6. http://www.gotyour6.org

Kania, J., & Kramer, M.., Collective Impact. (2011). *Stanford Social Innovation Review*, 38–40. Retrieved from http://www.nist.gov/ineap/upload/2011-Stanford-Article.pdf

Kudler, H., & Porter, R. I. (2013). Building communities of care for military children and families. *The Future of Children, Military Children and Families, 23*(2), 163–182.

Lerner, R. M., Zaff, J. F., & Lerner, J. V. (2009). *America's military youth: Towards a study of positive development in the face of challenge*, 2–3. Retrieved from http://www.militarychild. org/parents-and-students/resources

MacDermid Wadsworth, S. (2016). Civilian organizations that support military families. In K. R. Blaisure, T. Saath-Wells, A. Pereira, S. MacDermid Wadsworth, & A. L. Dombro (Eds.), *Serving military families* (pp. 287–306). New York, NY: Routledge.

Military Child Education Coalition. (2012). *Education of the military child in the 21st century: Current dimensions of the educational experiences for army children*, 8–9. Harker Heights, TX: Author. Retrieved from http://www.militarychild.org/emc21-report

Military Child Education Coalition. (2015). *College, career, and life readiness for military and veteran children*, 2. Harker Heights, TX: Author. Retrieved from http://www.militarychild.org/ public/upload/files/GE_Leaders_Guide-complete.pdf

Military Child Education Coalition. https://www.militarychild.org/professional/programs/ living-in-the-new-normal-public-engagement-linn-pe

National Council on Nonprofits. (2015). *Myths about nonprofits*. Retrieved from https://www. councilofnonprofits.org/myths-about-nonprofits

Points of Light | Community Blueprint. Retrieved from http://www.pointsoflight.org/programs/ military-initiatives/community-blueprint

Sherman, M. (2014). Children of military veterans: An overlooked population. *Commentary for Military and Veteran Families and Children: Policies and Programs for Health Maintenance and Positive Development Society for Research in Child Development, 28*(3), 15.

Springle, C., & Wilmer, C. M. (2014). Painting a moving train: Preparing civilian community providers to serve returning warriors and their families. In R. B. Everson & C. R. Figley (Eds.), *Families under fire* (pp. 239–240). New York, NY: Routledge.

The George W. Bush Institute & Institute for Veterans and Military Families (IVMF), Syracuse University. (2014). *Serving our post—9/11 Veterans, leading practices among non-profit organizations, i–iii, 2–5, 16–18, 24–28, 66, 73–77.* Retrieved from http://www.bushcenter.org/sites/ default.files/gwbi-msi-serving-our-vets-pdf

U.S. Chamber of Commerce Foundation. http://www.uschamberfoundation.org/hiring-our-heroes

United States Congress. (2015). Elementary and Secondary Education Act Reauthorization. *Every Student Succeeds Act.* "(ii) For all students and disaggregated by each subgroup of students described in subsection (b)(2)(B)(xi), homeless status, status as a child in foster care, and status as a student with a parent who is a member of the Armed Forces (as defined in section 101(a)(4) of title 10, United States Code) on active duty (as defined in section 101(d)(5) of such title), information on student achievement on the academic assessments described in subsection (b)(2) at each level of achievement, as determined by the State under subsection (b)(1)". Retrieved from http:// edworkforce.house.gov/uploadedfiles/every_student_succeeds_act_-_conference_report.pdf

United States Department of Veterans Affairs. National Center for Veterans Analysis and Statistics. Retrieved from http://www.va.gov/vetdata/Veteran_Population.asp

United States Government, Department of Defense. (2014). *Demographics report: Profile of the military community, 42*, 128.

United States Government, Department of Defense, Office of the Chairman of the Joint Chiefs of Staff, Office of Reintegration: Veterans/Families/Communities. (2014). *After the sea of goodwill: A collective approach to veteran reintegration.* Retrieved from http://www.jcs.mil/ Portals/36/Documents/CORe/After_the_Sea_of_Goodwill.pdf

United States Government, Department of Defense, Office of the Chairman of the Joint Chiefs of Staff, Warrior and Family Support. (2010). *Sea of goodwill: Matching the donor to the need.* Retrieved from http://www.slideshare.net/recruitdc/sea-of-goodwill

Chapter 13
Community Mobilization

Koby Langley and Leah Barber

13.1 Introduction

The military of today faces unique challenges, challenges which other generations did not encounter. Stark numbers support this claim. The military of the twenty-first century is all-volunteer, with less than 0.5% of the US population currently serving. This is in stark contrast to World War II, when more than 12% of the population served. Post-Vietnam, 70% of Congress had military service. Today, that number is only 20% (Eikenberry & Kennedy, 2013). These statistics will have a strong impact on the recruitment and retention of the future all-volunteer force, and the implications behind these statistics will be devastating to our national security if not addressed now. This has been referenced by many senior leaders in the community as the "civil/military divide," or more recently, "the civil/military drift" (Institute for Veterans and Military Families, 2013; Pew Research Center, 2011).

With the population of America hovering near 320 million, 0.5% is still 1.6 million people (United States Census Bureau, 2015). This means that approximately 1.6 million Americans are currently serving in some capacity in our armed forces and alongside those service members are spouses, children, parents, and other loved ones. While the percentage of those in the military is small, the number of those affected grows exponentially and in recent conflicts, it has become better understood that the family not only serves, but also suffers.

There is little argument that on September 11, 2001, the United States was not prepared for the extended conflict that we have now experienced. Our last major deployment of troops was in 1990–1991, with Operation Desert Storm (ODS). Unlike the conflicts in Iraq and Afghanistan, which meandered on for years, ODS was over in less than a year. Prior to ODS, the United States had not participated in

K. Langley (✉) • L. Barber
American Red Cross, Washington, DC, USA
e-mail: koby.langley@redcross.org; leah.barber@redcross.org

© Springer International Publishing AG 2018
L. Hughes-Kirchubel et al. (eds.), *A Battle Plan for Supporting Military Families*, Risk and Resilience in Military and Veteran Families,
https://doi.org/10.1007/978-3-319-68984-5_13

a major, multi-year conflict since Vietnam, which ended in 1975. When the Twin Towers fell, it had been over a quarter of a century since America had participated in a conflict that involved a large commitment of ground troops, air support, and an international coalition of joint forces.

Since September 2001, approximately 2.5 million members of the active duty services as well as the related Reserve and National Guard units have deployed to the Afghanistan and Iraq theaters. More than a third—over 833,000—have deployed more than once (Adams, 2013). Bilmes (2007) noted that their experience was also unique in that they had a much higher battlefield survival rate than twentieth century wars. In Iraq and Afghanistan, the ratio of wounded service members to those killed was 16 to 1. In Vietnam and Korea, there were 2.6 to 2.8 injuries for each fatality and World Wars I and II had even lower ratios (p. 2).

Other changes have also made these twenty-first century conflicts different from preceding wars. The multiple deployments have created a tail impact on family members and children and the increased number of women serving has also impacted families. Traditionally, women stayed home and took care of the "homefront" while their husbands went to war. In today's conflicts, women also deploy or both parents deploy, sometimes simultaneously. During the Gulf War, 41,000 women served. Over the course of the post-9/11 conflicts, that number rose to over 155,000 (Holder, 2010, p. 2). When these service members come home, they face a system that has not yet been developed sufficiently to provide the kind of caregiver and traumatic injury benefits specialized to these conflicts. By the Department of Veterans Affairs' (VA) own admission, they were ill-equipped and poorly prepared to serve not only our women veterans but also our veterans suffering from PTSD and TBI (Daly, 2014; Kashdan, 2014). Returning service members also face the long-lasting challenge of the lack of interoperability between military medical records and the civilian care provider network. The issues stemming from this are far-reaching, particularly when service members leave the service or, as activated Guardsmen and Reservists, deactivate. The gulf of disconnect between the civilian population and the military continues to be a growing issue, despite those larger numbers of citizen soldiers deploying to theaters of combat where "there are no front-lines anymore" (Woolf, 2015).

13.2   Key Landmark Events

When we look at Community Service Provider Mobilization, there are many issues that this sector was unprepared to meet in 2001. After more than 20 years of not having hundreds of thousands of deployed troops serving extended tours of duty over the course of a decade, no one really knew what to expect. And, of course, no one knew at that time that Operation Enduring Freedom would continue for more than a decade, unabated, and unfortunately, no one had a crystal ball that told them Operation Iraqi Freedom would begin 2 years later and last another 8 years. Here in 2015, we now have the luxury—and the ability—to look back and determine what key events and situations over the past 14-plus years inform our current model.

In 2002, however, then-Secretary of State Colin Powell came the closest to honestly foretelling of the scope of the commitment, arguing that, "US troops should join the small international peacekeeping force patrolling Kabul [...] and help Hamid Karzai extend his influence beyond just the capital of Kabul" ("Context of "February 2002: Powell's Proposal," 2002). His proposal was rejected. Four years later, even our inactive ready reserves would be activated at never-before-seen rates, throwing men and women—individuals with careers and lives completely separated and disconnected from their obligatory reserve status—into the conflict. These men and women did not even have an obligation to drill or train with a military reserve unit and during those years, most had not received any military training. This so-called inactive ready reserve activation was perhaps the most telling aspect of just how unready we really were ("U.S. Military Calling Back Troops," 2006).

According to a U.S. Government Accountability Office (GAO) report (2004), "with the high pace of operations since September 11, more than 51 percent of Army Guard members and 31 percent of Air Guard members have been activated to meet new homeland and overseas demands" ("Reserve Forces"). In 2005, we reached our peak of Guardsmen and Reservists in combat-deployed roles. At this time, they represented nearly 50% of the deployed force in Iraq (Tyson, 2006). This is unlike previous conflicts—those citizen soldiers had always deployed, but never in such high numbers. With the US military being an all-volunteer force, there were simply not enough active duty service members to support the needs of two simultaneous wars. Also, unlike their active duty brethren, these citizen soldiers did not come back to military-knowledgeable communities. Their families, by and large, did not have a frame of reference for their service members' experiences.

Particularly in the early years of OEF and OIF, the community resources and support for Reserve and Guard families were insufficient and even if some existed, the families did not necessarily know to seek them out. In a GAO report on the Federal Recovery Coordination Program (2011), one of the key issues identified was the limitations on information sharing between programs. Eighty-four percent of recovering service members and veterans were enrolled in more than one program, but because there was no coordination between programs, there was duplication of service and difficulties were created for the very people the program was created to help ("Federal Recovery Coordination Program," p. 6). Despite the support provided by these mass deployments of Guardsmen and Reservists, the force faced a dwell-time peak of 18–24 months. Service members had two or fewer years at home before deploying again, which in turn put more pressure on community resources. The families left behind still needed support and the service members needed support not only when they were deployed, but when they came home again.

Enter the "Sea of Goodwill" of American support—as Admiral Michael Mullen, the then-Chairman of the Joint Chiefs of Staff said, "The challenge… is how do you connect the sea of goodwill to the need?" (Copeland & Sutherland, 2010, p. 1). The issue was not a lack of organizations to provide services to these service members, veterans, and their family members. Instead, it was determining how to best connect those organizations and services to the people who needed them. That "Sea of Goodwill" can be overwhelming, particularly for those who are already facing other difficulties—personally, professionally, emotionally, mentally, physically—and many people give up because navigating those waters can seem like such an insurmountable task.

One of the most significant challenges for these service members, veterans, and family members was the lack of caregiver assistance for the catastrophically wounded, ill, or injured until 8 years into the conflict. This is one of the areas in which Community Mobilization stepped in. Organizations observed the lack of officially funded and provided caregiver assistance and many began to provide that assistance themselves. Because of the higher rate of survival due to better technology and faster medical care, many of those who would have perished in previous conflicts from their injuries instead survived. Some of those who survived were so severely injured that they need intensive care—often at home—for the rest of their lives.

13.3 Innovations and Key Strategies

An important step in strategically responding to the issue of military disconnectedness is identifying training for the caregiver outside of the support net of DoD and VA funding. While there is now DoD and VA support for caregivers, more is needed. Organizations need to invest in veteran and military family case management training—while the major conflicts are over, the needs of families and veterans will continue to increase as the effects of decades at war continue to ripple across those communities. Initial steps to "wrangle" this "Sea of Goodwill" were undertaken by the DoD and the VA with the creation of an online resource aggregator—the National Resource Directory. In 2014, the Government Accountability Office (GAO) identified publicly available sources containing lists of relevant programs, e.g., the National Resource Directory or the Catalog of Federal Domestic Assistance and highlighted them as a best practice, stating:

> The NRD is a partnership among DoD, VA and the Department of Labor that seeks to connect wounded and other servicemembers, veterans, their families and caregivers to programs and services that support them. Information contained within the NRD website is from federal, state and local government agencies; veteran and military service organizations; non-profit and community-based organizations; academic institutions and professional associations that provide assistance to wounded warriors and their families ("Military and Veteran Support").

By being caught unaware on that long-ago September day, we failed to create a clear and easy network of access to community resources and we are still trying to correct this problem. The "Sea of Goodwill" is vast, but in its vastness it is easy to get lost and overwhelmed. By focusing on direct services, such as caregiver training, complementary and alternative therapies, and volunteer management and engagement on military installations and VA facilities, as well as investing significant resources in integrated case management training, we will ensure that we continue to meet the changing needs of those communities and also remain prepared to face the realities of the next conflict.

Investing in behavioral health support services for military spouses and children is another key innovation. When the conflict began, there was no thought as to the psychological and emotional impact on family members. In 2001, we had no idea that we would be sending service members out on multiple deployments with minimal dwell time. This goes hand-in-hand with the importance of expanding National Guard and Reserve engagement efforts and support as those service members and families do not have the same level of support as do active duty service members and families stationed on regular military installations.

Currently, as defined by the GAO, there are over 50 mental health programs run by the DoD and the military service branches ("Military and Veteran Support," 2014). However, the Substance Abuse and Mental Health Services Administration (SAMHSA) found that approximately 50% of returning service members in need of mental health treatment sought it, but of that 50%, only half received adequate care. In 2014, it was noted that a significant number of active duty troops and their families opt to not access these services provided by the DoD and military services branches because they fear discrimination or harm to their military career for seeking treatment for behavioral health issues. Additionally, National Guardsmen and Reservists who served in Iraq and Afghanistan are also eligible for behavioral health care services from the VA, but many of them are also unable or unwilling to utilize those services ("Veterans and Military Families," 2014).

The issue of mental health services for military families will continue to be a legacy impact of military service. Cultural biases often run counter to command's intentional desire to have a healthy and deployable force, general biases and stigma related to mental health issues in general, and the inherent conflict of mental health care providers who value and understand the importance of confidentiality in treatment and a commander's right to know about the health and welfare of their troops.Many commanders I have spoken to state that mental health challenges are not conducive to military service. Right or wrong, too many of our military leaders hold steadfast to this belief, which in turn drives many service members and their families to seek care (if they seek it at all) outside of the military medical health system and into the community.

Organizations like the American Red Cross, with thousands of volunteers—including mental health care professionals—were not prepared to re-deploy those volunteers to serve the military family community until nearly 5 years into the conflict. Other nonprofit organizations, such as Give an Hour, saw the need very early on and began recruiting mental health professionals to provide free mental health services as early as 2007. Today, they have thousands of registered mental health professionals providing free counseling services to military families and still turn many away due to the demand.

13.4   Needs and Lessons Learned

With the benefit of hindsight, it is easy to see how we could have done things better, how we could have anticipated the needs more successfully. But we did not have that hindsight and as we were plunged into a faraway conflict in Afghanistan, we had to react instead of preparing. So we, just as the DoD and the VA did, reacted.

We reacted to those unexpectedly high numbers of citizen soldiers being deployed. Not just deployed, but deployed multiple times. Organizations saw that the DoD and the VA did not have the ability to meet those needs at that time, so they stepped in. The "Sea of Goodwill" went into overdrive.

We did not anticipate the effect on family members. Without intervention, multiple deployments can negatively affect a marriage and a child's relationship with their constantly deployed parent can become fraught with misunderstanding, resentment, and confusion. A study by James and Countryman (2012) finds that these children have problems with sleeping, have higher levels of stress and anxiety, declining grades and increased behavioral issues (p. 17).

Furthermore, we did not anticipate the increased medical needs. With more severely injured service members surviving, the existing medical facilities and caregiver support were insufficient. The VA was not prepared for an influx of veterans with such a wide range of physical, mental, and emotional injuries. Even now, we do not comprehend the full extent or cost of these conflicts. The demand for volunteer clinical and non-clinical volunteers at military treatment facilities and VA hospitals rose dramatically, increasing the demand on non-profit organizations to recruit, place, manage, and supervise a large number of volunteers in hundreds of military installations and VA hospitals around the globe. As an example, at its height, the Red Cross at Landstuhl Regional Medical Center had more than 400 volunteers contributing more than 40,000 h in a year. To volunteer, these individuals went through a rigorous screening process to include a Red Cross background check, a health and wellness clearance, HIPAA training, and a DoD security clearance. Managing that volunteer workforce was a tremendous endeavor and the voluntary contributions of those hundreds of volunteers contributed hugely to the care and treatment of the wounded, ill, and injured at Landstuhl.

13.5   Responses and Strategies

The Red Cross' response to the conflicts can be categorized into four main areas: the expansion of volunteer recruitment, placement, and management capabilities; the expansion of direct services that aligned with our organizational core competencies; the expansion of our presence on military installations overseas and in theaters of combat; and the expansion of our emergency communication capabilities.

The success of the American Red Cross has always been dependent on its volunteers. Even today, volunteers constitute roughly 90% of the organization's workforce ("Be a Disaster Volunteer," 2015). The expansion of our volunteer program in response to the conflicts in Iraq and Afghanistan was twofold: first, expand our volunteer presence on military installations and military treatment facilities. Second, expand that presence at VA facilities to ensure that Red Cross volunteers were alongside our service members every step of the way.

To maintain the integrity and viability of these volunteer programs within military and veteran treatment facilities, the organization focused on recruitment, placement, and onboarding. To volunteer in a military treatment facility is not just a matter of walking in 1 day and walking out again with a name tag. It is a process, a process created and developed to ensure not only the safety of the volunteer, but the safety and health of those they are there to help.

The expansion of direct services that are aligned with our organizational core competencies was another vital response to the conflicts in Iraq and Afghanistan. We were caught unawares in 2001, which meant that to be more effective, we needed to build upon our current strengths and develop what already existed into something that could meet the needs of a new fighting force.

So we focused on behavioral health support, creating programs such as Reconnection Workshops and Coping With Deployments. These two trainings were natural outgrowths of our current programs and focused on the needs of the population; what was needed were programs to help service members reconnect with their loved ones after a deployment and there needed to be more tools at the disposal of those left on the homefront to help them cope with their loved one being gone. We also focused on volunteer-supported morale and welfare support services, increasing our visits to the wounded, ill, and injured and distributing more comfort items to aid in recovery. Along with this, in several locations we created rest and recovery rooms to provide an oasis of peace not only for patients, but also for their caregivers. Finally, we expanded our financial assistance, reengineering emergency loans, and expanding our casualty assistance grants.

Next, the expansion of our presence on military installations overseas and in combat theaters was accomplished in several ways. First, we activated Red Cross reserve staff. Like reservists in the military, these were individuals who had normal lives and jobs, but signed up to deploy to a combat zone as a Red Cross staff member. By utilizing this reserve system, the organization was able to stabilize the deployments of its full-time staff and ensure continuity at Red Cross offices across the country and around the world.

The Red Cross continues to change and expand in response to the changing needs of the military. A significant part of this has been working with the DoD to ensure the success and integration of the organization on installations both in the United States and overseas. In recent years, an office has been opened in Djibouti and a second office opened in Kuwait, while at the same time an office in Afghanistan was closed due to troop drawdown in that theater. By placing Red Cross staff members in Kuwait, we are better able to meet the needs of a deployed military that is spread out geographically.

Finally, the expansion of clinical and non-clinical volunteers in military treatment facilities has played a significant role in expanding our presence. As stated previously, volunteers make up at least 90% of the Red Cross workforce. They are a force multiplier—from trauma surgeons to medical assistants, volunteer programs around the world have expanded our reach and ability to meet the needs of service members, veterans, and their families.

Lastly, the organization has made a huge push to expand our emergency communication capabilities. We have expanded the workforce, upgraded IT and telephony capabilities, and have redesigned the system to improve quality, timeliness, and consistency in service. Emergency communications are at the core of our service to the military and to do that job well in the twenty-first century, we need to ensure that our technology and workforce keeps up with the needs of the population we are here to serve.

13.6 Results/Evaluations

By being unprepared for the consequences of the conflicts in Iraq and Afghanistan, we were late to the game of providing appropriate and timely support to our service members, veterans, and their families. Most organizations and programs were in the same boat, but as everyone rushed to fill the gaps, we unknowingly created that "Sea of Goodwill." Everyone had the best intentions and good programs, but no one was communicating effectively. All that information was overwhelming, not just for those individuals and organizations in that space, but confusing for the very people we were there to help.

We are still continuing the process of having an information and referral process for all service members, veterans, and family members that is easy to use, up-to-date, and not overwhelming. With thousands of organizations to choose from, this confusion is not surprising. The result of the chaos post-9/11 was that all these organizations realized that they needed to improve and increase their programs and services. In evaluating the subsequent "Sea of Goodwill" today, in 2015, the main issue is not quality or quantity or a lack of assistance. It is simply getting the right assistance to the right person at the right time. As we move forward into 2016 and beyond, that needs to be the focus. We need to keep developing our programs and services to meet the ever-evolving needs of the population we serve, and we need to ensure that we provide a way to connect those in need with what is available.

13.7 Recommendations

I would make the following recommendations to ensure that we are prepared for whatever the next conflict may bring:

- We must expand to an integrated national case management network.
- Through volunteerism, we must bridge the civilian/military divide.
- We need to open our doors to the veteran community.
- We must leverage our global footprint.
- Wherever it is most needed, we have to provide measurable and impactful direct service.
- We need to publish data.
- We must communicate across multiple platforms and mediums.
- Finally, we need to anticipate needs for resources prior to the need dictating service delivery options.

13.8   Conclusion

The biggest challenge facing our nation in the next major armed conflict will be the reinvigoration and smart growth of the lean and tested strength of the all-volunteer force and their families. More specifically, the challenges will lie in the number of citizens who are willing to serve in uniform, our nation's temperament to fight and win a protracted conflict and our government's ability to meet the full long-tail costs of war. Community service organizations will play a critical role in helping to address these challenges. In some cases, we should be the de facto solution to what ails our national defense industrial complex. One of the most frequently cited contributor to all of these issues is the "civil/military drift" or the "civil/military divide." This well-known problem is ripe for a coordinated non-profit and community service organization-based strategy.

References

Adams, C. (2013, March 14). *Millions went to war in Iraq, Afghanistan, leaving many with lifelong scars.* Retrieved from http://www.mcclatchydc.com/news/nationworld/national/article24746680.html

American Red Cross. (2015). *Be a disaster volunteer.* Retrieved from http://www.redcross.org/support/volunteer/disaster-volunteer

Associated Press. (2006, August 20). U.S. military calling back troops who've been out of uniform for years. *USA Today.* Retrieved from http://usatoday30.usatoday.com/news/washington/2006-08-19-military-call-back_x.htm

Bilmes, L. (2007). *Soldiers returning from Iraq and Afghanistan: The long-term costs of providing veterans medical care and disability benefits.* KSG Faculty Research Working Paper Series RWP07–001. Retrieved from https://research.hks.harvard.edu/publications/workingpapers/citation.aspx?PubId=4329&t ype=WPN

Copeland, J., & Sutherland, D. (2010). *Sea of goodwill: Matching the donor to the need.* Retrieved from http://www.fifnc.org/programs/Sea_of_Goodwill.pdf

Daly, M. (2014, September 24). Report: Services for female veterans fall short. *Military Times.* Retrieved from http://www.militarytimes.com/story/military/benefits/health- care/2014/09/24/report-services-for-female-veterans-fall-short/16151527/.

Eikenberry, K., & Kennedy, D. (2013, May 26). Americans and their military, drifting apart. *The New York Times.* Retrieved from http://www.nytimes.com/2013/05/27/opinion/americans-and-their-military-drifting-apart.html?_r=0

History Commons. (2002). *Context of 'February 2002: Powell's proposal to secure all of Afghanistan is rejected by Rumsfeld.* Retrieved from http://www.historycommons.org/context.jsp?item=a0202powellreject

Holder, K. (2010). Presented at the 2010 Annual Meeting of the Population Association of America: *Post-9/11 Women Veterans.*

Institute for Veterans and Military Families and Institute for National Security and Counterterrorism. (2013). *A national veterans strategy: The economic, social and security imperative.* Syracuse, NY: Syracuse University.

James, T., & Countryman, J. (2012, February). Psychiatric effects of military deployment on children and families: The use of play therapy for assessment and treatment. *Innovative Clinical Neuroscience, 9*(2), 15–20.

Kashdan, T. (2014, September 9). 11 reasons that combat veterans with PTSD are being harmed. *Psychology Today*. Retrieved from https://www.psychologytoday.com/blog/curious/201409/11-reasons-combat-veterans-ptsd-are-being-harmed

Pew Research Center. (2011). *The military-civilian gap: War and sacrifice in the post-9/11 era.* Washington, DC: Pew Social and Demographic Trends.

Substance Abuse and Mental Health Services Administration. (2014). *Veterans and military families*. Retrieved from http://www.samhsa.gov/veterans-military-families

Tyson, A. (2006, November 5). Possible Iraq deployments would stretch reserve force. *The Washington Post*. Retrieved from http://www.washingtonpost.com/wp-dyn/content/article/2006/11/04/AR2006110401160.html

United States Census Bureau. (2015). *U.S. and world population clock*. Retrieved from http://www.census.gov/popclock

U.S. Government Accountability Office. (2004, April). *Reserve forces: Observations on recent National Guard use in overseas and homeland missions and future challenges* (Publication No. GAO-04-670T). Retrieved from http://www.gpo.gov/fdsys/pkg/GAOREPORTS-GAO-04-670T/content-detail.html

United States Government Accountability Office. (2011, May). *Federal Recovery Coordination Program: Enrollment, staffing, and care coordination pose significant challenges* (Publication No. GAO-11-572T). Retrieved from http://www.gao.gov/products/GAO-11-572T

U.S. Government Accountability Office. (2014, November). *Military and veteran support: DOD and VA programs that address the effects of combat and transition to civilian life* (Publication No. GAO-15-24). Retrieved from http://www.gao.gov/products/GAO-15-24

Woolf, C. (2015, August 20). *The US Army Rangers are about to have their first female members. What do vets think?* Retrieved from http://www.pri.org/stories/2015-08-20/us-army-rangers-are-about-have-their-first-female-members-what-do-vets-think

Chapter 14
Philanthropy for Military and Veteran Families: Challenges Past, Recommendations for Tomorrow

Linda Hughes-Kirchubel and Elizabeth Cline Johnson

The term philanthropy—"an act or gift done or made for humanitarian purposes" (Merriam-Webster, 2016)—evolved from the Greek *philanthropia*, which refers to benevolence and love of humankind. Over the centuries, philanthropists have been dedicated to local, national, and global issues. They have founded universities, supported medical institutions, and religious endeavors and worked to abolish slavery and establish civil rights. They have at times engaged with military and veteran communities. During the Civil War, for example, "the centerpiece of philanthropic efforts was the U.S. Sanitary Commission, a privately funded national federation that assumed responsibility for public health and relief measures on the battlefield and in military encampments" (Hall, 2006). During the Great Depression and World War II, philanthropists gave with a mission of promoting "science, scientific standards and professional values, as well as opportunity and personal responsibility" (Hammock, 2003). In 2014, individuals gave $358.4 billion—a year-over-year increase of more than 7%. Meanwhile, corporate giving increased to $17.77 billion, and foundation giving increased to $53.7 billion, increases of 13.7% and 8.2%, respectively (The National Philanthropic Trust, 2016). While some of the money was earmarked specifically for the military affiliated, giving specifically to veterans and military-affiliated families is a relatively novel endeavor (Meyer, 2013).

The purpose of this chapter is to describe philanthropic efforts that emerged after the terrorist attacks of Sept. 11, 2001, in support of service members, veterans, and their families. Concentrating broadly on corporations and foundations, it begins

L. Hughes-Kirchubel, M.A (✉)
Department of Human Development and Family Studies, Military Family Research Institute,
College of Health and Human Sciences, Purdue University, West Lafayette, IN, USA
e-mail: lhughesk@purdue.edu

E.C. Johnson, M.A
University of Houston, Sugar Land, TX, USA
e-mail: bethjohnson@uh.edu

© Springer International Publishing AG 2018

L. Hughes-Kirchubel et al. (eds.), *A Battle Plan for Supporting Military Families*, Risk and Resilience in Military and Veteran Families,
https://doi.org/10.1007/978-3-319-68984-5_14

with a background on the philanthropic sector before moving on to offer historical context on philanthropy's engagement with military families, as well as key events that helped to shape the post-9/11 response. Drawing on the expertise of leaders in the field, the chapter then details military and veteran families' needs and analyzes the philanthropic response, giving examples of efforts that succeeded as well as those that were less effective. After discussing gaps that remain, the chapter concludes with recommendations for future philanthropic leaders to consider when faced with responding to military and veteran family needs during an era of deployment, conflict, and combat.

14.1 Background

More than any other generation in history, the current one aims to support military members, veterans, and their families, according to a Department of Defense (DoD) white paper (Copeland & Sutherland, 2010). In the aftermath of 9/11, philanthropic organizations worked to address emerging needs of veterans, military members, and their families. Some worked on the national stage. Others were regional. Still others focused on local communities. Early on, some leaders emerged:

- Bob Woodruff Foundation (which focused on the needs of wounded warriors);
- Blue Shield of California Foundation (domestic violence prevention);
- The Bristol-Myers Squibb Foundation (mental health issues);
- The Dallas Foundation (military families and "shadow warriors");
- Fisher House Foundation (housing and scholarships);
- JP Morgan Chase Foundation (employment, financial capacity, and small businesses);
- The Lincoln Community Foundation (veteran reintegration);
- The Patterson Foundation (honoring and memorializing military members, veterans, and their families);
- The Robin Hood Foundation (economic, housing, and legal issues);
- Robert R. McCormick Foundation (education, employment, and behavioral health); and
- The Walmart Foundation (employment, education, and job training).

In the philanthropic ecosystem, these and other philanthropic organizations do not work in isolation. Foundations issue grants, but are buttressed by infrastructure that provides multiple kinds of support (Powers, 2015a, 2015b). For example, the Council on Foundations offers "opportunity, leadership, and tools" to more than 1750 member organizations and provides information, education, and occasions to network, exchange ideas, and share best practices (Council on Foundations, 2016a, 2016b). The Council established and maintains the Veterans Philanthropy Exchange, a clearinghouse in which organizations can connect and share ideas, challenges, and best practices. On the regional level, the Forum of Regional Associations of Grantmakers collaboratively links 33 regional associations of grant-making organizations, which together reach 5550 organizations, many of whom work in the military-affiliated space (Forum of Regional Associations and Grantmakers, 2016).

14.2 Historical Context and Key Events

Prior to Sept. 11, 2001, philanthropic foundations, like the American public, were largely disengaged with the military (Powers, 2015a, 2015b). However, in the aftermath of the attacks on the World Trade Center, United Airlines Flight 93, and the Pentagon, more than 1270 foundations, corporations, and other institutional donors gave an astonishing $1.1 billion for 9/11-related assistance (Renz & Marino, 2003). More than 70% of that went to relief efforts, survivors, and victim aid.

The attacks propelled the nation into conflicts in two countries, and between fiscal years 2002 and 2008, the number of troops located in Iraq and Afghanistan soared from about 5200 to more than 188,000 (Belasco, 2009). During this time of mobilization and deployment, communities and foundations began to take steps to support military members. But the lion's share of foundations did not have military or veteran family support as part of their mission. Early philanthropic efforts, largely uncoordinated, were tied to the communities that the funders served. Communities with high numbers of military or veteran families got more attention to military-specific issues; communities with fewer military or veteran families got less (Powers, 2015a, 2015b).

During this time, the public (and some funders with no experience in the space) assumed that military family needs would be handled first by the DoD and then by the Department of Veterans Affairs (VA). But it soon became clear that government agencies could not do it alone (Cooke, 2016; Nonprofit Quarterly, 2014; Powers, 2016a). Foundations were called upon by government leaders to help address these military family needs, not only during deployments and separations, but also after the conflicts ended (Wills, 2008). By 2008, service members were coming home to challenging economic scenarios. Many brought with them the visible and invisible wounds of war, including traumatic brain injury, posttraumatic stress disorder (PTSD) and life-changing physical limitations. Between December 2007 and June 2009, the Dow Jones Industrial Average fell 50%, with some of the hardest hit industries being the financial sector, construction, manufacturing, and real estate (Dividend.com, 2016). A seminal period in the philanthropy field had begun. It was a time of opportunity and change.

Philanthropic leaders determined that the only way to address military families' challenges would be through collaboration among funders, charities, and the government (Wills, 2008). However, recognizing the need for collaboration and implementing it were two very different things. Funders and foundations were not quite sure how they could help address the needs of this particular population, and how to weed through the ever-increasing numbers of charitable causes eager to serve. Then, in 2009, the California Community Foundation (CCF) released a report based on lessons learned through its Iraq Afghanistan Deployment Impact Fund, which awarded more than $243 million in grants to 53 nonprofits to meet the needs of men, women, and families affected by deployment to Iraq and Afghanistan. The report identified and explained challenges that military families faced upon reunion and offered advice to grant-makers who wanted to help. Suggestions included tackling issues regionally by collaborations between local government and private organizations to provide a community network of support, especially in places away from bases. Jack Amberg, senior director of the McCormick Foundation's veteran programs and a retired Army officer, explained at the time, "Working together can help foundations perform the critical role of identifying and plugging holes in the charity and government safety nets for veterans," (Blum, 2010).

14.3   Needs of Military-Affiliated Families

As leaders in the philanthropy domain worked to identify some of the most critical needs for military and veteran families, community foundations provided important guidance. They coordinated needs assessments to determine needs in local communities, and from there, larger foundations assessed funding gaps, determined if and when government agencies and others could respond, and prioritized opportunities for engagement. For example, the military's own transition programs were neither robust enough nor flexible enough to meet service member needs, causing unintended difficulties for the very individuals that they hoped to help. Funders began to look for solutions that could be adapted and used in multiple locations, believing that it did little to fund a localized community program that could not be successfully transferred elsewhere. "Our goal was to actually try to influence larger institutions … [by] really designing programs from that perspective" (Long, 2016).

However, foundations lacked a way to assess a global view of the needs of military and veteran families. Each foundation has its own sets of missions and funding priorities, so had to research, document, and understand military and veteran issues in order to best serve these families. Without an overarching understanding about the needs of military-affiliated families—it became difficult to find a strategic path forward. This revealed "the importance of advancing strategic philanthropy—not doing philanthropy that just feels good or charitable philanthropy, but philanthropy where there is either a systems goals or a broader outcome, beyond just an awareness raising campaign or something that's a kind of immediately meeting some needs" (Cooke, 2016). In many instances, foundations that were doing excellent work tackling social problems didn't even know that many of their clients were military connected.

Philanthropic foundations looked for smart intersections between their own missions and the needs of those who were military members, veterans, and their families. For example, foundations associated with the pharmaceutical industry began to focus on health care, while foundations associated with the financial industry focused on employment issues. Those foundations that were associated with behavioral healthcare issues soon recognized that these would be the signature wound of the war, a term first used by RAND Corporation. Like many physical wounds, mental health issues had their own associations with stigma. Researchers have found that there exist "negative stereotypes toward individuals with psychological problems" and that external stigmatization can be coupled with the experience of "self-stigma, leading to reduced self-esteem and motivation to seek help" (Green-Shortridge, Britt, & Castro, 2007). Such stigma can heighten military members' fears that help-seeking behaviors might imperil their job. Foundations thus recognized that they must walk a fine line of advocating for better mental health and creating a climate in which employers shied away from hiring veterans.

Meanwhile, foundations seeking to help with employment and career support began to see that while not all military members experienced transition-related problems, many did have difficulty finding a job and assimilating into the community—in part because many civilian hiring managers had limited understanding of how military skills could translate to the civilian world. "It's a very complex, difficult world to come back where almost nobody really knows what you have done if you've been a soldier or a sailor, because such a small percentage of the population has been in war or in the military," said Donald Cooke, vice president of philanthropy for the Robert R. McCormick Foundation (Cooke, 2016).

It also became clear that some philanthropic organizations needed to be educated about why they should get involved with military-affiliated issues, especially during the early part of this era. An apparent lack of motivation existed among some foundations about why military and veteran families deserved a portion of their philanthropic dollars. These organizations believed it was the government's job to take care of these families and failed to understand the extent to which governmental agencies could offer support. In addition, they did not see the breadth of military connections that existed in the populations they already served. For example, funders of faith-based organizations, healthcare providers, and K-12 education served military-connected families. And the term is very inclusive—families mean mothers, fathers, sisters, cousins, significant others, and grandparents in addition to the traditionally recognized spouse and children. But with so many others needing philanthropic support, these organizations needed convincing that military and veteran families were a good investment (Powers 2015a, 2015b).

14.4 Responses and Strategies: Successes and Challenges

One of the earliest philanthropies to focus efforts on addressing the needs of military families was the Chicago-based Robert R. McCormick Foundation. In 2008, the foundation created a new program aimed at making grants to charities that assisted veterans. It also gathered other grant-makers together to address the regional response in Chicago (Blum, 2010), supporting transitioning veterans in the areas of employment, behavioral health, and coordination of services (Robert R. McCormick Foundation, 2016). By 2015, 57 of its grants (ranging from $3,750 to $600,000) supported a host of community projects, not just in Chicago but in surrounding states as well.

238 L. Hughes-Kirchubel and E.C. Johnson

Certain comprehensive community solutions succeeded in effectively addressing problems that military and veteran families faced. One example, Points of Light's Community Blueprint initiative was a "call to action for communities to unite together, collaborate, and share tools and resources to build stronger communities by serving and engaging service members, veterans, and their families" (Points of Light, 2016). The initiative worked to bridge the civilian-military divide, and aimed to be sustainable over time—an important characteristic of successful philanthropic endeavors. Other community-oriented approaches throughout the country—in places like San Diego, San Antonio, and South Florida—became strong examples of success at the micro-level (Long, 2016). In addition, some funders who worked deeply on single issues such as mental health, drove progress forward over time by developing relationships with a variety of partners. A combination of "a good idea, long-term support and some really strong relationships...has worked very well," said Peter Long, president and CEO of Blue Shield of California Foundation.

Working on a multiplicity of issues, funders helped to change inadequate narratives surrounding military-affiliated families. Got Your 6, the Bristol-Myers Squibb Foundation and other organizations made a concerted effort to replace the "broken veteran" narrative with one that prioritized strength and resilience. "Just because our foundation is focusing on mental health, and we feel there's a need to do so, it does not mean that we're saying that all the veterans are broken," said Catharine Grimes, director of corporate philanthropy at the Bristol-Myers Squibb Foundation. "We're saying that there's very clear data showing that approximately one-third of these veterans are coming back with some pretty significant challenges from a mental health perspective and there is a need and role philanthropy can play for that subset of the veterans who need it" (Grimes, 2016). Organizations began to frame help-seeking behaviors as examples of military and veteran family resiliency and strength. They also worked to retrain the public to think about veterans as a more diverse—and younger—demographic, and to think about the unique needs faced by women veterans in conversations about issues such as education, health care, and financial security. Many programs that used peers to work with targeted groups, such as younger veterans, were also successful.

Working together became the hallmark of initiatives associated with Joining Forces, created in 2011 by First Lady Michelle Obama and Dr. Jill Biden, wife of the Vice President, to mobilize the nation in support of military and veteran families. Joining Forces focused on employment, education, and wellness issues as it aimed to raise the nation's awareness about military-affiliated families, as well as to generate volunteerism, activism, and support. In March 2013, the National Guard launched its own version of the program, Joining Community Forces, which leveraged the strengths of the National Guard—including its location in every single state—to create more supportive communities for military families. The convening power of leadership was important. These related initiatives provided a catalyst for seeing philanthropic opportunities differently. Joining Forces also provided a mechanism for government agencies to engage with funders in a responsible way.

In 2014, four foundations[1] helped to initiate the Philanthropy-Joining Forces Impact Pledge. A grassroots effort, the pledge began with the help of a group of funders that were already working in the veteran/military space. It prioritized collaboration and aimed to mobilize and sustain philanthropic support. At the same time, it encouraged funders to join in order to "strengthen services and support for millions of veterans and military families throughout America" (Council on Foundations, 2014). In the context of the pledge, the Council on Foundations offered input to policy makers as well as the VA, DoD, and White House. In addition, the Council acted as a communicative liaison between NGOs and VSOs that sought philanthropic partners while connecting Council members to new collaborative efforts. There were certainly successes; since its creation, the pledge "has cumulatively resulted in investments of nearly $282 million" in private funds through grants and other forms of support (Council on Foundations 2016a, 2016b). The pledge represents a unique opportunity for philanthropy to focus joint efforts on helping military and veteran families. However, its potential remains unreached, and it remains difficult to convince some to sign on to the pledge if they do not see themselves as military or veteran funders.

Within the philanthropic space, collaboration was a challenge. Nationally, large organizations struggled to work together, identify lessons learned, and then leverage projects for greater impact. It was difficult to clarify and embrace lessons learned, and then replicate the best programs, scaling them up or down as needed. Organizations were doing good work, but largely worked in silos. Though Joining Forces helped to address these challenges, competition for resources was and still is high. For example, in 2016 the Bob Woodward Foundation received more than 500 proposals for $22 million in funding (Carstensen, Director, National Collaboration Initiative, Bob Woodruff Foundation, 2016). On the other end of the spectrum, many small programs "from horse whispering to fly tying" were unsustainable (Cooke, 2016). Faith communities, often expert at attending to the moral wounds of war, struggled to find traction and become part of existing coalitions. Specialized military and veteran communities, such as female veterans, were underserved.

From a philanthropic perspective, other issues became problematic. For example, funding large national organizations that lacked tight community ties and "boots on the ground" relationships created less impact than desired. At best, effectiveness suffered due to organizational distance from its communities; at worst, organizations failed to deliver on commitments. In one instance, the leadership of a large, national organization received critical media attention and two top-level employees were fired after accusations of financial misconduct. For some organizations that lacked capacity to properly absorb the dollars, "overfunding" became problematic (Carstensen, 2016). It was also hard for some community foundations to justify setting aside any significant amount of money for veterans and families when they existed in such small numbers within the wider community. Understanding a potential grant recipient's business model and examining board members' relationships

---

[1] Blue Shield of California Foundation; the Bristol-Myers Squibb Foundation; the Lincoln Community Foundation; the Robert R. McCormick Foundation.

and expertise also provides a window into oversight capacity; so does training grant officers as "subject matter experts" about the population and needs the award is attempting to address (Carstensen, 2016).

Lastly, true partnerships between private foundations and the VA remained a source of untapped potential. Some funders believe this is because VA had to find a way to work through or around its own barriers to such partnerships, which existed within VA's bureaucratic structure as well as within its congressionally mandated policies. Philanthropic leaders believe, however, that it is "only a matter of time" until true public/private philanthropic efforts with the VA emerges. "Hopefully, we will be seeing that in the future," Grimes said. Smaller public/private partnerships are already being forged through community efforts with local VA centers; these are community-based models of success, where the veteran comes home, and "where the community wraps around the veteran" (Cooke, 2016). Finally, building relationship between philanthropy and the VA is key. This will enable both to set outcomes and impact so that both can use funds to leverage change (Carstensen, 2016).

14.5   Evaluation and Lessons Learned

Since Sept. 11, 2001, the philanthropic sector has accomplished much on behalf of military and veteran families; but gaps remain. First, there still exists a gap of national leadership within philanthropy. While many organizations individually have taken leadership roles in the space, and the Council on Foundations has also contributed to the national conversation, it would be erroneous to suggest that nationally, a voice on veteran and military philanthropy exists to help guide the way with respect to new directions, new initiative, and new challenges. This needs to be addressed sooner, rather than later, and especially in advance of future conflicts, crises, or wars.

It is not unusual for foundations to struggle with identifying the demographics of the military and veteran families in the communities the foundations service, often due to the government's privacy constraints. For one thing, veterans don't always self-identify. For another, states that experienced military deployments almost exclusively by National Guard and Reserve units may have military families with unique needs because these families do not live on installations with built-in support structures. Also, privacy issues may make it difficult to identify the kinds of issues these families are facing. Those who deployed to combat zones and whose jobs put them on the front lines may have different challenges when compared to those who deployed to areas that were far removed from the chance of blast injury, IED exposure, or patrols that placed them in direct contact with enemy combatants. Even if service members did not deploy in the traditional sense of the word, they might deal with deployment-related issues (i.e., stateside-based pilots of drones were not exempt from symptoms of PTSD) (Carstensen, 2016). Figuring out how best to serve returning veterans is also complicated by the fact that it is difficult to get details about the kinds of needs unit members may have based on their demographics and family characteristics (Bartle, 2016).

Gaps remain with regard to philanthropic intersections with the very severely wounded, those with mental health issues and, in particular, military-connected suicides. One RAND study states that "at least" 20% of Iraq and Afghanistan veterans are suffering from PTSD and/or depression. "But then there's that really small percentage that are severely wounded…. They really need around-the-clock care," said Grimes. "They really can't live independently." This, and the issue of veteran and military suicide, remains an elusive issue for the philanthropic sector. A related issue is a focus on helping caregivers of the severely injured, whether they are young spouses or aging parents. These individuals—from Baby Boomers to millennials—may be caregivers for decades, with this role affecting their identity, their family structure, and the dreams they had for their future. This "is not fully developed" and philanthropic attention should be paid to these individuals.

Gaps also remained between private foundations and public organizations, especially with regard to creating collaborations that reduced barriers to care. These kinds of partnerships break traditional boundaries, and double each organization's impact. Yet there were knowledge barriers that affected philanthropy's efforts to respond. The difficulties in identifying where veterans lived created barriers to developing strategic investments. Engagement by DoD and VA, coupled with changes to the laws that govern these agencies, can better serve the needs of military and veteran families (Bartle, 2016; Carstensen, 2016; Cooke, 2016; Grimes, 2016; Long, 2016; Powers,2016).

During his tenure as Chairman of the Joint Chiefs, Admiral Mike Mullen repeatedly issued a call for communities of all kinds, including philanthropic organizations, to better collaborate and care for those who serve:

> There is a huge list of needs, growing needs. It cannot be met by the Pentagon. It cannot be met by the VA. It can only be met, I believe, by the community groups throughout the country joined together with the Pentagon and the VA to get it right for those who've sacrificed so much (Van Dahlen, 2011).

The Office of the Joint Chiefs also called on the creation of a strategic plan for philanthropic organizations that helped shape the sector with respect to service of military-affiliated families, an effort that did not come to fruition during the past 15 years, though hope remains high that it still will.

14.6 Recommendations

The purpose of this chapter is to provide guidance to the next generation of philanthropic leaders in the event our nation's military engages in lengthy deployments and faces the stressors associated with combat and family separations. Since 9/11, the philanthropic sector has taken steps to respond to the needs of military and veteran families and continues to do so today. Looking to the future, a number of lessons can be learned from recent experiences. The following recommendations are designed for the next generation of philanthropic leaders, with the understanding that they must be adapted to fit the context and needs of future situations, be they deployments in peacetime or in times of war.

1. *Philanthropic organizations must understand that the populations they serve are infused with military and veteran families already.* Every foundation should be able to pinpoint those clients who have a military affiliation; they do not exist in silos. There is a constant need for vigilance, reflection, and revision, and funders must always be listening to what is being said on the national stage as well as what military and veteran families are saying (Cox, 2017). In a mature philanthropy ecosystem, philanthropic organizations should be vigilant in understanding where they are connected to the military and veteran families. Their thinking, giving, and strategies must be ready to evolve as circumstances change. In this way, funders can respond to families' unique and changing needs within the context of the funder's mission and goals (Cooke, 2016; Cox, 2017; Long, 2016).

2. *Overlay military cultural competence on existing philanthropic services, programs and initiatives.* Even as each philanthropic organization should identify the military and veteran families it serves, so should it examine the usefulness of filtering its services, programs, and initiatives through the military and veteran lens. Issues of poverty, behavioral health care, child welfare, education—these are just a few examples of the many philanthropy focuses that can be filtered through the military and veteran lens, integrating work on their behalf with existing efforts for civilians.

3. *Work to develop true public/private partnerships with the DoD, the VA, and other organizations that serve military and veteran families exclusively at national and local levels.* Philanthropic leaders believe that now is the time to pursue the development of true public/private relationships among and between the DoD, the VA, and philanthropic funders. Leaders in the public sphere appear ready and willing to partner; so do philanthropy leaders. VA has a unique opportunity to lead this charge by transparently partnering at the local level and integrating into local systems when there are opportunities. It remains to be seen whether barriers that have been built into laws, regulations, and bureaucratic processes can be broken down or modified to accomplish this goal. It is crucial to our military families, who represent a mere 1% of the nation's population. The devil is in the details, and it will take time and commitment to hammer out the means to create smooth and effective collaborations.

4. *Scrupulously avoid duplication of projects. Instead, look for ways to augment and complement.* Often, projects were created without examining whether similar ones already existed within the community. Funders should urge their partners to replicate and scale the best, most successful programs using the lessons learned to improve and modify them as necessary. In addition, the philanthropic community should be educated about how best to avoid the overabundance of organizations in a specific area of the space, so that they are not competing for the same resources.

5. *Build and maintain relationships at all levels and develop a national strategy for philanthropic efforts.* Midway through the conflicts, high-level leaders in multiple domains, including philanthropy, met to critically evaluate current work in the military/veteran space, and to set ambitious goals for future work. Known as the White Oak meetings, these gatherings helped to spur collaborations and build relationships, which in turn impacted work on behalf of military families. Future leaders in the philanthropic domain should heed this example as one to be replicated. In addition, create opportunities to convene with policy makers and service providers to increase funders' understanding of challenges. These kinds of meetings are important avenues for creating strategies that are embraced by leadership across multiple domains. They create and sustain a generative space for reflection, goal-setting, and creative collaboration among the highest leaders. Likewise, relationships within philanthropy should be built across national, regional, and local organizations as well as across organizations with divergent foci. Within these contexts, philanthropists should work to set a national strategy behind which all funders could rally.

6. *Prioritize the use of data, evidence-informed practices, and needs assessments to drive deeper understandings of the military and veteran space.* As funders are confronted with multiple demands on their resources, they need to pursue data-driven information to assess priorities and evaluate outcomes. To do so, joining together is key. Working with experts on rigorous evaluation methods is one way to do this; requiring evaluation, needs assessments and use of evidence-informed practices from funding partners is another way. Evidence can help build comprehensive understandings of military and veteran families, their situations and the solutions that are working best; add context and depth; and ensure that funders' dollars are spent on the most effective programs, initiatives, and outcomes. It is crucial to create systems of evaluation and measurement. What, for example, do healthy transitions look like? Bringing researchers together with funders can help identify these and other issues, and while some funders are investing in research to help drive the conversation forward, more should be done to achieve deeper understandings of evolving military and veteran family needs.

14.7 Conclusion

Philanthropy cannot exist in a vacuum, and there is no such thing as a philanthropic effort on its own. Peter Long, president and CEO of Blue Shield of California Foundation put it succinctly: "We have to fund somebody. We have to work with somebody. We have to get ideas from somebody." In creating a battle plan to serve military families, philanthropic leaders must determine how to work effectively within this ecosystem and identify ways to serve military-connected families before new crises emerge.

Cooke, of the Robert R. McCormick Foundation, says there is "room for everybody in philanthropy" to serve military and veteran families (Cooke, 2016). Many of the funders are doing so without knowing that the military affiliated are receiving their services. It starts with military cultural competency, which has been absent in decades past, but now is on the rise. That, Cooke said, may be one of the biggest contributions that current philanthropic leaders have made to the wider philanthropic domain in the past 15 years.

"I think that maybe a great, lasting piece—that the cultural awareness and competency has increased for the decades ahead," Cooke said. "And that would be a great thing."

Acknowledgements Linda Hughes-Kirchubel is director of external relations at the Military Family Research Institute at Purdue University. The Institute is located in the College of Health and Human Science's Department of Human Development and Family Studies. Elizabeth Cline Johnson executive director of public relations and community partnerships at the University of Houston. This research was supported in part by a grant from Lilly Endowment Inc.

We are very grateful to all of the philanthropic leaders who contributed to the preparation of this chapter.

References

Bartle, B. (2016, January 27). President, Lincoln Community Foundation. (L. Hughes-Kirchubel, & E. Johnson, Interviewers).

Belasco, A. (2009). *Troop levels in Afghanistan and Iraq FY2001-FY2012: Cost and other potential issues*. Washington, DC: Congressional Research Service.

Blue Shield of California Foundation. (2016, March 24). *Preventing violence in the homes of military families*. Retrieved from Blue Shield of California Foundation: chrome-extension://oem mndcbldboiebfnladdacbdfmadadm/http://www.blueshieldcafoundation.org/sites/default/files/u9/Preventing_Violence_Military_Families_June_2013.pdf

Blum, D. (2010). Grant makers collaborate to help veterans. *The Chronicle of Philanthropy, 23*(3), 18.

Bob Woodruff Foundation. (2015). *2015 Woodruff Foundation annual report*. New York, NY: Author.

Bob Woodruff Foundation. (2016, March 17). *The Woodruffs' story*. Retrieved from Bob Woodruff Foundation: http://bobwoodrufffoundation.org/woodruff/

Carstensen, M. (2016, October 26). Director, National Collaboration Initiative, Bob Woodruff Foundation. (L. Hughes-Kirchubel, Interviewer).

Cooke, D. (2016, January 27). Senior vice president-philanthropy, the Robert R. McCormick Foundation. (L. H. Hughes-Kirchubel, & E. C. Johnson, Interviewers).

Copeland, J. W., & Sutherland, D. W. (2010). *Sea of goodwill: Matching the donor to the need*. Washington, DC: Joint Chiefs of Staff.

Council on Foundations. (2014, May 2). *Announcing the Philanthropy-Joining Forces Impact Pledge*. Retrieved from cof.org: http://www.cof.org/content/announcing-philanthropy-joining-forces-impact-pledge

Council on Foundations. (2016a). *About the council* . Retrieved from Council on Foundations: http://www.cof.org/about

Council on Foundations. (2016b, April 6). *Supporting veterans and military families*. Retrieved from Council on Foundations: http://www.cof.org/content/supporting-veterans-military-families

Cox, K. (2017). Senior manager, Walmart Giving. (S.M. MacDermid Wadsworth, Interviewer).

Dictionary.com. (2016, March 16). *Philanthropy*. Retrieved from Dictionary.com: http://www.dictionary.com/browse/philanthropy?s=t

Dividend.com. (2016). *The Dow 30: A look into the last five recessions*. Retrieved from Dividend.com: http://www.dividend.com/dividend-education/the-dow-30-a-look-into-the-last-five-recessions/

Forum of Regional Associations and Grantmakers. (2016, March 12). *About us*. Retrieved from The Forum of Regional Associations and Grantmakers: https://www.givingforum.org/about

Green-Shortridge, T. M., Britt, T. W., & Castro, C. A. (2007). The stigma of mental health problems in the military. *Miltary Medicine, 172*, 157–161. https://doi.org/10.7205/MILMED.172.2.157.

Grimes, C. (2016, January 27). Director, corporate philanthropy, Bristol-Myers Squibb Foundation. (L. H. Hughes-Kirchubel, & E. C. Johnson, Interviewers).

Hall, P. (2006). A historical overview of philanthropy, voluntary associations, and nonprofit organizations in the United States, 1600-200. In W. W. Powell & R. Steinberg (Eds.), *The nonprofit sector: A research handbook - Second Edition* (pp. 32–65). Yale University Press.

Hammock, D. C. (2003). Failure and resilience: Pushing the limits in Depression and war. In L. J. Friedman & M. D. McGarvie (Eds.), *Charity, philanthropy and civility in American history* (pp. 263–280). Cambridge, UK: Cambridge University Press.

Long, P. (2016, January 27). President and CEO, Blue Shield of California. (L. Hughes-Kirchubel, & E. Johnson, Interviewers).

Merriam-Webster. (2016, March 16). *Philanthropy*. Retrieved from Merriam-Webster.com: http://www.merriam-webster.com/dictionary/philanthropy

Meyer, T. (2013). In K. Zinsmeister (Ed.), *Serving those who served: A wise giver's guide to assisting veterans and military famliies*. Washington, DC: The Philanthropy Roundtable.

Nonprofit Quarterly. (2014, May 5). *Major foundation initiative for returning veterans unveiled by White House*. Retrieved from Nonprofit Quarterly: https://nonprofitquarterly.org/2014/05/05/major-foundation-initiative-for-returning-veterans-announced-at-white-house/

Points of Light. (2016, April 2). *Community blueprint* . Retrieved from Points of Light: http://survey.clicktools.com/app/survey/response.jsp

Powers, S. (2015a, December 8). Senior director for policy and partnerships, Council on Foundations. (L. Hughes-Kirchubel, & E. C. Johnson, Interviewers).

Powers, S. (2015b, December 15). A battle plan for supporting miltary families: Efforts in the philanthropy domain. (Hughes-Kirchubel, L.H., & E. Johnson, Interviewers).

Renz, L., & Marino, L. (2003). *Giving in the aftermath of 9/11*. New York: The Foundation Center.

Robert R. McCormick Foundation. (2016, March 17). *Veterans program*. Retrieved from McCormick Foundation: http://www.mccormickfoundation.org/veterans

Robin Hood Foundation. (2016, March 23). *Robin Hood Veterans*. Retrieved from Robin Hood Foundation: https://www.robinhood.org/veterans

The National Philanthropic Trust. (2016, March 16). *Philanthropy timeline: The roots of giving*. Retrieved from The National Philanthropic Trust: http://www.nptrust.org/history-of-giving/timeline/roots/

Van Dahlen, B. (2011, May 25). *Keeping faith with our military communiity*. Retrieved from Veterans Advantage: https://www.veteransadvantage.com/va/coverstory/keeping-faith-our-military-community

Wills, D. K. (2008). Charities scramble to provide housing and health care to veterans. *The Chronicle of Philanthropy, 20*(11), 3.

Chapter 15
The White Oak Retreat: Iterative Retreats as a Uniquely Effective Mechanism for Building Consensus and Coordinating Support in the Military Community 2010–2016

Jennifer L. Hurwitz, Cristin Orr Shiffer, and Hisako Sonethavilay

15.1 Context Leading to White Oak

The concept of a collaborative retreat among government and nonprofit actors in support of service members, veterans, and their families emerged following the 2008 election amid a rising consensus in the military and veteran support community that support for the challenges facing the American military in wartime required cross-sector solutions, and the perception that a new president presented an opportunity to engage the new Administration and increase the Commander in Chief's understanding of military family and veteran concerns. No one sector or organization had the ability to identify, organize, and fund solutions to the problems arising as a result of, at that time, nearly 8 years of continuous war in a post-9/11 world. Active duty service members and veterans who had served in Iraq and Afghanistan were returning to their local communities with high and increasing rates of depression, brain injury, and suicide; their families were trying to cope with the disruption of family life by repeated deployments (Berglass, 2010). As the public became more aware of these issues impacting military and veteran families, support for the all-volunteer force and veterans increased substantially. Philanthropic funders, corporate entities, and nonprofit organizations began trying to piece together services within local communities that would meet the growing needs. However, this vast "sea of goodwill" that included more than 40,000 philanthropic organizations across the United States was in need of coordination (Carter & Kidder, 2015) and while recognition of the need for support had increased among national governmental actors such as Congress

J.L. Hurwitz, Ph.D. (✉) • C.O. Shiffer • H. Sonethavilay
Research and Policy Department, Blue Star Families, Encinitas, CA, USA
e-mail: jhurwitz@bluestarfam.org; cristin@bluestarfam.org; hsonethavilay@bluestarfam.org

© Springer International Publishing AG 2018   247
L. Hughes-Kirchubel et al. (eds.), *A Battle Plan for Supporting Military Families*, Risk and Resilience in Military and Veteran Families,
https://doi.org/10.1007/978-3-319-68984-5_15

and the new Obama Administration, identifying and prioritizing ways to provide that support required guidance from the "front lines"—the warfighters, veterans, and their families.

15.2 Background of White Oak

In light of this conclusion, military family and veteran support organization leaders envisioned a candid retreat under Chatham House Rule to incubate creative thinking and collaboration among participants across government, nonprofit, and philanthropic sectors; this is where the story of White Oak begins. In the fall of 2009, with the Obama Administration's transition more firmly in place, deliberation over a renewed Afghanistan engagement or "surge," emerged. A new Afghanistan policy for a new Administration, along with a number of critical assessments of "on the ground" progress suggested that significant American military engagement in Iraq and Afghanistan would be continuing for the foreseeable future—and it also generated interest on developing improved and expanded support for the military and veteran community. Doug Wilson, a leader in the veteran community support space who was also serving as a board member of a large philanthropic foundation, was able to obtain use of one of the foundation's assets, the White Oak Conference Center, and connected with Kathy Roth-Douquet, CEO of Blue Star Families, with the aim of convening a cross-sector retreat that could focus attention on the need for increased military family and veteran support and incubate an effective, collaborative strategy to that end. Together they formed a core team comprised of senior government, nonprofit, and philanthropic leaders to design a conference to bring the required actors together to address the concerns described above. Given that many of the challenges required cross-sector solutions, a retreat-like conference was felt to be the best structure to facilitate the needed coordination. The retreat would bring together public and private sector leaders for a weekend of focused discussions aimed at developing a common agenda without interfering with the ongoing individual efforts being pursued by participants and a date was set for January 2010.

15.3 Importance of Format at White Oak

During his time as executive vice president for policy at the Howard Gilman Foundation, Wilson established the Leaders Project, which brought together innovative, next-generation policy leaders from around the world to discuss global challenges. Using his insights from and experiences with this project, he envisioned a specific format for White Oak.

> I proposed a format that would minimize formal presentations and maximize interactivity, informal discussion, and extracurricular bonding in an environment that was conducive to strengthening personal ties and to listening to each other, rather than talking at each other.

To that end, White Oak participants began a tradition of everyone around the same table; opening with very brief introductions to give all involved a sense of belonging, inclusion, and openness to different approaches for common issues; identifying springboard questions that would frame discussion of the issues to emphasize new and creative thinking rather than "show and tell" presentations; informal dress to reinforce a relaxed atmosphere; breakout sessions to provide venues for more focused discussion and brainstorming of general session discussions; and final report sessions in a very informal atmosphere (couches and chairs in a big lodge) at the end to help foster a sense of productivity and teamwork (Wilson, 2016).

15.4 Historical View of White Oak Responses and Strategies

15.4.1 White Oak I

Although the retreat's formal title was "America Joins Forces with Military Families," the simplified "White Oak" title was, and continues to be, more commonly used. At the inaugural meeting in January 2010, 55 participants from key military family and government organizations convened at White Oak Plantation. The group included both subject matter experts and generalists with considerable impact on the development and implementation of government policies and private sector programs. The retreat was designed to highlight new thinking, develop networks, and update frameworks within which many of those invited were already addressing independently. Individuals at the first White Oak participated in an agenda specifically designed to build cross-sector partnerships in order to foster innovative public–private strategies that would better meet the needs of veteran and military families and establish a common approach moving forward. Three central themes of community, empowerment, and asset mapping structured this agenda at White Oak I.

15.4.2 White Oak II

Throughout White Oak II, participants were buoyed by the progress that was being made at the Federal level and the refocusing of efforts for the military and veteran communities through the Presidential Study Directive-9, Strengthening Our Military Families: Meeting America's Commitment, and Joining Forces[1]; however, participants also recognized that much more needed to be accomplished. The objectives of White Oak II included: (1) continuing to address gaps in military family and veteran support; (2) highlighting areas where the private sector could be more effectively

---

[1] For more information, please refer to Results.

engaged; and (3) exploring ways to reduce competition and overlap while promoting joint efforts toward realizing common goals. Both government and nongovernmental representatives cited miscommunication, confusing messaging, a myriad of barriers to public–private cooperation, and lack of access to military community populations as the main hurdles to collaboration across sectors. Additionally, education, employment, and wellness were discussed as key concerns.

15.4.3   White Oak III

By the time of White Oak III, several of the original White Oak organizers and participants were serving in key positions at the White House, on Congressional staffs, and at the Defense Department. Other participants had established significant collaborative initiatives, yet many new challenges loomed on the horizon. With the majority of combat troops removed from Iraq and Afghanistan, the public's attention to military and veteran issues was waning while at the same time the Department of Defense's (DoD) spending was significantly curtailed due to 2013's Budget Control Act. Amid this financially constrained environment, White Oak III was an important opportunity to evaluate progress and discuss ways to preserve public support.

White Oak III was structured around three objectives: (1) sharing knowledge, perspectives, needs, and opportunities in working for the benefit of military families; (2) creating new relationships and building upon existing ones in support of operational and intellectual partnerships; and (3) achieving consensus in identifying new, scalable "big ideas" that could serve as galvanizing actions moving forward. The following priorities for moving the community forward were established during White Oak III: (1) resource multipliers are needed to counteract declining resources; (2) resource mapping is needed to improve knowledge and delivery of services; (3) decentralized services needed to foster local community integration; and (4) positive messaging to counteract "damaged service members and veterans" narrative and draw attention to the significant contributions military and veteran members bring to the communities in which they live must be an accompanying part of initiatives.

15.4.4   White Oak IV

During White Oak IV, the participants continued their line of forward thinking in the military and veteran community space, while strategizing how to maintain interest and awareness after almost 15 years of war. Three key issues were discussed: collaboration, communication and strategy, and gaps and solutions. Based on these discussions, the following topics were viewed as joint impact areas with collective support and viable solutions: (1) continue to develop shared best practices for funders and their communities; (2) record and maintain data to better prepare for support during future conflicts; (3) formulate a 2016 Government Transition Strategy that presents a nonpartisan, united message of support for military and veteran families; (4) ensure asset mapping for maximum impact; (5) synchronize and align positive messaging; and (6) formalize the White Oak Consortium.

15.4.5   White Oak V

At White Oak V, dialogue and collaboration continued working toward the ultimate goal of providing military members, transitioning veterans, and their families with comprehensive support networks and superior care. Three themes structured the retreat: (1) defining priorities, opportunities, and challenges; (2) improving support through policy, specifically considering retention, the voice of military families, and personnel management; and (3) communicating a collective agenda and strategy to ensure the preservation of the Joining Forces initiative to continue support and partnership with the next administration, not on the basis of politics, but rather on the foundation of bipartisan civic responsibility to serve those who serve our great country.

15.5   Research Methodology and Themes from Participant Interviews

15.5.1   Research Methodology

The research team, consisting of two independent research contractors, used qualitative research methods to conduct interviews, analyze data, and develop themes from White Oak participant interviews (Miles & Huberman, 1994). Qualitative data "often have been advocated as the best strategy for discovery, exploring a new area, and developing hypotheses" (Miles & Huberman, 1994, p. 10) and as such was determined to be the best strategy for a more formal evaluation of the White Oak process. Out of 32 possible White Oak participants identified by the research team in conjunction with Blue Star Families, 19 agreed to be interviewed by phone or by email in August and September 2016. The purpose of the interviews was to explore the White Oak process and gain a better understanding of the outcomes. With five White Oak conferences completed and a new administration on its way into power, the timing seemed well suited for an evaluation. Structured formal interviews using phone or email were based on participant preference. The interview questions were developed by the research team and the same questions were asked of each participant.

Interview Questions

(1) What is your favorite memory or outcome from White Oak? (2) What are some examples of efforts that your organization has been involved in because of your participation in White Oak? (i.e., partnerships, collaborative programs, events, research) (3) What progress that has been made for military families do you believe can be attributed directly to White Oak? (4) Had White Oak not occurred, what progress might have been lost?

   Additionally, respondents had the opportunity to make additional comments if desired; however, specific follow-up questions were not asked.

Qualitative Data Analysis

Following the collection of interview data, interviews were transcribed and entered into a spreadsheet. The qualitative data were imported into NVivo, a Qualitative Data Analysis Software (QDAS), to further assist with data analysis (Bazeley & Jackson, 2013). Designed for applied policy research, Spencer and Ritchie's (2002) framework approach for the qualitative data analysis was employed. The framework provides a structured process that systematically analyzes the qualitative data through a process of five stages: familiarization, identifying a thematic framework, indexing, charting, and mapping and interpretation (Spencer & Ritchie, 2002).

15.5.2   White Oak Themes

Based on the qualitative analysis of the interview responses, three central themes surfaced to provide a clear picture of the White Oak process and how it works to achieve outcomes: (1) harnessing the power of the community; (2) collaborating for maximum impact; and (3) expanding perspective and innovating solutions. Each of these themes will be described in more detail in the following sections.

Harnessing the Power of the Community

Harnessing the power of the community is viewed as a critical element for the White Oak retreats among the interview participants. Six supporting themes illuminated the overarching theme (Fig. 15.1). Participant quotes will be used to illustrate and support the theme.

   First, White Oak provides a safe space for dialogue on key issues facing military and veteran families, face-to-face networking, and an environment where all participants feel respected and welcomed. One respondent reported, "I am very appreciative of the thought that has gone into the invite list…everyone is there with such

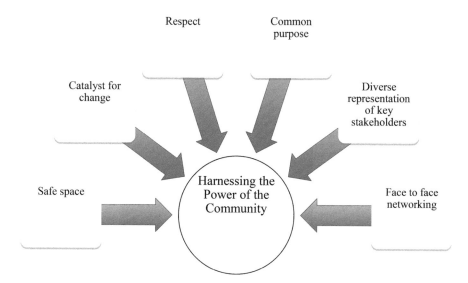

Fig. 15.1 Harnessing the Power of the Community

great intent. The ground rules are very important so everyone has clear expectations and a safe space is created to have tough conversations" (personal communication, September 1, 2016). Another member added, "I entered the 2015 evening reception a complete stranger to all organizers and participants, and I left the function feeling like part of the long-standing team. Everyone was very welcoming…" (personal communication, August 31, 2016).

Moreover, White Oak participants share a common purpose yet diverse representation of key stakeholders is also carefully considered. As one respondent explained,

> I have been to every White Oak, and I feel that its strengths are the diversity of the people asked to join the conversation. It seems there was a concerted effort to ensure all stakeholders were included. For someone who works for the government, it was incredible to hear from people in philanthropy and nonprofits, who all work for a common cause. The diversity was the strength of the conference and made it so successful. (personal communication, August 18, 2016).

White Oak is also a catalyst for change, "Had White Oak not occurred, it would have been years longer before many initiatives like the [U.S. Chamber of Commerce Foundation's] Hiring Our Heroes program, close collaboration with the government offices, or the engagement of the funding community would have taken place…White Oak has served as a catalyst to make things happen quickly" (personal communication, August 17, 2016). Respondents agree that harnessing the power of the community is a key ingredient in making White Oak a process that evoked action.

Collaboration for Maximum Impact

The White Oak participants also cite the importance of collaboration for maximum impact. Six sub-themes provide further support for this primary theme (Fig. 15.2). Statements taken from the participant interviews are utilized to offer insight into how this collaboration works.

The White Oak process is distinctive in that few attempts at military support work on so many levels and across sectors in a collaborative, iterative, retreat process that allows for natural development of relationships. It is "a process by which positive transformation is made possible…a rare blend of national, regional and grassroots efforts working toward the ultimate goal" (White Oak V Summary Report, p. 6). One interview participant emphasizes that the retreat "has been wonderful at building partnerships…it is collaborative, not competitive…people really do follow through and want to work with each other" (personal communication, September 1, 2016). White Oak also carves out the time and environment for "collaboration of people who work together frequently [but] never have the chance to connect reflectively…White Oak establishes side bar conversations that lead to relationship building" (personal communication, August 19, 2016). Moreover, the White Oak retreat and its associated outcomes are "a testament to the power of the private sector to help federal agencies see inefficiencies in duplicative, disparate, and sometimes ineffective programs…to better align programs and services for maximum impact" (personal communication, August 18, 2016). The collaborative opportunities that begin at White Oak and continue after the retreat are viewed by interview participants as critical for achieving timely outcomes and the greatest effect.

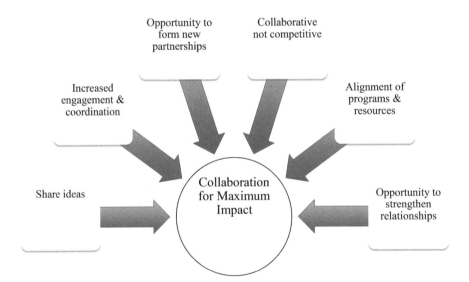

Fig. 15.2 Collaboration for Maximum Impact

Expanding Perspective and Innovating Solutions

Expanding perspective and innovating solutions is the third and final overarching theme developed from the interview transcripts. Again, this theme is illuminated by six supporting themes (Fig. 15.3). Quotes from the interview responses are used to provide further support for the theme.

Participants appreciate the White Oak process because it provides the opportunity to learn from one another. "Access to such a wide array of perspectives taught me more than six months of listening tours…it has greatly expanded my knowledge and perspective" (personal communication, August 17, 2016). Moreover, the retreat is a forum where understanding is shaped, philanthropy is informed, and messaging is focused on the positive. One interview participant explained, "It shaped my understanding of the military person. I had been adding to the narrative of the down and out service member, but I have learned, and we have changed our approach…. it educated us and improved the way we engage in military philanthropy" (personal communication, September 8, 2016). Finally, White Oak provides disparate sectors with a big picture view and the critical inspiration needed for continuing what can be difficult work. "To see what was happening on the national front, as a small local organization, was very helpful" (personal communication, September 7, 2016). Maintaining perspective and feeling inspired can be challenging at times, but White Oak is "powerful and inspirational, and that helps folks who have been in the space for a long time…a little inspiration" (personal communication, August 17, 2016). By expanding perspective and reminding participants of the reasons they initially committed to military family and veteran work, White Oak creates conditions necessary for continuing and innovative support.

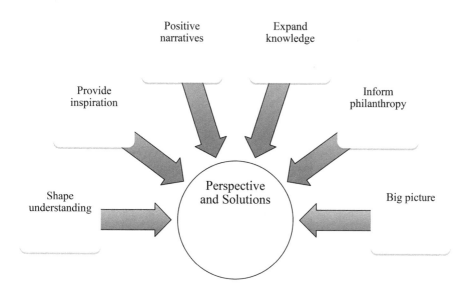

Fig. 15.3 Perspective and Solutions

15.6   Lessons Learned

Examining what has worked well and what could be improved in the White Oak process is crucial after five retreats. A number of participants feel White Oak should be formalized into an annual gathering of key stakeholders. The size of the White Oak gathering is also considered a strength yet a possible limitation to impact. The total number of participants is kept at roughly 70 people each year to foster an intimate experience while significant attention is paid to ensuring the most representative group possible. The smaller forum is perceived as essential for creating an environment conducive to building the necessary trust through small group discussion and development of personal relationships. Moreover, participants indicate that the use of the Chatham House Rule for non-attribution is critical to the success of the retreats. This confidentiality has allowed participants to share openly; by stepping out of their organizational paradigms, discussions among cross-sector participants are candid and a myriad of solutions to frequently politically contentious problems are more earnestly considered. It also allows military family and veteran support actors to build personal networks through which they are able to share information from their respective sectors and organizations, thus advancing the collaboration necessary to successfully address military family and veteran support.

Institutionalizing a process like White Oak provides the military and veteran family support community with a venue where individual relationships are created, nurtured, and mature in the form of collaborative partnerships and cross-sector solutions. In the retreat format, participants commit to a dedicated 2-day period, making them more likely to shed organizational paradigms which tend to favor competition for scarce resources in the military and family support space, they are better able to evaluate the problem as it is, rather than as they would like it to be. This type of environment facilitates interaction among individuals who would not normally find themselves in the same space to develop a mutual understanding without institutional pressure or explicit support.

A future White Oak process would benefit from increased institutionalization should it bring more reliable funding and a commitment among key organizations to collaborate on the event planning, attendee selection, and topic selection working groups. Independent and reliable funding would also reduce the risk of disproportionate influence from individual sectors or organizations. The retreat is only one weekend; time is precious and effective planning is critical. Further success is likely to be achieved through development of working groups who continue collaboration efforts throughout the year. Topic areas found to be most challenging and in need of continual, rather than ad hoc attention include: post-traumatic stress, military spouse employment, modernizing defense personnel policy, government integration and support, increasing morale and resilience during deployments, and caregiver support.

15.7   Results

White Oak provides a unique forum where participants can harness the power of the community, collaborate for maximum impact, and expand their perspective while innovating solutions. The genesis of ideas takes root at White Oak and grows through post-convening interactions. Five key achievements resulted from the first five White Oak retreats and should be considered as crucial steps for support during a future large-scale military conflict.

15.7.1   *Presidential Study Directive-9 (2010)*

White Oak I participants contributed research that prompted action resulting in the Presidential Study Directive (PSD-9), titled Strengthening Our Military Families: Meeting America's Commitment. The policy focused the Federal approach to supporting military families to ensure that government agencies and organizations worked collaboratively. This directive facilitated a "Whole of Government" approach to military family support that will be a critical early step in obtaining federal government support in future wars. For example, the DoD's Military Spouse Employment Program was created, an outdated and ineffective Transition Assistance Program was updated and expanded to include the needs of transitioning military spouses, coordination and information sharing when possible between the DoD, the Department of Labor, and the VA was prioritized, and the Defense State Liaison Office undertook an examination of state-specific legislative fixes in support of military families and transitioning veteran families.

15.7.2   *Joining Forces (2011)*

The First Lady Michelle Obama and Dr. Jill Biden developed the "Joining Forces" initiative to raise awareness and channel support for military members, veterans, and their families among the American public. White Oak participants recognized the need for a "bully pulpit" in educating and engaging the broader U.S. society about the nature and challenges the armed services face during wartime. The prioritization of military and veteran support via the First Lady's office and the Joining Forces initiative also served to galvanize the DoD to increase military family support and quantify progress, as success metrics were reported back to the East Wing. Hearing the First Lady and Dr. Biden prioritize military and veteran issues opened doors to increased funding and in kind support from major philanthropic foundations, corporate America and other sectors not traditionally involved, but critically needed, in military and veteran support.

White Oak retreats provided a "crash course" on military cultural competency, educating and engaging some of these non-traditional actors whose resources and ideas were extremely helpful to the military and veteran support community. The retreat setting enabled both more formal research briefs and more informal community input that provided guidance, real world context, and feedback that supported the crucial Executive branch Joining Forces efforts. For example, identifying the need for a national dialogue about the skills, value, and service of military personnel and their families as a method to increase public awareness of the positive role military families play in their communities was initiated at White Oak.

15.7.3 Community Blueprint (2012)

Engaging local communities is central to ensuring support for military and veteran families during future conflicts. The first two White Oak retreats led to the Community Blueprint: a program that emphasizes local grassroots level action where community leaders and military families work together toward positive change. Military families will all eventually become civilian families; as such civilian communities need to be understood as the first and best line of support as the most important resources used by military and veteran families tend to be located at the local and state level. Early state and local integration and collaboration with the Departments of Defense, Labor, and Veterans Affairs is critical to successful support in future wartime.

15.7.4 Non-Governmental Organization Consortium

Future military and veteran support initiatives should consider the benefit of a voluntary consortium of veteran and military family nonprofits. The United Kingdom's British Confederation of Service Charities (COBSEO) served as one example along with similar institutions. A DoD policy memorandum signed by the Secretary of Defense in 2015 was designed to ensure smooth pathways for nonprofits' provision of benefits or assistance to active duty members and their families on military installations, and further steps are required to ensure nonprofit organizations are able to reach military families.

15.7.5 Philanthropy-Joining Forces Impact Pledge (2014)

The philanthropic community must be educated and included early in future wartime. The landmark Philanthropy-Joining Forces pledge initiated by Blue Shield of California Foundation, the Bristol-Myers Squibb Foundation, the Lincoln Community Foundation, and the Robert R. McCormick Foundation united the philanthropic community in prioritizing and providing funding for programs supporting service members, veterans, and their families. The Council on Foundations took leadership for the pledge and developed the Veterans Philanthropy Exchange to share resources and data and encourage smart, collaborative funding in the military family and veteran landscape. This structure or one similar must be nurtured and maintained so that the philanthropic community is able to respond early during future large-scale national conflict.

15.8   White Oak Themes in Context

Additional collaborations and projects found their genesis in the White Oak retreats; three examples of collaborative efforts will be discussed to illustrate the interview themes in context and demonstrate how White Oak participants addressed specific areas of need. These examples could be used to inform collaboration during future wartime. However, new wars will bring new problems; thus, new solutions may need to be developed also.

15.8.1   *Harnessing the Power of the Community to Increase Community-Level Engagement*

White Oak participants benefit from a diverse representation of key stakeholders; government representatives along with veterans' service organizations, military service organizations, and other nonprofits use the White Oak retreat as a catalyst for change. For this example, community-level engagement is used to provide context. A number of resources and support programs do not always need to be done by the DoD or the VA. They are frequently already performed by local organizations, so it is not always necessary to replicate support programs already offered outside of the installation. However, the responsibility for ensuring cultural competency and connecting military families to these community resources is critical to their success and should remain with the DoD and the VA. White Oak participants understood the need for increased community-level engagement, which led to the idea for and formation of Vets' Community Connections, a community-based initiative focused on supporting veteran reintegration, which has led to relationships with San Diego 2-1-1, Vista, Salesforce, and the Chamber of Commerce, as well as a partnership with the National Association of Counties.

15.8.2   *Collaborating for Maximum Impact Through Coordinated Philanthropy*

As mentioned at the beginning of this chapter, before White Oak began, philanthropic funders, corporate entities, and nonprofit organizations were struggling as they tried to coordinate efforts and piece together support services within local communities for military and veteran families. White Oak provided the opportunity to assess the "sea of goodwill" that included more than 40,000 philanthropic organizations and to discuss methods for better coordination. The "Spouseforce" program, a partnership between Blue Star Families and the Clinton Foundation's Health Matters Initiative, is one example that could be used as a future model. Salesforce, a cloud-based technology company, donated the training for "Spouseforce," while the Walmart Foundation provided programmatic funding, and San Diego 2-1-1 offered to host the "Spouseforce" classes. By providing the time to share ideas and the opportunity for discussions of possible partnerships, White Oak has started paving the way to more coordinated philanthropic efforts that will benefit military and veteran families.

15.8.3 Expanding Perspective and Innovating Solutions for Military Spouse Employment

Military families are less likely to field two incomes than average U.S. families and the majority of military spouses want and need to work (Blue Star Families, 2014; U.S. Department of Labor, 2016). Employed military spouses also appear to experience less distress than their counterparts who do not work (Blue Star Families, 2015). In recognition of this, the expansion of the U.S. Chamber of Commerce Foundation's Hiring Our Heroes program to include military spouses was also explored at White Oak and launched in 2011. This program hosts hiring and networking events across the country throughout the year and continues to grow and address military spouse employment issues. Without White Oak, the expansion of the Hiring Our Heroes program to include military spouses may not have happened, or at least it would not have happened as quickly; the inclusion of military spouses occurred due to White Oak participants shaping the understanding of military spouse employment challenges.

15.9 General Recommendations

Much has been accomplished since the first White Oak in 2010; however, focus must be maintained in order to preserve the results achieved. With every new administration, new priorities arise, and attention given to veteran and military families can decrease in times of perceived peace. The White Oak process has illustrated the need for continuous cross-sector, multi-organizational relationship building to collectively support America's military and veteran communities. If participants work together regularly, we create the opportunity for programs and services to be in place to meet the needs of veteran and military families. Thus, when the next war happens, the hope is that there will not be a need to build services from square one or recreate programs.

Another area that will benefit from continued focus is positive, shared messaging. White Oak participants have strived to coordinate messaging, but more work needs to be done. With a unified and representative voice, there will be more opportunities to influence policy on the national stage and shape understanding for philanthropic efforts.

Going forward, White Oak participants and those seeking to learn from the White Oak process could consider the value of identifying communities where veteran and military families are integrating with less difficulty. These communities could be used as models when developing additional programs and services. In order to further reduce the civilian-military divide, focused education regarding the value of veteran and military families in local communities should be encouraged. By garnering the investment of local entities in the integration process, programs will have a greater chance of success.

15.10   Conclusion

This chapter has provided the background of White Oak, a historical view of responses and strategies employed, a discussion of the themes developed from participant interviews, a review of lessons learned and results achieved, and recommendations to consider for the future. The White Oak process has led to coordination of national, regional, and grassroots efforts focused on providing beneficial programs and services to veteran and military families. White Oak participants understand that their voice is more likely to resonate and be heard when they present a unified message. As one interview participant articulated, "The issues and challenges have to be approached from a holistic perspective, and having a group with expertise in so many areas where there is need, working together towards common solutions, is critical" (personal communication, August 17, 2016).

References

Bazeley, P., & Jackson, K. (Eds.). (2013). *Qualitative data analysis with NVivo*. Thousand Oaks, CA: Sage Publications Limited.

Berglass, N. (2010). *America's duty: The imperative of a new approach to warrior and Veteran care*. Center for a New American Security. Retrieved from https://s3.amazonaws.com/files.cnas.org/documents/CNAS_AmericasDuty_Berglass_0.pdf

Blue Star Families, Department of Research and Policy. (2014). *2014 Military Family Lifestyle Survey Comprehensive Report*. Washington, DC. Retrieved from https://www.scribd.com/document/239928121/Blue-Star-Families-2014-Military-Family-Lifestyle-Survey-Comprehensive-Report

Blue Star Families, Department of Research and Policy. (2015). *2015 Military Family Lifestyle Survey Comprehensive Report*. Washington, DC. Retrieved from https://bluestarfam.org/wp-content/uploads/2016/04/bsf_2015_comprehensive_report.pdf

Carter, P., & Kidder, K. (2015). *Charting the Sea of Goodwill*. Center for a New American Security. Retrieved from https://s3.amazonaws.com/files.cnas.org/documents/VeteransPhilanthropy_151207_rev.pdf

Miles, M. B., & Huberman, A. M. (1994). *Qualitative data analysis: An expanded sourcebook*. Thousand Oaks: Sage Publications.

Spencer, L., & Ritchie, J. (2002). Qualitative data analysis for applied policy research. In A. Michael Huberman & M. B. Miles (Eds.), *The Qualitative Researcher's Companion*. Thousand Oaks, CA: Sage Publications.

U.S. Department of Labor. (2016). *Labor Force Statistics from the Current Population Survey*. Bureau of Labor Statistics. Retrieved from http://www.bls.gov/web/empsit/cpseea10.htm

Wilson, D. (2016). Personal communication of August 18.

Part IV
Knowledge Generation and Dissemination

Chapter 16
Lessons Learned and Future Recommendations for Conducting Research with Military Children and Families

Stephen J. Cozza, Leanne K. Knobloch, Abigail H. Gewirtz, Ellen R. DeVoe, Lisa A. Gorman, Eric M. Flake, Patricia E. Lester, Michelle R. Kees, and Richard M. Lerner

16.1 Background

The recent wars in Iraq and Afghanistan ushered in a period of heightened, near continuous stress for military communities. As a result, at no other time has there been such an opportunity and responsibility to understand the challenges faced by military children and families in order to better meet their needs. Prior to the start of combat operations in 2001, the scientific knowledge base about the impact of wartime service on children was extremely limited. It included less than 10 peer reviewed publications. Providers, senior leaders, and policymakers had to rely on outdated or limited research based on dissimilar populations (such as research on Vietnam era veterans with posttraumatic stress disorder (PTSD) and their families, and civilian traumatic brain injury (TBI)). Systems of care, both military health care facilities and community support programs, had not been developed to support a

S.J. Cozza, M.D. (✉)
Center for the Study of Traumatic Stress, Department of Psychiatry, Uniformed Services University of the Health Sciences, Bethesda, MD, USA
e-mail: stephen.cozza@usuhs.edu

L.K. Knobloch, Ph.D.
Department of Communication, University of Illinois, Urbana, IL, USA
e-mail: knobl@illinois.edu

A.H. Gewirtz, Ph.D.
Department of Family Social Science & Institute of Child Development, & Institute for Translational Research in Children's Mental Health, University of Minnesota, St Paul, MN, USA
e-mail: agewirtz@umn.edu

E.R. DeVoe, Ph.D.
School of Social Work, Boston University, Boston, MA, USA
e-mail: edevoe@bu.edu

© Springer International Publishing AG 2018
L. Hughes-Kirchubel et al. (eds.), *A Battle Plan for Supporting Military Families*, Risk and Resilience in Military and Veteran Families,
https://doi.org/10.1007/978-3-319-68984-5_16

highly stressed population of families facing combat-related challenges. Existing services were characterized by general child psychiatry evaluation and treatment (provided by military treatment facilities (MTFs) or by TRICARE-funded civilian health care) and general child social service programs or universal prevention efforts. There was no system in place for comprehensive screening, early identification, or prevention programs for an all-volunteer, professional military with large numbers of dependent spouses and children engaged in a sustained war.

A broad range of individuals and organizations, both within and outside of the military, worked together in common interest to address the needs of this unique population. Key players included military and civilian health care providers (e.g., pediatricians and family physicians), behavioral health specialists (e.g., child and adult psychiatrists, psychologists, and social workers), and military community support professionals (e.g., chaplains, New Parent Support Program providers, Family Advocacy Program providers, and Military Family Life Counselors). Professional organizations (e.g., American Academy of Pediatrics, American Academy of Child and Adolescent Psychiatry, American Psychiatric Association, American Psychological Association, National Association of Social Workers) educated their members, developing both the interest and capacity of these professional disciplines to support military children and families. Other invested entities included senior military commanders, congressional leaders, the White House Joining Forces program, federal and state agencies (e.g., the Substance Abuse and Mental Health Services Administration (SAMHSA), its National Child Traumatic Stress Network (NCTSN), and the Department of Education (DoE)), consulting firms and think tanks, policymakers, military family support organizations (e.g., National Military Family Association, Military Child Education Coalition, Blue Star Families, Tragedy Assistance Program for Survivors), other not for profit and non-governmental organizations (e.g., Sesame Workshop, Zero to Three), as well as military families themselves.

L.A. Gorman, Ph.D.
Michigan Public Health Institute, Okemos, MI, USA
e-mail: lgorman@mphi.org

E.M. Flake, M.D.
Developmental Pediatrics, Madigan Army Medical Center, Tacoma, WA, USA
e-mail: eric.m.flake2.mil@mail.mil

P.E. Lester, M.D.
Nathanson Family Resilience Center, University of California Los Angeles,
Los Angeles, CA, USA
e-mail: plester@mednet.ucla.edu

M.R. Kees, Ph.D.
Military Support Programs and Networks, Department of Psychiatry, University of Michigan,
Ann Arbor, MI, USA
e-mail: mkees@umich.edu

R.M. Lerner, Ph.D.
Institute for Applied Research in Youth Development, Tufts University, Medford, MA, USA
e-mail: richard.lerner@tufts.edu

Critical to this community response were the roles of scientists and researchers, whose major goals included the development and dissemination of knowledge to support military children and families. Early in the war, the research task involved playing "catch up" in understanding how best to sustain the health of a distressed population of military families facing the consequences of repeated combat deployments. Family exposures included extended deployment separations, reintegration challenges, combat-related physical and mental health conditions and, in rare circumstances, service member death. Scientists from public and private agencies, federal institutions, and higher education joined this community of professionals to bring the most effective science to policy and practice. Researchers played critical roles in educating the clinical and support community by translating existing studies of civilian populations and by informing and refining the methodology of research needed to fill in the gaps in science in order to inform and expand evidence-based practice. In fact, the partnerships that evolved between military and civilian academic researchers, clinicians, families, and leadership have arguably been the greatest accomplishment of the last 10 years in advancing the health of military families. Despite these advances, there continue to be challenges to conducting high-quality research with military children and families, and many scientific questions remain. The remainder of this chapter focuses on historical perspectives related to research on military children and families, challenges faced by researchers, strategies that support successful research, and a summary of lessons learned and future recommendations for researchers, military leaders, policymakers, and funders in anticipation of future combat operations.

16.2 Historical Events

The general public, as well as the scientific community, became increasingly interested in the health and well-being of the children and families of military service members after the start of combat operations in Iraq and Afghanistan. However, well-intentioned interest was commonly affected by media reports that told only one side of the story—vulnerable military families were suffering. Conclusions were drawn due to misinterpretation and bias based upon a lack of understanding of the military community or a stereotyped, rather than a nuanced, perception of this heterogeneous population (Cozza, Chun, & Polo, 2005). In fact, prior peacetime studies had shown that military children functioned comparably to their civilian counterparts. Several existing studies had examined the impact of parental deployment on military children during Operation Desert Storm (ODS), a conflict that was relatively short lived and resulted in few casualties and deaths. While moderate increases in internalizing and externalizing symptoms were noted in children whose parents were deployed to combat areas (Rosen, Teitelbaum, & Wethuis, 1993), those children rarely required clinical attention and those who did were more likely to have a past history of mental health treatment (Rosen et al., 1993). It remained to be seen how the more recent highly stressful and diverse war experiences would variably impact children and families.

The challenge of war presented several conditions (e.g., lengthy and repeated deployments, prolonged period of war, resultant combat-related physical and psychiatric illnesses) that created inherently novel scientific questions for collaborative study and planning. A new level of connection for families to the front lines modified the context of combat deployments. The Internet and cellular telephone service made it feasible to maintain daily contact between service members and their families, resulting in both positive and negative consequences for families and mission readiness.

Over the past several decades, a robust civilian research base on developmental systems, resilience, traumatic stress, and family-based prevention science has developed to help inform planning and guide research questions and opportunities (Cozza & Lerner, 2013a), but scant efforts had been made to apply this knowledge to the military community prior to 2001. To what degree would these findings from the civilian community apply to the military population? In addition to basic understanding of community responses to war, the adaptation and testing of empirically supported interventions for military children and families became a major task of the last decade.

16.3 Challenges

The recent period of combat deployments revealed significant challenges to conducting research with military children and families, which are described below.

16.3.1 Structural Challenges to Research

Multiple structural barriers have slowed the field in effectively conducting research. For example, regulatory policies often required that research protocols be reviewed and approved by multiple institutional review boards (IRBs), both within the DoD, as well as civilian academic institutions. Since DoD—civilian university collaborative efforts were relatively new, there were few satisfactory models for collaborative or partnering studies. As IRBs are autonomous agencies, differences of opinion between IRBs were not uncommon. But there were few mechanisms for resolving these disagreements, placing research scientists in the difficult position of arbitrating satisfactory solutions, slowing the research process. In addition to institutional IRB reviews, DoD-funded research required second-level regulatory review that added time to protocol approval. Moreover, at the start of the war, military IRBs had less experience than their civilian academic counterparts with protocols involving children, and were often hamstrung by more stringent federal regulations governing research with children, making the progress of protocol acceptance even more cumbersome.

16.3.2   Challenges Related to Wartime Research

The nature of war, similar to disaster scenarios, creates a highly dynamic environment, making it challenging to conduct "just-in-time," responsive research. At the start of the war, military leadership was challenged with rolling out evidence-based programs to respond to the evolving needs of military families. Whereas civilian models were available to help inform planning and to guide research questions and opportunities, little research had been conducted testing these programs with military families. The adaptation and testing of empirically supported interventions became a major task of the last decade, creating a constant tension between an urgency to gather rigorous evidence and a pressure to offer solutions to the community. In addition, research funding and regulatory procedures lacked the ability to flexibly respond to evolving needs in this dynamic environment. One author (SC) related his example of a comprehensive intervention trial funded by DoD entitled FOCUS-CI (a refinement of the FOCUS program—see below—for combat injured families) that intended to recruit combat injured families from two large DoD medical centers. Changes in the constellation and numbers of combat injured families during the grant period made it necessary to make changes to the original DoD grant statement of work and the research protocol. Given the inability of regulatory agencies to rapidly make these required changes, the population of injured families dwindled, recruitment became untenable, and the study was prematurely closed before the intervention could be adequately tested.

16.3.3   Challenges Engaging Military Communities

Other research challenges were related to difficulties in engaging the military family population. Cultural differences existed between civilian researchers and military organizations and personnel. Even though most civilian researchers were sensitive to military cultural uniqueness, experience with and understanding of the population required time. Military populations not infrequently harbored distrust of researchers' (both military and civilian) motivations or questioned their perceptions of military family life (e.g., "they see us as victims rather than as serving by choice."). In addition, commanders were not always comfortable with the scientific method, particularly when their interest was to provide programs to support their families. As a result, installation culture viewed control conditions as unacceptable alternatives to experimental conditions, and randomized control trials (RCTs) were viewed skeptically by military partners. It became far more acceptable to conduct RCTs (e.g., After Deployment: Adaptive Parenting Tools/ADAPT, Families OverComing Under Stress—Early Childhood/FOCUS-EC, Strong Bonds, and Strong Families Strong Forces) in civilian-dwelling military populations rather than through on-installation trials, limiting access to research populations and slowing science that could support evidence-based programs. Of note, most federally (i.e.,

National Institutes of Health/NIH) funded research with military children and families has been conducted in civilian-dwelling military populations rather than those living on installations. These populations are not equivalent in their demographics, structure, or needs, to installation-based military families.

16.3.4 Challenges Related to Military Population Mobility

Although the military is often viewed as a monolithic and unchanging organization, it is quite dynamic in both its composition as well as geographic locations. Approximately 11% of active duty service members leave the military each year, either through retirement or expiration of term of service (ETS). In addition, National Guard (NG) and reserve service members typically activate for periods of 4–12 months, after which they deactivate for unspecified periods of time and return to their civilian homes and jobs. Even when service members remain in the active duty, they and their families incur routine residential moves, or permanent changes of station (PCS), every 2–4 years to installations both within and outside of the continental US. As a result, military families are a highly transient population, moving from active to veteran status and from one geographic location to another, making involvement in research challenging. Family transitions are also greatly impacted by the deployments of a partner/parent, during which up to 50% of families choose to relocate in proximity to extended families (Flake, Davis, Johnson, & Middleton, 2009).

Rapid transitions among military personnel can result in a lack of continuity in research, especially in longitudinal studies or intervention trials. Service or veteran families affected by combat injury, combat-related psychiatric illness (e.g., PTSD), or service member death may be particularly hard to reach. Ethnic minority families, non-English speaking families, or single parent families pose additional recruitment and retention challenges. Changes in authorities (e.g., commanders) who partner with researchers in support of scientific studies can also complicate study completion. After a change of command, the new commander may be hesitant or unwilling to support the research agenda that was developed in collaboration with the prior commander.

16.3.5 Funding Challenges

It remains unclear to what degree funding for research focusing on military children and families will be sustained, especially as combat deployment tempo decreases. Beginning in 2002, the DoD supported several studies of military children and families. Although such funding continues, it is unclear to what degree the DoD will continue to support family research in the future. Alternate sources of funding are critically important. Early in the war, non-DoD federal funding (e.g., Institutes within the NIH, such as National Institute on Drug Abuse/NIDA, National Institute of Child Health and Development/NICHD, and National Center for Complementary and Integrative Health/NCCIH) of projects was less robust for several reasons. First, many such agencies did not have military children and families "on their radar." They may have considered military family health concerns as the responsibility of the DoD, reserving their own agency funding for research relevant to the broader health needs of the nation's children. In addition, early answers to questions about the impact of parental deployment on children were not adequately substantial to support the need for intervention trials. Furthermore, military cultural and systems issues that are difficult for civilian scientific review panels to appreciate may have reduced the number of funded applications in this area.

More recently, active collaborations have emerged across federal funding agencies to focus on military children. For example, the Substance Abuse and Mental Health Services Administration's/SAMHSA's National Child Traumatic Stress Network/NCTSN has added military communities as a population of interest, and has partnered with the DoD (e.g., DoD's Military Community and Family Policy office and the Uniformed Services University of the Health Sciences/USUHS Center for the Study of Traumatic Stress) to highlight military family needs, and to bring evidence-based trauma-focused efforts to the DoD. In addition, since 2014, DoD and NIH have been collaborating to develop joint portfolios of military family research and have convened NIH and DoD-funded researchers to present in-progress reviews of their projects. The NCCIH Council Working Group Report, *Strengthening Collaborations with the U.S. Department of Defense and U.S. Department of Veterans Affairs: Effectiveness Research on Mind and Body Interventions* (https:// nccih.nih.gov/about/naccih/military-report)), provides another example of a cross-agency federal effort. Despite progress, military child and family research would still benefit from the development of a broad and coordinated federally funded portfolio.

16.4 Responses, Strategies, and Scenarios

16.4.1 Collaborative Relationships

Several strategies have contributed to successful research outcomes with military and veteran families. Most importantly, active networking among scientific and military professionals allowed researchers to develop understanding of populations-of-interest, gain access to study samples, and develop mechanisms of funding to support research, ultimately producing collaborative research opportunities. As an example, one author (LG) described how the University of Michigan (UM) joined with Michigan State University and the Michigan National Guard in 2008 through a UM affiliated philanthropic opportunity. The philanthropist's initiative, **Welcome Back Veterans**, sought to involve the general population in a nationwide campaign to support Centers of Excellence in developing and providing services for returning OIF and OEF veterans. UM brought additional clinicians and researchers to the project, ensuring a robust clinical and research opportunity (Dalack et al., 2010).

Other partnerships between research scientists at civilian universities and military organizations were similarly fruitful. Another author (PL), a UCLA expert in the area of family prevention research, partnered with senior program managers in the Department of the Navy to develop and implement a military family resilience program to support Navy and Marine Corps families who were challenged with ongoing deployments and military life transitions. Families OverComing Under Stress (project FOCUS) incorporated existing family resilience science from evidence-based preventive interventions that had been conducted with families managing parental depression and HIV. Researchers successfully adapted and implemented this work for at-risk military families. Program data evidenced positive effects for family members (Lester et al., 2016) and, as a result, FOCUS has now been incorporated as part of family support programming across the DoD. Program success led to NICHD funding for an RCT of FOCUS-Early Childhood (FOCUS-EC), a study of FOCUS in military families with younger children.

In collaboration with the Minnesota National Guard (MN NG), another author (AG) developed and tested a group-based parenting program: After Deployment: Adaptive Parenting Tools (ADAPT) for NG and reserve families (Gewirtz, Pinna, Hanson, & Brockberg, 2014). ADAPT is based on social interaction learning theory and draws from family stress models; the program is an adaptation of the evidence-based parent management training-Oregon model. NIH (NIDA) funded a randomized controlled trial of the program, and results indicated that ADAPT was effective in improving observed and reported parenting, and in reducing child behavioral and emotional problems (by parent, teacher, and child report; Gewirtz, DeGarmo, & Zamir, 2017). Moreover, improvements in parenting self-efficacy as a result of the program led to reductions in parents' own depression, PTSD symptoms, and suicidality (Gewirtz, DeGarmo, & Zamir, 2016) as well as improvements in children's peer adjustment (Piehler, Ausherbauer, Gewirtz, & Gliske, 2016). These findings have resulted in two subsequent DoD-funded studies, one of which, ADAPT4U, compares three different versions of the ADAPT program including an online-only program format, as well as a virtual interaction (telehealth) option so that the program will be able to reach families who are unable to travel to a group program. A recently funded study will extend ADAPT for active duty service members, including Special Operations personnel, who continue to deploy frequently. Both the MN NG and active duty components have requested broader implementation of the ADAPT program for military families. Both the FOCUS and ADAPT programs demonstrate the success of partnered studies conducted by established researchers utilizing multiple funding options to promote long-term programs of research in military families.

16.4.2 Community-Based "Grassroots" Efforts

The application of grassroots, community-based methods in research design for military populations represents an important innovation for military-related research. But, there is a need for more "out of the box" thinking to address sustainability and implementation issues. Such community-based methods incorporate active communication and engagement with supportive commanders, as well as military family service recipients. Successful researchers provided ongoing consultation to commanders and their staff, as well as education, outreach, and other support services for military families, making recruitment more successful. In developing Strong Families Strong Forces, a family-based reintegration program, another author (ED) described an effective "bottom up" community-based approach that was very successful for engagement and outreach in military families with young children. The study team used a home-based approach for all research and intervention sessions—which resulted in very low no-show/missed appointments and high dose of intervention. Findings from the first efficacy trial of Strong Families were promising with reductions in service member parent distress and parenting stress (DeVoe, Paris, Emmert-Aronson, Ross, & Acker, 2016). With additional DoD funding, this author has partnered with the STRONG STAR Consortium at Ft. Hood Army installation to conduct a second RCT assessing Strong Families with active duty families with upcoming deployments.

This same author also stated that their project was highly subscribed by families interested in participating in Strong Families Strong Forces (Ross & DeVoe, 2014). However, families not eligible for their research study were unable to be offered programmatic support. Given the magnitude of need in some populations of military families (especially in the first years of the war), researchers were sometimes challenged by maintaining positive engagement with communities while conducting their studies. The NG placed a greater priority on providing programs to their populations-in-need, rather than focusing on science.

Researchers in Michigan faced similar challenges. Early in the war, the National Guard recognized the need for additional supports and reintegration programs but did not have the resources in family programs to support the operational tempo. Between 2006 and 2008, faculty and doctoral students from Michigan State University volunteered hundreds if not thousands of hours to address existing needs. Often, research was of secondary interest to military communities, making evaluation of programs difficult, if not impossible. The use of a randomized control group was largely unacceptable in these circumstances.

16.5 Results

16.5.1 Embracing Quality Methodology

A recent edition of the Princeton University and Brookings Institution's *Future of Children* series reviewed the evidence base regarding military children and families (Cozza & Lerner, 2013a). There have been several limitations of existing scientific studies of military children and families. For example, most studies have employed small convenience samples, groups of easily accessible people who volunteer their participation, but who may not be representative of the broader population. In addition, most studies have focused on children's deficits rather than their strengths. Research on the development of military children that focuses on the potential risks of a parent's deployment to their well-being does not describe how these experiences can also contribute to strength and resilience in facing such challenging circumstances. Approaches that move beyond military children's purported deficits to recognize and examine the broad impacts of both challenges as well as strengths in military children, families, and communities are required. Moreover, researchers have yet to fully identify and assess the resources for positive development that exist in these children's families, in their schools, in the military, and in their civilian communities. Existing reports of military children and families offer only a limited depiction across their respective life courses, and certainly not a representative one (Cozza & Lerner, 2013b).

16.5.2 Suggested Research Strategies

Chandra and London (2013) reviewed several strategies to advance research on military children and provide a more comprehensive picture of their strengths, vulnerabilities, and responses to challenging circumstances in a broader and more representative fashion. They suggest that three types of data could help researchers examine military children's health, cognitive and academic development, and social and emotional well-being: large national surveys, administrative records, and smaller studies that focus on unique populations or circumstances.

The National Survey of Children's Health and the National Education Longitudinal Study are examples of large national surveys that could incorporate questions pertaining to military status, deployments, and other military exposures, to examine these effects on military children. Similarly, administrative databases, such as TRICARE-dependent health care data, can be linked to data within the Defense Manpower Data Center. Some studies have incorporated these methods, providing important information about the impact of deployment on the mental health of military spouses (Mansfield et al., 2010) and children (Mansfield, Kaufman, Engel, & Gaynes, 2011). The California Healthy Kids Survey, another administrative data set, is the largest statewide survey of resilience, protective factors, risk behaviors, and school climate in the nation and includes information about military affiliation. Results have been used to compare military to civilian children regarding well-being, suicidal ideation, victimization, and weapons carrying (Cederbaum et al., 2014; Gilreath et al., 2013, 2016).

Two promising longitudinal research studies focusing on military families include the Millennium Cohort Family Study and the Deployment Life Study. The Millennium Cohort Study (Crum-Cianflone, Fairbank, Marmar, & Schlenger, 2014) is a DoD-sponsored study under the direction of a multidisciplinary team of investigators at the Naval Health Research Center, Abt Associates, Duke University, and New York University. Its major objective is to "evaluate prospectively the associations between military experiences (including deployments) and service member readjustment on families' health and well-being" (Crum-Cianflone et al., 2014, p. 322). The strength of the study includes its size (>10,000 military service member and spouse dyads), broad representation (including military family members from all services across the globe), and its planned extended period of follow-up (21+ years) that will include time when the service member is within the military, as well as after the service member departs the military.

The Deployment Life Study, conducted by the Rand Corporation (Tanielian et al., 2014), was jointly sponsored by the Office of the Surgeon General, US Army, and the Defense Centers of Excellence for Psychological Health and Traumatic Brain Injury (DCoE) in 2009. The study surveyed military family members at varying intervals throughout the deployment cycle (before, during, and after deployment) specifically assessing marital and parental relationships, physical and psychological health of family members (both adults and children), as well as attitudes toward the military. A summary of findings of the longitudinal assessment of 2742 military families is available through the Rand Corporation (Meadows, Tanielian, & Karney, 2016).

Relevant to our purposes, the Deployment Life Study offered several suggestions for future research related to military families: data should be collected from multiple family members at the same time; future resources should prioritize longitudinal studies of military families; studies should collect real-time data—data that are "capable of tracking changes in the historical, political, and social climates"; research methods should be developed and implemented that better address unique and complex relationships between deployments and their outcomes; and future research should examine the interactions between military life (e.g., promotions, deployments) and other family-timed events (e.g., marriages, births; see Meadows et al., 2016).

16.5.3 Opportunities for Primary Data Studies

Considerable information can be gleaned from work that makes use of large data bases or data from national studies; however, smaller primary data studies can explore important niche areas, as well as enrich, expand, and inform future efforts while incorporating rigorous science (e.g., longitudinal design, multiple-methods, multi-informant data, developmentally informed methodology). Opportunities for smaller studies also allow scientists to bring established lines of research to the military family populations and are likely to encourage the development and mentoring of future military family researchers that will enhance the field. Such opportunities could encourage collaboration with land-grant universities by leveraging their extension offices as well.

There are other arguments in support of smaller primary data studies. Large or national studies typically cannot include a range of variables or methods (e.g., behavioral observations, physiological data) that may be required to address questions or processes specific to military families. For example, examination of communication dynamics in military couples affected by mental health issues might be better addressed in a study using specialized measures that are not practical for larger scale studies (e.g., Knobloch, Ebata, McGlaughlin, & Theiss, 2013). Other populations of interest are unique, smaller, and harder to access. Those individuals are not likely to be reached through a large national study or through an existing data set. Families impacted by combat injury, TBI, PTSD, or service member death are faced with unique challenges that would be better understood by studies that can more carefully address those conditions.

In addition, there are populations within the military that are not well represented in the overall community, but may be uniquely affected by military life—such as nontraditional families (e.g., Gay, Lesbian, Bisexual, Transgendered, Queer/GLBTQ, single parent families), or families in which English is not the primary language. In addition, young children (infants, toddlers, or preschoolers), or children with developmental, learning or medical conditions are important members of the military family community, but underrepresented in research studies. Participants from all of these groups would need to be carefully recruited and data collection should be uniquely tailored to answer research questions of interest. Special research methods, including observational assessment of very young children and caregiving relationships, should be employed, when appropriate.

16.5.4 Implications for Developmental Studies

The study of development involves describing changes within people across their lives, as well as comparisons among people in how they change across life (Baltes, Reese, & Nesselroade, 1977; Lerner, 2012). Obviously, the methods that are used to study development need to be appropriate for assessing change. For instance, measures should be designed to be sensitive to changes across age levels and research must be designed in manners that allow the collection of information about change. Longitudinal designs, which involve repeated testing of individuals across different times in their lives, are necessary. Unfortunately, there are few examples of the use of change-sensitive measures and designs in the study of military children. In fact, there has never been a national longitudinal study of the normative development of these youth. There are many different types of longitudinal designs that generate the multiple observation points necessary to index change (e.g., see Baltes et al., 1977; Nesselroade & Baltes, 1979). Other types of designs of research (e.g., assessing one group of people at one point in time, or assessing groups of differently aged people at one point in time, that is, using a cross-sectional design) are not useful for measuring change. These latter designs do not assess change and, therefore, provide no data about development (Baltes et al., 1977; Molenaar & Nesselroade, 2013). Simply, change can only be detected across multiple times of measurement, and therefore longitudinal research is essential.

However, selection of a longitudinal design is not the only research design consideration. Researchers should also determine when in life individuals should be observed. Time (usually age) is the x-axis in developmental research, and the facet of development that is assessed in a study is displayed along the y-axis. Most developmental research that has been conducted divides the x-axis on the basis of convenience or feasibility (Lerner, Schwartz, & Phelps, 2009). In many studies of youth development annual time points are used (e.g., youth may be sampled at the beginning of Grades 5, 6, and 7). These selections are often made because the budget of a project may not allow more frequent assessments or because the size of a sample may make it difficult to collect data more often. However, the processes of development do not necessarily unfold in ways that correspond to these x-axis divisions.

For example, consider military youth involved in an out-of-school-time program designed to enhance their academic skills. To assess the development of an individual's sense of mastery of these skills, theory or past research might suggest that x-axis divisions be spaced on the basis of phases of her involvement in the program (e.g., attending an information session to learn about the program, the beginning of the curriculum, midway through the program, at the end of the program, and in long-term follow-ups). The point is that theory or inferences from past research should dictate the design of times of observation; however, such bases for x-axis selections rarely occur (Lerner et al., 2009). Furthermore, in studying the developmental process as it may evolve in the context of a specific set of experiences (e.g., the deployment, return, and redeployment of a parent, or the engagement of a young person in an academic program versus a sports or community service program), selections of temporal division should also take into account variables such as the nature of the experience and any special characteristics of the youth being sampled (e.g., children of wounded warriors or children with special needs).

Clearly, the issues involved in using a change-sensitive design in regard to studying positive youth development raise issues of sampling as well. Samples must be selected on the basis of their potential to change during particular portions of development and/or because they are involved in experiences (e.g., intervention programs involving participation in sports) wherein it is appropriate to expect systematic change (plasticity) due to the experiences. For instance, if one wanted to study the effect of menarche on youth development, one would not select a sample of high school seniors to study. Similarly, if one wished to appraise the impact of a specific academic-enhancement program, one would need to select youth who are beginning their first such program as compared to youth who have long and diverse histories of involvement in such programs. Sampling within a military family context might incorporate the timing of deployments, moves, and transitions as they affect family life.

Research must also analyze scores derived from change-sensitive measures with statistical procedures suitable for identifying within-personal change. Statistics that assess if groups remain the same or change are of use in studying change. However, whether individuals within a group all change in the same way cannot be known by just looking at changes in average scores for a group. In the current study of human development, methods are being developed to focus first on the study of patterns of change for each individual in a group. These person-centered analyses, which are also termed idiographic analyses, are then used in subsequent, group-oriented analyses of change (Molenaar, 2014; Molenaar & Nesselroade, 2013; Rose, 2015). These statistical procedures enable researchers to describe both group changes and, as well, the specific changes for the individuals in a group. In short, then, contemporary research methods in the study of development are combining change-sensitive measures, change-sensitive research designs, and change-sensitive statistical analysis procedures that, together, enable the changes within individuals to be described and compared to the changes seen among other individuals. [LRM1].

Other innovations in developmental research are also occurring. For instance, researchers are increasingly interested in using multiple-informants and multiple-methods of data collection (e.g., Cicchetti & Valentino, 2007). Military family studies to-date have often focused on single informants within a family (e.g., one parent, typically a mother; Gewirtz & Youssef, 2016). Concerns about the complexities of IRB approval may have stymied researchers interested in gathering self-report data from children. However, high-quality developmental research requires an understanding of the child from as many perspectives as possible—and gathering data from multiple-informants (e.g., parents, children, teachers, peers) also lessens shared method variance.

It is also far more robust to gather multiple method data that can be analyzed at multiple levels both within and beyond the individual (Cicchetti & Dawson, 2002). As an example, understanding emotion communication within families is important for examining how parents with PTSD symptoms might socialize their children's emotions. Asking parents and/or children (via self-report) might only access one aspect of this construct (i.e., parents'/children's perceptions of their emotional communication). Gathering parent–child observations would enable an understanding of observable dyadic or triadic communication (via, for example, facial or relational emotion coding of emotionally challenging discussions). Simultaneous measurement of aspects of physiology, such as heart-rate variability, allow for an understanding of what is happening "beneath the skin" for parents as they attempt to navigate potentially challenging emotional interactions with their children. Objective measures of executive functioning, such as inhibitory control or working memory, would also help shed light on whether individual differences in executive functioning might serve as vulnerability or protective factors both for parenting, and for PTSD. Studies of one of the authors (AG/ADAPT) have incorporated all these measures in efforts to understand child and family functioning at multiple levels across time in the wake of deployment and related stressors.

16.6 Lessons Learned

More than a decade of experience building a broad, collaborative, multidisciplinary program of research to better understand and meet the needs of military children and families has resulted in several "lessons learned" that should guide future efforts in this field. We believe that these lessons will sustain the collaborative efforts; they should not be forgotten.

16.6.1 Understanding and Respecting Military Family Culture

Researchers who work with military populations should recognize the unique and rich culture of military family life which can also be military branch specific (e.g., Knobloch & Wehrman, 2014). Dependent spouses and children, like their military service members, serve their country and do so with a sense of dignity and purpose. Recognizing and respecting this unique culture, being mindful of one's own biases (e.g., expecting a sense of victimization among military family members), and understanding that this population possesses multiple strengths (while it faces challenges) will support a fair and effective research agenda. Given the ever-evolving nature of military life, military family needs are likely to change, as well, and the research agenda should reflect those changes.

16.6.2 Building Trust Within the Community

Military family researchers have responsibilities to both themselves and the military community. During the last decade, sizeable funding was made available to researchers to develop and implement studies that would further understanding of military children and families. Those funds also provide incentives for researchers to sustain their own programs of research. While there are no inherent conflicts between these two goals, researchers must be prepared to answer to their intentions and to promote trust within the communities that they plan to study. Military community values emphasize service and, as a result, principles of service need to be effectively communicated by researchers who choose to study these populations. Indeed, one of the authors (AG) examined the motivation of families to join a military family prevention study; the majority of families reported that their primary motivation for participating was to help other military families. Even experienced researchers may be viewed (fairly or not) as opportunistic in their approaches and may inspire little trust in their studies or promote little willingness to participate. Trust is best developed by communicating with all members of the community (command and community partners, as well as potential study participants) about the purpose of the study and the expectation that the study will benefit the community that supports it.

16.6.3   Fostering Lasting Relationships Within the Community

The most successful military family researchers have developed relationships with communities that have extended beyond the specific activities of an individual study. Researchers who support the community beyond the study objectives (e.g., by providing information, giving lectures, offering consultation, and/or reporting findings back to the community) are far more likely to be successful in recruiting participants. Several of us have had success using community and command participatory models where research objectives are shaped in collaboration with members of the community, building a sense of shared purpose and commitment to completion of a study. Collaborations are best developed when researchers and community members share study objectives. Most rewarding, the establishment of community–research partnerships often leads to a series of successful research studies within those communities, progressing the science that feels most relevant to the study population.

16.6.4   Building Collaborative Multidisciplinary Academic Research Teams

The last decade of military family research has led to opportunities for highly successful collaborations among academicians who possess a broad range of experiences, knowledge, approaches, and skill sets. Professional experiences include time in the active duty military (Army, Navy, Air Force, and Marines), civilian and military academic expertise, as well as clinical and research experience with both military and non-military populations. Collaborations have incorporated interdisciplinary input from military personnel, service providers, pediatricians, family practitioners, psychiatrists, clinical psychologists, researchers, social workers, nurses, and chaplains, bringing a richness to discussion, research, and scientific products. The breadth of the resultant research agenda reflects the diverse backgrounds of the collaborators: epidemiology, basic science, family and relationship studies, resilience, developmental sciences (including infancy, early childhood, and adolescence), positive youth development, prevention, traumatology, and intervention sciences. The collaborative academic network that has developed across public and private organizations over the last decade is as much an important product as the research studies themselves. Partnerships and team efforts that draw from leveraged expertise more capably address the research agenda and require the collaboration of active duty military experience. Efforts between civilian researchers and military researchers are vital to the proximal success of the scientific enterprise, as are partnerships between established scholars and junior scholars. A key task is to nurture subsequent generations of scholars focused on military family issues so that the field remains innovative in the face of the future conflicts. In sum, an interdependent network of expertise must be sustained, developed, and mentored into the future.

16.6.5 *Sustaining a Scientific Military Family Program of Research*

As described throughout this chapter, a considerable amount of work has been accomplished in developing an initial scientific military family program of research. Much of its future depends upon the continuation of funding to support the effort. Multi-sourced funding should be encouraged and pursued. The well-being of military children and families is of national interest, and not solely a concern of the DoD. In addition to DoD funding, monies from NIH, and other federal sources (e.g., SAMHSA, DoE), as well as public and private research or granting agencies, should be sought. Even within a disciplined research agenda, science advances in a patchwork fashion. However, efforts should be systematic, and move from small to large studies, and from basic science to intervention science, always incorporating the most rigorous methodology. Existing evidence (including both military-specific as well as non-military relevant) should inform the research agenda, as well as policy and practice. Military family researchers must work collaboratively with command, policymakers and funders to bring the best science to practice in support of military children and families during wartime.

16.7 Recommendations and Future Directions

We conclude this chapter by offering recommendations for child and family researchers; military leaders and policymakers; and private and public funders of research who will face future wars. Their joint task must be a collaborative one—to foster both the development and the dissemination of science that sustains military children and families through wartime and other challenges of military life, and that contextualizes that work within the broader body of research on American children and families.

16.7.1 Recommendations for Researchers

With respect to researchers, we encourage military family scientists to examine the variety of transitions that occur throughout military life. The US military is a dynamic and evolving organization. The nature of duty-related responsibilities and family member experiences are likely to change. As a result, the military family research agenda needs to incorporate studies of those evolving needs. Although sustained attention to the various stages of the deployment cycle is warranted, other areas relevant to military children and families must be addressed. For example, how military families navigate the process of leaving the military and adapting to veteran family life in the civilian community is, to-date, an understudied transition. Moreover, it would be helpful to understand the life course experiences of military children as they age, whether their pathways include vocational training, college, military service, or employment. We might expect, given their experiences, that military children uniquely contribute as US citizens; however, we currently cannot determine that effect. Longitudinal studies currently underway (the Millennium Cohort Family Study, for example) may answer some of these questions, but additional research is needed to examine positive growth in military-connected youth and their parents.

Significant gaps in the literature require targeted research focusing on nontraditional family forms. Military family configurations in particular need of attention include GLBTQ military families; single parent military families; military families including female service members, especially those military families in which mothers deploy; military families with infants and young children (0–3 years); military families with at-risk children, especially children with medical, developmental, or learning disorders; non-English fluent military families; and ethnic minority military families. Work along these lines will serve to enrich our understanding of all military families.

A third recommendation is to complement basic research with applied scholarship and translational efforts, including program evaluation research. Applied work is needed to investigate how existing support programs are used and whether such programs benefit the population. Are programs accessible? Are they grounded in evidence-based practices? Do they effectively accomplish their aims? What barriers stand in the way of their maximum effectiveness? Given the geographic dispersion and transitory nature of military families, we see particular value in employing technology for intervention delivery and collection of assessment data. Of course, the use of technology requires careful design, execution, and evaluation to determine its effectiveness among military families. Second, translational work is important for connecting research to policy. Although military family researchers may be well versed in publishing their findings for academic audiences, they may need assistance translating their results into policy recommendations and identifying the appropriate channels of dissemination. We encourage researchers to seek the counsel of key stakeholders to ensure that their results make a difference for military families.

Finally, further collaborations between researchers who study adults and those who study children and families are required. We should be leveraging ongoing and new studies of military-connected adults to further our understanding of military children. For example, dozens of PTSD-related studies have investigated military service members and veterans, but they do not typically consider family-level data, nor the impact of PTSD on parenting or other family structure or functioning. Researchers could learn a great deal about children whose parents are suffering from PTSD, TBI, or other combat-related conditions if they collaborated with adult researchers in studies that were informed by family ecology. Adding value, this kind of collaboration could include mentoring of new investigators from multiple disciplines across child, adult, and family research arenas.

16.7.2 Recommendations for Military Leaders and Policymakers

Of primary importance, military leaders and policymakers must sustain interest in and support of military child and family research. Historically, military leaders have focused on service members. The recent wars have clarified that service members, veterans, and their spouses/partners and children share linked lives, and their experiences and stresses are mutually impactful (Cozza & Lerner, 2013a). Family-based research must continue to guide DoD leadership and policymakers in recognizing the interconnected effects of combat, families, and mission readiness. These areas of focus will minimize existing gaps of knowledge and empower military leaders to make informed decisions regarding the needs of military families to help promote service member readiness and family wellness.

Military leaders and policymakers must understand that research involves both the active development and dissemination of knowledge in support of practice. Whenever possible, they should implement programs with a rigorous evidence base that incorporate established outcome measures included in a well-designed and funded evaluation process. However, scientific evidence regarding program effectiveness is rarely present, and even well-tested civilian programs have not been systematically examined in military populations. Leaders and policymakers must be comfortable with simultaneously introducing evidence informed programs to meet the needs of their constituents, while supporting the randomized controlled study of other, newly proposed programs. As a result, not all programs can be available to everyone, nor should they be until they demonstrate their effectiveness. Service members and families within different branches, locations, and missions have distinct needs that cannot be addressed by DoD one-size-fits-all programming. Support to develop and adapt policies and programs that are specific to local cultural context, behavioral health problem, special populations (e.g., combat injured or grieving families) and military role are likely to be most productive.

Military leaders and policymakers are also in a unique position to break down barriers and positively impact studies by minimizing challenges faced by researchers. For example, they can develop connections with military families and communicate trust of researchers within military communities. Military leaders and policymakers should facilitate access and utilization of large DoD archival databases that would allow scientists to aggregate population-based data in order to answer military relevant questions (e.g., "how does deployment exposure interact with other military family variables to predict child maltreatment events?"). They should also advocate for the use of military identifiers in other large, national data sets that would allow researchers to compare military children with their civilian peers. Leaders and policymakers have the capacity to best support the collaborative efforts of military and civilian researchers, bringing civilian and academic expertise to bear in the military community, as well as encouraging the exportation of science from military families to the understanding and support of civilian families. In addition, leaders and policymakers could further facilitate timely response to wartime research efforts by employing established mechanisms for time-sensitive research incorporated by the NIH in disaster research settings, as well as simplifying research regulatory (IRB) procedures for collaborative efforts between military and civilian agencies.

16.7.3   Recommendations for Public and Private Funders

An underlying theme of this chapter is that science requires sufficient resources to make innovative and lasting contributions to military family readiness. Continued progress depends on the degree to which financial and social capital is available to support research. Of course, grant mechanisms can pave the way for more sophisticated research designs, longer observation windows, more representative samples, and ultimately, stronger scientific claims. At a broader level, programs of research benefit most when funding opportunities, particularly large grants from public/federal agencies, reflect coordinated efforts across multiple agencies. As stated earlier in this chapter, research focused on military children would greatly benefit from the development of a federally funded portfolio of research activities. Specifically, we see value in collaborative mechanisms that serve both military populations and civilian populations. Not only can research on military children and families provide valuable information about US families as a whole, but it also can generate insight into the dynamics of civilian families who face stressful circumstances, as well as the mechanisms that support resilience.

Private research funding from foundations, not-for-profit groups, individual or family donors and other contributors provide alternate sources of research support that lend unique opportunities for military family studies. Not infrequently, these funds come with guidelines that reflect special interests of the organization or individual donors, who may not always recognize needs within the field or understand how their contributions can bring the greatest good. Under such circumstances, advisory boards can serve a useful role by allowing researchers, military leaders, policymakers, and representatives of the community (clinicians, community service providers, and family members) to guide privately funded contributions to efforts that can best serve the military community. Private funding often best assists by partnering with researchers or universities in targeting shared research interests or specialized populations in which studies have not been previously funded.

Money is not the only resource that funding agencies can provide to facilitate research on military families. Social capital, particularly in terms of interdisciplinary networking opportunities, mentoring and apprenticeship programs, and training mechanisms, would be exceedingly valuable for sustaining the momentum of the scientific enterprise. Both public and private funding have the opportunity to build research collaboratives, creating networks of military and civilian researchers with capacity for sustained research efforts. Examples of model programs include opportunities for interdisciplinary conference grants and multi-site or cross-agency research collaborative grants. The ability of military family science to address the pressing questions of the next major conflict depends—in no small measure—on the strength of the partnerships formed by key stakeholders in a position to provide resources, including DoD units, civilian funding agencies, private foundations, and nonprofit organizations.

References

Baltes, P. B., Reese, H. W., & Nesselroade, J. R. (1977). *Life-span developmental psychology: Introduction to research methods.* Monterey, CA: Brooks/Cole.

Cederbaum, J. A., Gilreath, T. D., Benbenishty, R., Astor, R. A., Pineda, D., DePedro, K. T., et al. (2014). Well-being and suicidal ideation of secondary school students from military families. *Journal of Adolescent Health, 54*(6), 672–677.

Chandra, A., & London, A. S. (2013). Unlocking insights about military children and families. *The Future of Children, 23*(2), 187–198.

Cicchetti, D., & Dawson, G. (2002). Editorial: Multiple levels of analysis. *Development and Psychopathology, 14*(03), 417–420.

Cicchetti, D., & Valentino, K. (2007, January). Toward the application of a multiple-levels-of-analysis perspective to research in development and psychopathology. In *Multilevel dynamics in developmental psychology, Minnesota Symposia on Child Development* (Vol. 34, pp. 243–284).

Cozza, S. J., Chun, R. S., & Polo, J. A. (2005). Military families and children during Operation Iraqi Freedom. *Psychiatric Quarterly, 76*(4), 371–378.

Cozza, S. J., & Lerner, R. M. (2013a). Military children and families: Introducing the issue. *The Future of Children, 23*(2), 3–11.

Cozza, S.J. & Lerner, R.M. (2013b). Eds;. Military children and families. *The Future of Children, 23*(2), Princeton University and the Brookings Institution.

Crum-Cianflone, N. F., Fairbank, J. A., Marmar, C. R., & Schlenger, W. (2014). The Millennium Cohort Family Study: A prospective evaluation of the health and well-being of military service members and their families. *International Journal of Methods in Psychiatric Research, 23*(3), 320–330.

Dalack, G. W., Blow, A. J., Valenstein, M., Gorman, L., Spinner, J., Marcus, S., Kees, M., McDonough, S., Greden, J., Ames, B., Francisco, B., Anderson, J. R., Bartolacci, J., & Lagrou,

R. (2010). Public-Academic Partnerships: Working together to meet the needs of Army National Guard soldiers: An academic-military partnership. *Psychiatric Services, 61*, 1069–1071.

DeVoe, E. R., Paris, R., Emmert-Aronson, B., Ross, A., & Acker, M. A. (2016). A Randomized clinical trial of a post-deployment parenting intervention for service members and their families with very young children. *Psychological Trauma: Theory, Research, Policy, Practice.* https://doi.org/10.1037/tra0000196.

Flake, E., Davis, B., Johnson, P., & Middleton, L. (2009). The psychosocial effects of deployment on military children. *Journal of Developmental & Behavioral Pediatrics, 30*(4), 271.

Gewirtz, A. H., & Youssef, A. M. (2016). Conclusions and a research agenda for parenting in military families. In A. H. Gewirtz & A. M. Youssef (Eds.), *Parenting and children's resilience in military families* (pp. 299–306). Basel: Springer International Publishing.

Gewirtz, A. H., DeGarmo, D. S., & Zamir, O. (2016). Effects of a military parenting program on parental distress and suicidal ideation: After Deployment Adaptive Parenting Tools. *Suicide & Life-Threatening Behavior, 46*(Suppl. 1), S23–S31. https://doi.org/10.1111/sltb.12255.

Gewirtz, A.H., DeGarmo, D.S., & Zamir, O. (resubmitted, *Prevention Science*). After Deployment, Adaptive Parenting Tools: One-year outcomes of an evidence-based parenting program for military families following deployment.

Gewirtz A.H., DeGarmo D.S., Zamir O. (2017) After deployment, adaptive parenting tools: 1-year outcomes of an evidence-based parenting program for military families following deployment. *Prevention Science,* https://doi.org/10.1007/s11121-017-0839-4.

Gewirtz, A. H., Pinna, K., Hanson, S. K., & Brockberg, D. (2014). Promoting parenting to support reintegrating military families: After Deployment, Adaptive Parenting Tools. *Psychological Services, 11*, 31–40. https://doi.org/10.1037/a0034134.

Gilreath, T. D., Cederbaum, J. A., Astor, R. A., Benbenishty, R., Pineda, D., & Atuel, H. (2013). Substance use among military-connected youth: The California Healthy Kids survey. *American Journal of Preventive Medicine, 44*(2), 150–153.

Gilreath, T. D., Wrabel, S. L., Sullivan, K. S., Capp, G. P., Roziner, I., Benbenishty, R., & Astor, R. A. (2016). Suicidality among military-connected adolescents in California schools. *European Child and Adolescent Psychiatry, 25*(1), 61–66.

Knobloch, L. K., Ebata, A. T., McGlaughlin, P. C., & Theiss, J. A. (2013). Generalized anxiety and relational uncertainty as predictors of topic avoidance during reintegration following military deployment. *Communication Monographs, 80*, 452–477.

Knobloch, L. K., & Wehrman, E. C. (2014). Family relationships embedded in United States military culture. In C. R. Agnew (Ed.), *Social influences on close relationships: Beyond the dyad* (pp. 58–82). Cambridge, UK: Cambridge University Press.

Lerner, R. M. (2012). Essay review: Developmental science: Past, present, and future. *International Journal of Developmental Science, 6*, 29–36.

Lerner, R. M., Schwartz, S. J., & Phelps, E. (2009). Problematics of time and timing in the longitudinal study of human development: Theoretical and methodological issues. *Human Development, 52*, 44–68.

Lester, P., Liang, L. J., Milburn, N., Mogil, C., Woodward, K., Nash, W., et al. (2016). Evaluation of a family-centered preventive intervention for military families: Parent and child longitudinal outcomes. *Journal of the American Academy of Child and Adolescent Psychiatry, 55*(1), 14–24.

Mansfield, A. J., Kaufman, J. S., Marshall, S. W., Gaynes, B. N., Morrissey, J. P., & Engel, C. C. (2010). Deployment and the use of mental health services among U.S. Army wives. *New England Journal of Medicine, 362*(2), 101–109.

Mansfield, A. J., Kaufman, J. S., Engel, C. C., & Gaynes, B. N. (2011). Deployment and mental health diagnoses among children of US Army personnel. *Archives of Pediatrics and Adolescent Medicine, 165*(11), 999–1005.

Meadows, S. O., Tanielian, T., & Karney, B. R. (Eds.). (2016). *The Deployment Life Study: Longitudinal analysis of military families across the deployment cycle.* Santa Monica: The RAND Corporation.

Molenaar, P. C. (2014). Dynamic models of biological pattern formation have surprising implications for understanding the epigenetics of development. *Research in Human Development,* *11*(1), 50–62.

Molenaar, P. C. M., & Nesselroade, J. R. (2013). New trends in the inductive use of relational developmental systems theory: Ergodicity, nonstationarity, and heterogeneity. In P. C. M. Molenaar, R. M. Lerner, & K. M. Newell (Eds.), *Handbook of developmental systems theory and methodology.* New York: Guilford Press.

Nesselroade, J. R., & Baltes, P. B. (Eds.). (1979). *Longitudinal research in the study of behavior and development.* New York: Academic Press.

Piehler, T. F., Ausherbauer, K., Gewirtz, A., & Gliske, K. (2016). Improving child peer adjustment in military families through parent training: the mediational role of parental locus of control. *The Journal of Early Adolescence,* 0272431616678990.

Rose, T. (2015). The end of average. New York: Harper One.

Rosen, L. N., Teitelbaum, J. M., & Wethuis, D. J. (1993). Children's reactions to the Desert Storm deployment: Initial findings from a survey of Army families. *Military Medicine, 158,* 465–469.

Ross, A., & DeVoe, E. R. (2014). Engaging OEF/OIF/OND military parents in a home-based reintegration program. Special Issue on Service Members, Veterans, and Their Families. *Health & Social Work, 39*(1), 47–54.

Tanielian, T., Karney, B. R., Chandra, A., Meadows, S. O., & the Deployment Life Study Team. (2014). *The Deployment Life Study: Methodological overview and baseline sample description.* Santa Monica: The RAND Corporation.

Chapter 17
Serving Military Families Through Research: The View from the Ivory Tower

Meredith Kleykamp

17.1 The Academic Sector: An Introduction

Much as we work to become more interdisciplinary, academics are bound by their disciplinary cultures, norms, and mores. Because we are experts in our own disciplines, trying to provide a comprehensive view from the perspective of "an academic" is nearly impossible. As a result, the perspective reflected in this chapter stems from my experiences as a social rather than behavioral scientist, specifically a sociologist. By focusing on the part of academia I know best, there will naturally be a lack of attention to the experiences of researchers in other disciplines. I hope it resonates with those in other fields, but there may be points of disagreement originating from the different kinds of work we do, and the different ways we do our work.

Sociology is one of many disciplines that engage in research on military families. Some come from the social sciences like economics, political science, anthropology, and sociology. Many come from the behavioral sciences, especially clinical, developmental, and industrial-organizational psychology, while still others come from the helping professions like nursing, medicine, and social work. Based on their particular domain of expert knowledge, researchers from different disciplines bring a variety of theoretical interests, methodological tools, and research questions to research on military families. Academic research tends to fall along a spectrum from pure, fundamental or basic research, intended to advance new knowledge about phenomena, to applied research intended to apply the insights from basic science to solve practical problems. Some of the research related to military families of immediate and obvious practical relevance, while other research may fall further toward the basic science side, with application of the knowledge being of secondary

M. Kleykamp, Ph.D. (✉)
Department of Sociology, University of Maryland, College Park, MD, USA
e-mail: kleykamp@umd.edu

© Springer International Publishing AG 2018
L. Hughes-Kirchubel et al. (eds.), *A Battle Plan for Supporting Military Families*, Risk and Resilience in Military and Veteran Families,
https://doi.org/10.1007/978-3-319-68984-5_17

importance. But even the scholarship having less immediate practical relevance falls within the notion of "use-inspired basic science" (Stokes, 1997). All these forms of knowledge production are important, but they are often important to different consumers.

For example, some psychologists may work directly with patients, and their research may involve the testing and evaluation of different treatment interventions with a client or clients (e.g., Bowen, Mancini, Martin, Ware, & Nelson, 2003; Sautter, Glynn, Thompson, Franklin, & Han, 2009). The knowledge generated from this kind of research may immediately translate to better therapies for military families in crisis. Other scholars might study how parental deployment affects military children by increasing ambiguity in their lives (Huebner, Mancini, Wilcox, Grass, & Grass, 2007) or by leading to child maltreatment (Gibbs, Martin, Kupper, & Johnson, 2007). Other research may examine mental health related behaviors and treatment among military wives (Mansfield et al., 2010), or marital satisfaction among those who deployed and were exposed to combat (Renshaw, Rodrigues, & Jones, 2009). Still other academic research involves reviewing the unique aspects of military families for clinical providers (Savitsky, Illingworth, & DuLaney, 2009). Each of these kinds of research seems fairly immediately informative for serving military families.

Other social scientists like economists or sociologists may conduct research that doesn't always involve direct interactions with military families, but relies on available nationally representative data to inform us about military families' lives. This might mean studying marriage and divorce trends among military members (Hogan & Seifert, 2009; Lundquist, 2004, 2006). It may also offer theoretical or conceptual models for approaching the study of military families (Segal, 1986). Even if the research does involve primary data collection through new surveys or interviews, these researchers may not engage in the delivery of treatments, programs, or services, and their disciplinary approach would not consider that to be a goal or desired outcome of their research. Scholars in all disciplines often conduct a mix of basic and applied research even if their discipline tends toward one side or the other. But all of this research serves military families in different ways.

Sociological research often "problematizes" aspects of the military family experience by applying a critical lens to what otherwise may be seen as normal or routine (McGarry, Walklate, & Mythen, 2014). Our research informs the public and policymakers about the real challenges military families face, and some of the reasons why. But this kind of work does not always involve the development of the solutions to those problems. It can sometimes be difficult for nonacademic researchers to understand just how focused within disciplines many of us are. Thus, it is important for policymakers, and those interested in serving military families to understand the disciplinary approaches of their academic partners or the researchers in their domain, and to recognize both the benefits and limitations of the variety of academic approaches to research on military families.

Within the academic sector, a number of inter- and multidisciplinary research centers have developed over the past few decades. These centers offer the opportunity to bridge disciplinary divides. Research centers serve to connect scholars with overlapping research interests in military families, veterans, and military service-members. Perhaps the most visible of these for military families is the Military Family Research Institute (MFRI) at Purdue University, led by the editor of this volume, Shelley MacDermid Wadsworth. Under her leadership, MFRI has helped to coalesce a field of study around military families, and to connect academic researchers, policy researchers, policymakers, service providers, and military family advocates so that each can learn from the other to serve the needs of military families. Through annual conferences and symposia, and published volumes of the work stemming from those events, MFRI has helped to build and grow the intellectual community around military families. And these activities connect different sectors and stakeholders. The rise of MFRI presents an important case study for how to build an intellectual community around a topic of vital importance. Most notably, the center began with core funding from Department of Defense (DoD) and has been sustained with support from philanthropic partners, research grants, and contracts for programs. The Institute for Veteran and Military Families (IVMF) at Syracuse University represents another academic center that has experienced phenomenal growth in the past decade. It began with a mission to educate veterans about entrepreneurship and rapidly evolved to a large, well-funded organization with multiple missions. It follows a similar model to MFRI in bringing together research and service to military-connected populations. This is an important distinction from many other types of University centers which exist primarily as research-oriented centers with limited teaching or service missions.

However, most academic researchers do not have the benefit of affiliation with one of these major research centers. As a result, many scholars work in an environment without a community of like-minded scholars in residence, access to shared resources, or deep connections to military policymakers or "insiders." These researchers may or may not be well integrated into dense networks of scholars with expertise on military families, or have close access to military family populations or data for study. And without strong ties to sources of research support and access to military families to study, these scholars can find the climate for doing impactful research on military families quite challenging. As a scholar at a research-intensive university, I see many eager and interested graduate students become discouraged from their interest in researching military families owing to the daunting task of gaining access to data and study populations. Many move on to productive research careers in fields with fewer impediments to conducting research. But our community, and ultimately military families, loses out when promising scholars feel there are few opportunities for them to pursue research on military families.

When nonacademics think about the academic world, what often distinguishes us is our tenure policies. It is important for other sectors to understand what tenure means to academics and why it can be a driving force especially for young scholars. Tenure provides protections to scholars so they can pursue the advancement of knowledge in ways that may be unpopular, or unfashionable (AAUP, 2001). It does not guarantee a job for life, and it doesn't protect incompetence, but it does allow researchers to continue to pursue research unfettered by politics and it protects scholars from dismissal because of unpopularity. These protections are not given to everyone. They must be earned by producing high enough quality research for peers in the discipline. Because of the demands of the tenure process, academic researchers must first and foremost produce quality research that satisfies the peers who will evaluate us for tenure. If we are denied tenure, we are not able to continue employment at our institution.

The research that is most compelling for our academic community may not always be the research most desired by policymakers, practitioners, advocates, or military families. Some academics, those in land grant institutions and those with forward-thinking administrators, do understand the vital importance of community engagement and translation into practice, but this isn't necessarily the norm across institutions, nor across disciplines (Boyer, 1990; Hernandez, Rosenstock, & Gebbie, 2003). Even when outreach and engagement work is valued and rewarded by our institutions, it is not typically our primary focus. Thus, academics try to work on research projects that have the potential to accomplish both the demands of their careers and the needs of military family community whenever possible, but will privilege career demands, especially if they want to earn tenure.

One of the great challenges for academics who are advocates for military families then is to produce research that is useful to our scientific colleagues *and* to the military and policy communities. Academics researching military family issues want to do important work that is beneficial to the policy community. We do not see ourselves as disinterested elites working from the security of our ivory tower. We care about this community and these issues, but we also have to do work that aligns with OUR sector's mission, or we may be unemployed. We typically approach topics with a critical lens and seek to understand the broader context, structures, and systems that generate problems for military families. But we are not fighting against or criticizing military families, even if we sometime critique the systems and structures that add stress to their lives. Our work may seem esoteric to those who want to solve immediate and practical problems. But, this is the work our sector demands. What we do, however, provides the foundational knowledge for what is likely to work and why when serving families. Thus, those who wish to engage with academic research must understand the professional interests and constraints academics face in researching military families.

Academic researchers on the whole do a poor job of writing for our policy audience, of identifying what in our research is likely to be useful to them, and of connecting our work to those who might develop applications from it. This is a long-standing challenge, but stems from what was just discussed. The primary audience for academic research is our peer scientists, and there is little professional reward for doing additional work to translate our research for others including for policymakers, or stakeholders. Academic researchers should be better at this, but we are not trained in how to communicate our findings to a variety of audiences. Our "mission" may not involve an expectation of translating our findings into practical or applied outcomes, but communicating in more plain language what we find and how it might apply to policy and practice would be an important step to bridge the gaps between academics and others serving military families (cf. the work of the Alan Alda Center for Communicating Science for one example of working to train scientists to better communicate outside their disciplinary audience). We academics would benefit from learning what is of most interest to our nonacademic audiences, how to present our work in the most effective way, and how to gain the attention of those who make decisions and could use our expert knowledge to make better ones. Academic researchers sometimes have the (mis)perception that those in the policy community are actively reading the latest scholarship in our disciplines. But many outside academia don't even have full access to our publications housed behind paywalls on publisher websites. For our scholarship to be useful we need to help others access our research to make the best use of that knowledge. By taking seriously the need to engage our various communities and audiences, academics might be better positioned to be more responsive to the needs of military families in the future.

17.2 How Academic Research Serves Military Families

Academic research has constraints and limitations in serving military families, but academic researchers have gotten a number of things right over the past 15 years. First and foremost, we are *constantly* thinking about how to generate better knowledge. The community of scholars interested in military families remains interested and expert in this area regardless of the geopolitical situation or pace of deployments. Our purpose is to constantly assess the landscape of ideas, to identify gaps and holes in our knowledge, and wrestle with the limits of our science and data as we try to fill those gaps in knowledge. We are ever-vigilant in this respect. When the challenges facing military families grow, and public attention turns to these issues, more scholars may become interested. But the core experts in the field typically maintain an active research agenda that can weather the ups and downs of public attention. Internal researchers in DoD may turn attention away from military families as new challenges emerge and overtake attention and resources. Think tanks must turn attention toward areas with funding. Academic researchers have the luxury to continue to work on what is important to them, even as public attention and resources shift to other concerns. Without funding for larger scale studies, this work may be smaller in scale, and more incremental, but it persists. In many ways, the scholarly research community IS the continuity plan for understanding military families' needs. Our constant focus, even if among a small group of researchers, is the most important way academic researchers serve military families.

Sustained research attention to military families generated numerous published studies that have been influential in helping to serve military families. While a comprehensive review of all of the research is beyond the scope and purpose of this chapter, many of these studies can be found in some of the systematic reviews conducted in the past two decades, or in the special journal volumes or edited works produced to synthesize research and establish a research agenda around military families. A recent volume of *The Future of Children* (2013) focused on military children and their families. Papers in this journal volume were authored by some of the top researchers in and out of academia. The volumes in the *Risk and Resilience in Military Families* series also offer an interdisciplinary and inter-sector look at research on issues facing military families (cf. Wadsworth & Riggs, 2010, 2014). There are many, many more individual studies and review papers or chapters produced by the work of academic researchers. But collectively, this work is making a difference, even if slowly, in the lives of military families.

17.3   Challenges Facing Academic Researchers

Since the wars in Afghanistan and Iraq, academic researchers have continued to wrestle with several gaps in our knowledge and data that impede effective service to military families. These challenges are not unique to academic researchers but extend to researchers from all sectors. They appear repeatedly over time in the published literature from multiple disciplines. The main challenges facing scholars come from limited access to high-quality data. In this section, I detail the kinds of data sources academics need to produce useful research about military families.

A common refrain among researchers is the need for more and better data (for recent examples, see Chandra & London, 2013 or Teachman, 2012). The research we produce is only as good as the data that go into that research. This chapter joins the chorus to argue that knowledge generation about military families is limited by the data (not) made available to external researchers. The data challenges take several forms. Academic social scientists need information about both military and nonmilitary cases to compare what is unique and different about military, veteran, and civilian experiences. Those who serve military families want to know about dynamics within the military family, but our communities of scholars often find such a focus too limiting. Scholars often have primary interest in understanding how and why military life affects family outcomes, compared to the experiences of nonmilitary families. Data that includes civilians usually lacks detailed military information, or even military service indicators. Good data on military families' experiences either from primary data collection or administrative records lacks comparable data on civilian families. These comparisons are crucial to distinguish what characteristics and experiences are unique to military families that shape well-being. It may seem obvious that things like deployments, intensive training, and frequent relocations might be stressors for military families that civilian families don't experience. But the military also provides important sources of family support through housing, pay stability, and healthcare that civilian employers may not provide. Thus, comparisons with nonmilitary families must address the full range of benefits and burdens of military life on families.

Military-only data are also limited. These sources are too often confined to active duty populations, to a single branch of service, or a specific family type, such as a heterosexual male servicemember with a female wife and children for convenience, or because these reflect the largest category of military families. To generate new knowledge, our data needs to acknowledge the changing nature of the military family. The widespread activation and deployment of reserve component forces presents a particular challenge to researchers, as most military family research has focused on active duty families. Similarly, routine ship and shore duty experiences among Navy families differ from the kinds of combat deployments experienced by Army and Marine families. These two branches differ from each other in the normative lengths of deployments as well. Ignoring women servicemembers' families, LGBT families, and others has impeded our understanding of these growing segments of the population. It also symbolically suggests these families are less important than those family types that receive the most study. Ignoring single servicemembers and their families of origin, or their unmarried partners, means we don't measure how military stressors may impede family formation, or challenge relationships with siblings and parents. And it leads us to ignore a large segment of the military population as if they don't have a family yet. Accessing and generating the kinds of data that can inform us about the dynamics within the full diversity of military family types has been a challenge, but will be of increasing importance into the future.

Because academic researchers have limited access to the data collected by the DoD, or by private entities like think tanks, they often make use of publically available data sources like the Census. But many of our nationally representative data sources do not identify military families well, if at all. If they do indicate military service, and offer the ability to link family members' data together, they typically do not include much detail about that service experience, such as dates of service, rank, branch, etc… (Chandra & London, 2013). And since rates of service are declining in the population, a truly nationally representative sample may have less than 5% of the sample who serves in the military in contemporary cohorts.

Another form of "available" data comes from administrative data. "Big data" conjures thoughts of terabytes and petabytes of information, but it refers to a variety of forms of data, including information not intended originally for research but with potential research value. This data includes administrative records such as administrative data on servicemembers and their families (Einav & Levin, 2014). Such information can be a cost-effective source of data for research because it already exists. When linked with multiple sources of administrative data, there is the potential for compelling insights into military family life. Yet, access to such data is severely restricted to those outside the administrative systems that house such information because it typically includes personally identifying information. This could be stripped in order to share it with external researchers, but access is rarely granted to those outside the government (Institute of Medicine, 2013). Even administrative data don't solve all research problems because such data typically offers no ability to compare to nonmilitary populations.

Researchers have been especially challenged by a lack of longitudinal data. Such data are needed to identify how military families adapt to military life over time and how important events like a protracted conflict and repeated deployments impact military families. Longitudinal data allows us to understand how military families before and after these important events unfold. We have long understood the need for ongoing, prospective research designs that are longitudinal or panel studies of cohorts (multiple cohorts) that allow for sophisticated treatments of things like the selectivity of who joins the military, who stays in the force, who they marry, and how a whole host of complex experiences during military service generate the "outcomes" that we are interested in. These data collection mechanisms need to be in place before critical events happen, because it's too late to gather a baseline once a crucial event like an attack, a deployment, or an injury does happen. Policymakers want *causal* evidence. If we want to craft good programs and policies to support military families through deployments, or even PCS moves, we really need to understand lives before these events, so we can understand how and why key events change lives. The optimal scientific means to study the effects of events might be a randomized experiment, but we don't randomly assign families to deployments. We can compare families who do and do not deploy. But if these families differ in key ways, such a strategy may be misleading. But having information on the same families over time, seeing how they are functioning before and after key events, provides a better understanding of the impacts of a whole range of unanticipated events. Academic researchers have been pushing for years for a comprehensive longitudinal data collection effort so that there are data collection mechanisms in place already when the next big event occurs. There are existing longitudinal data collections, but it is unclear whether these will be made widely available to the research community.

17.4   Lessons Learned and Recommendations for the Next Event

How do academics work to resolve these challenges to conducting high-quality research on military families? Here, I provide some examples from my own discipline, again recognizing there will be similarities and differences across disciplines and scholars. These strategies would fall under two colloquialisms: "don't let the perfect be the enemy of the good," but "keep up the good fight" for better data. There are core research needs that would significantly advance our knowledge of military families. These suggestions have been repeated time and again, by multiple communities to a variety of audiences. Nevertheless, we all continue to push for them in order to make advancements in knowledge. But, if we waited for the optimal solution, there would be no research on military families. While we fight for the optimal, we make do with the available and accessible. These efforts have taken different forms and have had varying levels of success.

A group of scholars worked to augment existing data collection efforts in order to add military variables or military samples to these efforts. In most available data there are very few active duty, veterans, or military spouses if they can be identified at all. For example we explored whether there might be potential to add items and a military oversample to the latest National Longitudinal Survey of Youth (NLSY), and the Panel Study of Income Dynamics (PSID). These efforts stalled due to lack of a clear path for funding, particularly from military sources. As part of an IOM panel, scholars from multiple disciplines tried building administrative data linkages to be able to address the research questions mandated by Congress (IOM, 2013). After a long delay establishing data use agreements, financial support for the analysis dried up. I have intentionally avoided discussions of funding for research, knowing that all sectors feel under-resourced. But the lack of resourcing for high-quality research means that high-quality data are not able to be collected on key topics.

Some social scientists also have worked to reframe our theoretical approach to the study of military families to emphasize a lifecourse perspective (Chandra & London, 2013; Wilmoth & London, 2012). In changing how we frame the scientific merit of this research, we have been able to broaden interest in the topic, and convince civilian funding agencies of the merits of studying military populations. The lifecourse framework emphasizes that there isn't a sharp divide between active duty and veteran, and soldier and family from a research perspective. Even if institutionally, programmatically, and administratively, these are very different populations served by different agencies, research should view the influence of the military experience in lives across time, and through family linkages.

In the end, we tried to more creatively use what is available, as incomplete and limited as it may be. Many scholars engaged in smaller scale, primary data collection because "big," national, representative, or comprehensive data weren't available. Due to limitations, the research generated was narrower in scope, and more fragmented, based on doing what was possible, rather than what was optimal. But these slowly accumulate to build knowledge. Still others have moved on to different research agendas entirely. This is a real loss. There are excellent researchers who want to work in this area, and we often lose them due to the extreme challenges of doing this work from the outside and with available data. Today we make the case that hiring veterans capitalizes on a potentially hidden talent pool. The research community loses a talent pool when there are such barriers to doing research on military families.

17.4.1 Recommendations

I conclude with five major recommendations for how to ensure quality research is in place to support military families. When the next big conflict erupts, those in the government should recognize that any large-scale deployment and mobilization of forces (both active and reserve components) should be matched with a "mobilization" of the research community. If we expect to commit significant resources and personnel into a conflict, we must recognize the responsibility to invest in research to understand the impact of that choice on our servicemembers and military families. Knowing there will be a need for programs and service for families, and not investing in the research necessary to understand which of them are effective is shortsighted. One of the most important lessons learned in trying to research the impact of nearly 15 years at war is that we started investing in research too late.

A second and related recommendation is to sustain and maintain the community of researchers that have developed expertise in military families over the past 15 or more years. This is the research community to mobilize in times of conflict. But just as the National Guard and Reserves have to train, and be maintained, this community must be supported. Building a consortium or working group of experts, "mustering" them regularly through conferences or convenings provides for ongoing conversation about research needs and the state of knowledge in the field. If this research community is sustained, there is no need to have to "stand up" or start up this community because it already exists and persists (with varying members) regardless of war or conflict. There will always be newcomers with good intentions who seek to capitalize on studying military families during times of stress. We should be welcoming of their efforts and expertise. But that expertise is lost if there is nothing to sustain the initial investment of time, energy, and their own institutional and personal resources. Such a group should convene experts regularly, but especially at the outset of large-scale military actions to lay out a research agenda so that research efforts can be coordinated rather than duplicative, and to ensure critical needs are not lost or ignored.

Third, while academic researchers can serve as the continuity plan, maintaining research agendas through the ups and downs of funding, they cannot be expected to do this important work without resources forever. Resources are not just large-scale grant or contract funds, although these are needed to support ambitious programs of research. Support also includes access to study populations and data, and collaborations and partnerships to provide such resources. Academic researchers can bring deep expertise in methods and theory to a partnership with internal government researchers. Academic researchers are exposed to the latest methodologies and theories because these innovations are being developed among academic researchers. We are always learning of new developments as peer reviewers, members of scientific panels, and through our teaching at our institutions. If statutory authority cannot grant us an ability to "touch" data for research (which we would prefer), partner with us. By connecting our respective strengths we can together improve science, AND improve policy. We also have an important resource—our students. We can help you to generate the next generation of experts and policymakers in your sector. We have veterans in our classes who will be looking for meaningful work and still want to serve the military population. We have graduate students who become very enthusiastic about serving military families once introduced to the area. Civilian students want to help military families but they are often scared away once they actually find out how little data is available to them, or they face distrust from the military community. Research shows that diverse teams produce better work (Page, 2008). We all benefit when the barriers to entry are reduced for doing research about military families.

The fourth and fifth recommendations are related, and center on developing better data resources of two types. One way to improve research on military families is to ensure that ongoing nationally representative data collection efforts include information about military service and military families to the greatest extent possible. The second way is to respond to the many voices calling for a large-scale longitudinal data collection and administrative data linkages, and to ensure those data are available to all researchers, not just those in the government or think tanks.

With respect to the first point, many national data sources, funded with public dollars, do not include indicators of military service experience, key details about that experience, or large enough samples of military personnel to be useful to researchers. DoD, Department of Veterans Affairs (VA), and other large agencies should work with entities managing large datasets to encourage the inclusion of important military-service variables, and to reconsider whether the exclusion of military populations from sampling frames continues to be warranted. The American Community Survey is the primary source of data that identifies currently serving individuals, but has little additional information about the nature of that service, deployment, rank, or other key variables for understanding military families. One way to quickly collect data as needed would be to supplement an ongoing data collection with a military oversample, as was done with the 1979 NLSY (NLS, n.d.). Once funds were no longer provided to pay for the military oversample, data collection on that oversample was suspended, however.

On the second point, researchers in all sectors have understood the need for high-quality, longitudinal data on military families. They have also made clear the value of administrative data for answering key policy questions (IOM, 2013). Administrative data, especially when linked across sources can build in a longitudinal element, observing individuals as they pass through the military into, for example, the VA system. Some researchers have access to these kinds of data. Government researchers have access to administrative data, and researchers in think tanks or contracting firms may have access to contracted data collections. Yet these data, often paid for with public funds, are not typically made publicly available. Thus, the value of these datasets is limited because the scientific community cannot replicate the work published from them, and other scholars cannot build on this work. In other areas, research supported with public funds must be shared with other scientists and researchers (National Science Foundation grants, for example, must include a data management plan detailing how data from the research will be shared). While there is a need for operational security and protections of personally identifying information, research on military families should become much more transparent by requiring broader release of data paid for with public funds used for research.

In conclusion, academic researchers have a wealth of knowledge and skills to offer the community of interest around military families. Research is sometimes seen as an unnecessary luxury, rather than a critical expense. But the programs and services developed for assist military families are only as good as the knowledge base used to develop and evaluate them. While academics operate within their own culture that rewards certain kinds of research, they also have the skills and resources to help identify knowledge gaps, to design effective data collections, and to produce high-quality research that draws on state-of-the-art methods and theories. All sectors serving military families benefit when we work together, including academics working in partnership with other researchers.

References

American Association of University Professors. (2001). *Policy documents and reports* (9th ed.). Johns Hopkins University Press: Baltimore.

Bowen, G. L., Mancini, J. A., Martin, J. A., Ware, W. B., & Nelson, J. P. (2003). Promoting the adaptation of military families: An empirical test of a community practice model. *Family Relations, 52*(1), 33–44.

Boyer, E. L.(1990). Scholarship reconsidered: Priorities of the professoriate.

Chandra, A., & London, A. S. (2013). Unlocking insights about military children and families. *The Future of Children, 23*(2), 187–198.

Einav, L., & Levin, J. (2014). Economics in the age of big data. *Science, 346*(6210), 1243089.

Gibbs, D. A., Martin, S. L., Kupper, L. L., & Johnson, R. E. (2007). Child maltreatment in enlisted soldiers' families during combat-related deployments. *Journal of the American Medical Association, 298*(5), 528–535.

Hernandez, L. M., Rosenstock, L., & Gebbie, K. (2003). *Who will keep the public healthy?: Educating public health professionals for the 21st century*. Washington, DC: National Academies Press.

Hogan, P. F., & Seifert, R. F. (2009). Marriage and the military: Evidence that those who serve marry earlier and divorce earlier. *Armed Forces & Society, 36*, 420–438.

Huebner, A. J., Mancini, J. A., Wilcox, R. M., Grass, S. R., & Grass, G. A. (2007). Parental deployment and youth in military families: Exploring uncertainty and ambiguous loss. *Family Relations, 56*(2), 112–122.

Institute of Medicine (US). (2013). *Returning home from Iraq and Afghanistan: Assessment of readjustment needs of veterans, service members, and their families*. National Academies Press.

Lundquist, J. H. (2004). When race makes no difference: Marriage and the military. *Social Forces, 83*(2), 731–757.

Lundquist, J. H. (2006). Black-White gap in marital dissolution among young adults: What can a counterfactual scenario tell us? *Social Problems, 53*, 421.

Mansfield, A. J., Kaufman, J. S., Marshall, S. W., Gaynes, B. N., Morrissey, J. P., & Engel, C. C. (2010). Deployment and the use of mental health services among US Army wives. *New England Journal of Medicine, 362*(2), 101–109.

McGarry, R., Walklate, S., & Mythen, G. (2014). A sociological analysis of military resilience: Opening up the debate. *Armed Forces & Society, 41*(2), 352–378. https://doi.org/10.1177/0095327X13513452.

National Longitudinal Surveys. (n.d.). NLSY79 "Introduction to the sample." Retrieved March 30, 2016, from https://www.nlsinfo.org/content/cohorts/nlsy79/intro-to-the-sample/nlsy79-sample-introduction

Page, S. E. (2008). *The difference: How the power of diversity creates better groups, firms, schools, and societies*. Princeton: Princeton University Press.

Renshaw, K. D., Rodrigues, C. S., & Jones, D. H. (2009). Combat exposure, psychological symptoms, and marital satisfaction in National Guard soldiers who served in Operation Iraqi Freedom from 2005 to 2006. *Anxiety, Stress, and Coping, 22*(1), 101–115.

Sautter, F. J., Glynn, S. M., Thompson, K. E., Franklin, L., & Han, X. (2009). A couple-based approach to the reduction of PTSD avoidance symptoms: Preliminary findings. *Journal of Marital and Family Therapy, 35*(3), 343–349.

Savitsky, L., Illingworth, M., & DuLaney, M. (2009). Civilian social work: Serving the military and veteran populations. *Social Work, 54*(4), 327–339.

Segal, M. W. (1986). The military and the family as greedy institutions. *Armed Forces & Society, 13*(1), 9–38.

Stokes, D. E. (1997). *Pasteur's quadrant: Basic science and technological innovation*. Washington, DC: Brookings Institution Press.

Teachman, J. D. (2012). Setting an agenda for future research on military service and the life course. *Life Course Perspectives on Military Service, 83*, 275.

Wadsworth, S. M. D., & Riggs, D. S. (2010). *Risk and resilience in US military families*. New York: Springer.

Wadsworth, S. M. D., & Riggs, D. S. (2014). *Military deployment and its consequences for families*. New York: Springer.

Wilmoth, J. M., & London, A. S. (2012). 1 Life-course perspectives on military service. *Life Course Perspectives on Military Service, 83*, 1.

Chapter 18
Designing and Implementing Strategic Research Studies to Support Military Families

Terri Tanielian, Thomas E. Trail, and Nida Corry

18.1 Introduction

Making sound evidence-based policy decisions is critically important, not only to effectively meet the needs of military families and maintain overall force readiness but also to ensure that responses to those needs are strategic, impactful, and sustainable. Within the research and policy institute sector, several organizations have designed and conducted large-scale studies to help assess the needs of military families and to inform such program and policy solutions. This sector includes research organizations and think tanks who conduct studies and analyses through sponsored research portfolios that include contract and grant funding from governmental and nongovernmental sources. These research organizations range in size; however, all maintain professionally trained research staff with subject matter expertise as well as methodological expertise and sophisticated capabilities needed to conduct small- to large-scale assessments as well as to disseminate findings to the appropriate stakeholder audiences.

Over recent decades, private research organizations like RAND, Westat, ICF International, RTI, and Abt Associates have been at the forefront of implementing surveys and studies on behalf of the Department of Defense (DoD) to understand issues affecting military families. Many of these organizations have engaged in grants and contracts from other federal agencies as well, including the Department of Veterans Affairs (VA), Department of Health and Human Services, and the Department of Labor. Also among this sector are some of the DoD Policy Analysis Federally Funded Research and Development Centers (FFRDCs) whose primary

T. Tanielian, M.A. (✉) • T.E. Trail, Ph.D.
RAND Corporation, Arlington, VA, USA
e-mail: Terri_Tanielian@rand.org; Thomas_Trail@rand.org

N. Corry
Abt Associates, Durham, NC, USA
e-mail: Nida_Corry@abtassoc.com

© Springer International Publishing AG 2018
L. Hughes-Kirchubel et al. (eds.), *A Battle Plan for Supporting Military Families*, Risk and Resilience in Military and Veteran Families, https://doi.org/10.1007/978-3-319-68984-5_18

objective and mandate from Congress is to conduct independent studies and analyses to inform decision-making on defense and national security matters. These organizations, which include the Institute for Defense Analysis, Center for Naval Analysis, and the RAND Corporation's three FFRDCs—the Arroyo Center, Project Air Force, and the National Defense Research Institute (NDRI), not only conduct work through the FFRDC vehicles but have other sponsor relationships, like the research organizations listed above. RAND Corporation in particular has a significant portfolio of research related to supporting military families that has been both federally and privately funded through philanthropic organizations.

The role of the research and policy institute sector is instrumental in generating and disseminating critical knowledge for supporting military families; not only because of their significant contributions to the field but also for their ability to sustain institutional knowledge, expertise, and engagement in these matters over time and to support large-scale studies that have the potential of informing public policy. As a result, their work and contributions in the field extend well beyond the contributions of the individual researchers. While researchers at each of the institutions publish papers in refereed journals, these research and policy institutes also produce organizationally branded reports and prioritize briefing senior leaders and stakeholders about the findings and implications of their work on a regular basis. Thus, these research and policy institute organizations are in a unique position to continue to inform efforts that will support military families not only during times of extended conflict, but also during the times in between.

18.2 Historical Perspectives

As the US Armed Forces began deploying troops to Afghanistan in support of Operation Enduring Freedom in 2001, most in the military community expected swift and conclusive results. When the USA also launched Operation Iraqi Freedom, more troops were deployed and uncertainties grew about the timeline for these operations. In the early years of the "Global War on Terrorism," daily news coverage provided updates on the extent of US casualties as well as progress in diminishing the capabilities of the enemies (Allen, 2003; Loeb, 2003). Yet, as we faced periods of high demand for troops in light of the changing security conditions on the ground, the military was forced to extend tours, issue stop loss orders to retain needed personnel, and deploy the same units multiple times with little "dwell" time in between (Davis, Polich, Hix, Greenberg, & Brady, 2005; Ross, 2010). During this same time, news media also began sharing the stories of the families left behind, highlighting their service and sacrifice (e.g., Glod, 2008; McIntyre, 2005). As the deployments began to protract and more troops were sent to the combat theater, the nation's interest in and appreciation for the importance of supporting their loved ones back at home increased significantly.

As the USA looks back on its longest period of combat operations, there is common agreement among scholars, policymakers, and Defense officials, that the high OPTEMPO and PERSTEMO that has characterized the past 15 years has taken its toll on military families. However, it is still not clear exactly how to quantify or characterize this toll with certainty. Over the past decade, the need to understand the impact of these particular deployments became increasingly important. In the early years of the conflicts, however, the primary goal was to implement programs in a traditional reactive policy making stance rather than to undertake large studies or assessments of the population. If there was a perceived demand or need based upon anecdotal evidence or ongoing experiences, a new program would be created and implemented. Usually, and particularly in the early part of the GWOT, this was done without empirical evidence about the nature and scope of the need among military families. Certainly, smaller scale research studies, for example those within specific operational units, as well as evidence from research on prior deployments or communities exposed to stress, informed these early interventions but often representative datasets were unable to guide larger scale responses.

As programs began to proliferate in the mid-2000s, new research studies were also initiated. At the time, however, there was also significant variation across the field in terms of defining key terms, constructs, processes, and outcomes of interest for these studies. For example, in the middle part of the deployments there was great attention to constructs like readiness and resilience. As time evolved, these constructs of interest widened to embrace more holistic concepts of fitness, and eventually well-being. Similarly, the focus on populations widened as well. Initially policy researchers were primarily focused on military spouses and children of active duty and Guard/Reserve members, and then by natural extension of the concern for the severely wounded, ill, and injured, policymakers concerns turned to caregivers (who were largely believed to be spouses). Overtime, studies and programs also tried to look more comprehensively at the family, to include parents, siblings, and significant others of service members.

Over the course of the conflicts, our sector also became interested in a larger set of outcomes. Initially, researchers were focused primarily on identifying deficits or problems that were associated with deployment, and indeed most of the military family studies focused on looking for negative outcomes like marital dissolution, mental health problems, school-related challenges for children, and spousal unemployment (e.g., Engel, Hyams, & Scott, 2006; Karney & Crown, 2010; SteelFisher, Zaslavsky, & Blendon, 2008). Largely driven by the nature of how research funding is made available (e.g., identify, define, and measure a problem), more studies were focused on understanding the deployment-related harm to families and unfortunately, the potential positive aspects of deployment and military life received little scientific attention particularly in the early years of OEF/OIF/OND.

As more troops returned home from the war, concerns shifted from supporting families during deployment to ensuring successful transitions for service members and their families to civilian settings and communities for a new generation of veterans. This brought an increased focus on reintegration as an important process affecting outcomes and a priority research topic. Just as earlier questions focused on "how can we promote family resilience and readiness for a deployment," later questions began to ask "how can we facilitate successful reintegration for service members and their families." All throughout this time, we saw a proliferation of support programs, first those to help families preparing for deployment, then programs to support coping during deployment, and then finally, new programs to improve transition processes (e.g., TAP) and enhance benefits for service members returning to civilian life (e.g., post-9/11 GI benefits, Yellow Ribbon Reintegration Program). Yet, these policy changes and new programs continued to outpace the ability of the field to generate the empirical data to strategically inform the solutions.

18.3 Responses and Strategies Employed to Understand and Support Military Families

Demographic changes in the composition of the force and policymakers' growing interest in military families resulted in several major policy and program initiatives. These initiatives focused greater attention to the needs of military families and increased the demand for rigorous studies. For example, the Military and Family Life Counseling (MFLC) program was established in 2004, at the height of OEF/OIF operations, to address the need for no-cost, accessible, and confidential counseling for service members and their families. The 2007 Congressional Task Force on Mental Health stressed the importance of families as integral for service member readiness and resilience. Recommendations from the Task Force led to the creation of the Defense Center of Excellence for Psychological Health and Traumatic Brain Injury, which provides outreach and education to mental health providers, service members, and families about mental health issues—particularly Traumatic Brain Injury (TBI) and PTSD—and a 24/7 hotline for military family members and caregivers dealing with psychological issues or TBI. In addition, the Caregivers and Veterans Omnibus Health Benefits Act of 2010 established the Caregiver Support Program within the VA which has multiple benefits for military caregivers including respite care, travel assistance, caregiving training, a financial stipend, and a Peer Support Mentoring Program for eligible caregivers. The 2011 White House report "Strengthening Military Families and Veterans" and subsequent founding of the Joining Forces Initiative further heightened awareness of the needs of military families at a national level and spurred new program and policy initiative to help military families and veterans with access to mental health care, as well as other benefits such as job training and education.

With the new programs also came a proliferation of studies of military family members. As discussed in more detail below, most studies focused on the spouse of a service member, but some studies examined military children or the family as a whole. Studies conducted over this period typically used survey methodology and were cross-sectional in nature (gathering data at one point in time, offering a "snapshot"), but interest grew in longitudinal cohort studies that might help understand how families were faring over time. Administrative data were utilized to address research questions, but the data available were limited and findings were sometimes conflicting. Many studies were either carried out by the Defense Manpower Data Center (DMDC) or used data collected by DMDC. Other studies were funded by the DoD or the VA and carried out by public policy institutes or academic centers, although institutes within NIH have become increasingly interested in funding research on service members and military families (Table 18.1).

Table 18.1 Overview of major studies of military families

Study name	Population and sampling method	Sponsor	Constructs assessed
2012 Survey of Active Duty Spouses (ADSS)	Stratified nonproportional sample of spouses of active duty Army, Navy, Marine Corps, and Air Force with at least 6 months of service up to and including paygrade O6, with over-sampling of small domains and population subgroups having low response rates	Defense Manpower Data Center	• Education and employment • PCS moves • Health and well-being • Family • Military life • Deployments and reintegration • Financial well-being
Millennium Cohort Family Study	A random sample of service members and spouses	Naval Health Research Center	• Physical and functional status • Psychosocial assessment • Medical conditions • Self-reported symptoms • PTSD • Alcohol and tobacco use • Alternative medicine use • Life events • Occupational exposure
Deployment Life Study	Stratified random sample of deployable married service members, and one-child	Army OTSG and Defense Centers of Excellence for PH and TBI	• Psychological, behavioral, and physical health of family members • Marital and parental relationships • Military integration • Child well-being • Financial well-being
Military Life Study	Random sample of spouses of service members	Military Community and Family Policy	• Health and well-being • Financial well-being • Military life • Deployment history • Child outcomes • Reunion and reunification
Blue Star Families Annual Family Lifestyle Survey	Convenience sample of service members, their spouses, and parents	Blue Star Families	• Pay, benefits, and changes to retirement • Family well-being • Satisfaction with military • Deployment and wellness • Financial security/readiness • Military/civilian connectedness • Spouse Employment • Transition

Of the studies on military families, the majority have focused on the married spouse of a service member. For example, the Survey of Active Duty Spouses conducted by DMDC, as well as the Millennium Cohort Study and Military Life Study have focused on the experiences of military spouses. The Millennium Cohort Study (MilCo) is a longitudinal cohort study of married service members and their spouses (Crum-Cianflone, Fairbank, Marmar, & Schlenger, 2014) funded by the DoD and administered by the Naval Health Research Center. First launched in October 2000, the study began enrolling military spouses in the fourth study panel, from 2011 to 2013. Participants will be surveyed every 3 years for a 21 year period, and survey instruments encompass a variety of topics and use standard, validated instruments to measure participant health, mental health, and family well-being. The study is designed so that survey data can be linked to DoD administrative records, and it will eventually include over 10,000 military couples (Crum-Cianflone et al., 2014). The Military Family Life Project specifically focuses on quality of life issues experienced by military families during and after deployments (IOM, 2013). Launched in May 2010, the study incorporates a random sample of service members and military spouses, who are surveyed at baseline and again a year later (IOM, 2013).

A less studied, but important group to understand, is military children. Military spouses are often asked survey questions about their child's well-being, but few studies gathered information directly from the military child, directly interviewing or observing military children. The Children on the Homefront project was one exception (Chandra et al., 2010). This project was a comprehensive study investigating the emotional, social, and academic functioning of military children and the challenges they faced with parental deployment (Chandra et al., 2011). Researchers conducted interviews at several time points with both the non-deployed caregiver (e.g., the spouse of the deployed service members) and the child (aged 11–17 years) using a sample of military youth applying to the Operation Purple summer camp (Chandra et al., 2010).

Even fewer studies have attempted to examine the family as a unit, with service members, spouses, and children from the same family providing data that can be analyzed to examine the shared impacts and downstream implications of military life, including deployments. This sort of "family systems" approach is labor intense and analytically complicated, but provides a more holistic perspective of the family and how individual family members affect one another. The Deployment Life Study is one example of this type of approach to understanding military families (Tanielian, Karney, Chandra, Meadows, & Deployment Life Study Team, 2014). Researchers sampled a service member, spouse, and child (if eligible) from the same family and conducted a longitudinal survey to examine the impact of deployment on individual and family outcomes. Participant families were surveyed every 4 months over 3 years so that outcomes could be measured before, during, and post deployment (Tanielian et al., 2014).

Finally, there have also been a number of cross-sectional studies conducted (e.g., not a cohort, longitudinal, or annual/biannual study), generally designed to answer a fairly narrow set of research questions. For example, a survey examining the relationship between deployment and intimate partner violence among married Army soldiers (McCarroll et al., 2010). Convenience samples are also sometimes used to study specific populations. For example, researchers interested in the experiences of spouses have recruited participants through Family Resource Groups, and studies of caregivers of veterans with TBI or other health issues have recruited participants through VA rehabilitation centers.

18.3.1 Difficulties and Missed Opportunities

One of the main difficulties faced by researchers over the past decade has been conducting timely studies to address policy questions in a rapidly changing operational and policy environment. There are several obstacles that researchers will have to overcome to conduct strategic, responsive research needed to understand the impact of ongoing developments (e.g., increases in deployments and/or changes in types of deployments) and inform policy decisions in the future. Some of the major difficulties in the field are outlined below.

Recruitment of Military Family Members for Research Is Cumbersome and Time Consuming

Although recruiting participants for any research study is difficult, recruiting military family members has some particular challenges. Two main obstacles arise when attempting to recruit military spouses or other military family members for research studies. First, the administrative process for acquiring human subjects approval to recruit family members can take an inordinate amount of time. All research studies that involve service members have to be approved by DoD and the relevant services IRBs, but studies that also recruit members of military families have to undergo an additional review under the Paperwork Reduction Act. This review typically requires 6 months or more to gain approval for the study. Second, once information collection approval is obtained, it is difficult to identify, contact, and recruit military spouses and other family members for research studies. Although the DoD maintains administrative records with contact information for service members (including email addresses), the records on service members' home addresses are often out of date. This problem is important because DoD administrative records do not contain an email address for spouses, so recruitment of the spouse is limited to data provided by the service member or hard copy mailings to the home address on record. Furthermore, records on service members' marital status can be incorrect or outdated for a sizable number of service members, so many more households need to be contacted to obtain an appropriate sample. These factors extend recruitment phases and are inefficient in terms of time and cost, which makes it difficult, if not impossible, to gather information to inform time-sensitive policy decisions and stay ahead of the curve.

Need Assessments and Program Evaluations Are Late or Nonexistent

Although there is clearly a great need for programs to help military families cope with military life, the abundance of programs implemented in the past 10 years has led to duplication of services and potential confusion about which programs to use to help with particular problems. It is unclear whether any policy analysis or needs assessment preceded the design and implementation of these programs, and evaluations of new programs are lagging. For example, a recent study identified 211 programs designed to address service member and family needs focused on psychological health and TBI (Weinick et al., 2011). The study determined that there was no central location within DoD or the services to track and coordinate these services and programs, and that few of the individual programs had conducted a formal needs assessment to provide empirical data to guide and tailor their programming to meet the spectrum of needs of service members and their families (Weinick et al., 2011). With so many family programs, evaluations of program effectiveness are sparse and can lag longer than typically recommended (Weinick et al., 2011). However, as the financial climate within the DoD has tightened, evaluations of some of the major program initiatives are in process.

The Meaning of Military "Family" Is Changing

Finally, most research on military families has focused on a narrow definition of "family"—typically a married service member and spouse with their dependent children—because that has been the definition used by the DoD and may be consistent with the practicalities of using administrative records to draw study samples (IOM, 2013). However, we recognize that other familial relationships may also be important to force readiness. Unfortunately, these relationships such as co-habiting unmarried couples, same-sex couples, and relationships with other family members, such as elderly parents, siblings, and children from prior relationships have been less explored (IOM, 2013). Moving forward, it will be important that stakeholders agree upon an expanded definition of "family" to guide future research on military families to ensure that we do not limit our understanding to only a subsection of families affected by military service.

18.4   Major Findings on Military Families and Remaining Knowledge Gaps

As described in the previous sections, several large-scale surveys have been implemented over recent years to better understand the challenges and most pressing needs among military families. Many of these studies have yielded important descriptive information about military families and the association of deployment and military life to familial outcomes, and others still in the analytic phase will soon provide important findings intended to guide national and local policy and practices. We summarize these here to serve as a frame of reference.

18.4.1 Findings from Completed Studies on Military Spouses, Children, and the Family Unit

Over the course of the past decade, the Defense Manpower Data Center conducted several surveys focused on military spouse and family outcomes. The 2012 Survey of Active Duty Spouses assessed satisfaction with military life, financial health, child well-being, and spousal education/employment among military spouses in the Army, Navy, Marine Corps, and Air Force (excluding National Guard and Reserve). The survey was administered in 2006, 2008, and 2012 with 65,000 spouses responding to the latest wave representing a weighted response rate of 23% (DMDC, 2012). Approximately 81% of spouses reported having experienced a deployment in their partner's career, the majority of which were to a combat zone. Approximately 60% reported a deployment within the past year and nearly 70% of spouses reported having children under 18 living in the home. Spouses most commonly reported experiencing the following problems during deployment: loneliness, dealing with issues/decisions alone, technical difficulties communicating with spouse, difficulty maintaining emotional connection with spouse, maintenance of the home, and emotional problems in the family. Upon the service member's return, spouses most commonly noted that their partner appreciated family, friends and life more, experienced trouble sleeping, got angry faster, and was more emotionally distant. Over 60% reported that their child was able to stay connected with the service member during separation, coped well, and easily reconnected and approximately 13% reported poor coping with deployment. Over half of the spouses reported that their child(ren) were close to family members, accepted responsibility, and felt pride in having a military parent. Just over a third of spouses were not in the labor force, in large part because they wanted to care for their children or child care was too costly. Overall these findings suggest that the majority of military spouses perceived their family to be coping well with the hardships of deployment and pointed to some specific areas where programs might support their families more effectively during deployments (DMDC, 2012).

The DMDC Military Family Life Project, commissioned by the Military Community and Family Policy (MCFP) office in 2010, was designed to longitudinally assess spousal and child well-being among a representative sample of families across military branches. The survey was administered in 2010, 2011, and 2012, with 6412 spouses completing all three waves. Overall, findings suggested that deployments are associated with greater spousal psychological distress and higher levels of "problematic" behaviors among children that are associated with greater difficulties reconnecting with the service member following deployment. Deployments were also associated with positive family financial outcomes. In contract, PCS moves were associated with reductions in spousal financial, educational, and employment outcomes but did not appear to negatively impact family psychosocial functioning (DMDC, 2015).

As was noted in the prior section, there was a growing recognition in the field that we know very little about how children are faring during the parent's deployment and return. In 2009, researchers at RAND interviewed approximately 1500 military children aged 11–17 and their non-deployed caregivers, drawing from the National Military Family Association's 2008 Operation Purple camp, to assess well-being and deployment-related difficulties (Chandra et al., 2010). Results suggest that military children experienced a higher frequency of emotional difficulties compared to civilian samples and that among military families, older children and girls were most likely to experience difficulties. Longer parental deployment and poorer overall caregiver mental health were associated with more challenges for children both during and after deployment (Chandra et al., 2010, 2011). These findings could help inform the identification of families "at risk" for targeted intervention/support across, namely those who experience extended deployments and/or whose primary caregiver experiences mental health issues.

18.4.2 New Knowledge on the Horizon: Overview of Epidemiological Military Family Studies Recently Out of the Field

In the past several months, two major military family studies completed data collection. At the time of this writing, both study teams are working on analyses and we expect new insights and knowledge from these studies to be disseminated in the near future. These studies are described briefly below.

The RAND Deployment Life Study (Tanielian et al., 2014) is a longitudinal study underway that follows military families from the Army, Navy, Air Force, and Marines over a 3 year period to examine how deployment affects the health and well-being of families. Multiple members of the military families responded to the survey at 4 month intervals, including the service member, spouse, and if eligible a child. Data collection ended in mid-2015 and RAND analyzed the data to identify characteristics of families who successfully manage the challenges of deployments as well as families who experience more difficulties. Primary outcomes examined psychological health of the family members, quality of the marital and parental relationships, child outcomes, military career outcomes, and financial well-being (Tanielian et al., 2014).

The MilCo Family Study completed the first wave of data collection with military spouses of participants in the first wave of the fourth panel of the MilCo survey cycle conducted in 2011. The target sample size was reached, with nearly 10,000 spouses completing the spousal survey (Crum-Cianflone et al., 2014). This sample represents the baseline cohort in the Family Study, on which longitudinal analyses will be based in future waves of the study. As previously described, the Family Study is designed to continue as an adjunct to MilCo over the coming two decades. The second wave of the Family Study spousal survey was administered in tandem with the second wave of the fourth panel survey of the MilCo survey in 2014 and the third wave will be administered in 2017. The research team is currently analyzing the baseline data to examine the prevalence of depression, anxiety, substance use, and health issues among spouses as well as behavioral and adjustment issues among the children. The quality of the marital relationship will also be examined, in relation to deployment features and other service member and spousal indices. Together, these results will provide an invaluable descriptive profile of military family adjustment, spousal and service member well-being in terms of psychosocial and health outcomes, and child outcomes. Not only will the study inform our understanding of risk and resilience factors among military families, it will serve as the basis for examining the trajectory of functioning and outcomes among these families over the coming years and potentially in future conflicts.

18.4.3   Remaining Knowledge Gaps

There remains a notable gap in our understanding of the deployment-related and readjustment challenges that face National Guard and Reserve families, which is even more pressing given that the Guard and Reserves were deployed at unprecedented rates in the OEF/OIF conflicts. A 2006 study conducted by the RAND Corporation provided valuable insight into how Guard and Reserve families prepare for and cope during deployment, and provided several implications for supporting and retaining Reserve and Guard members. However, it remains the only large-scale study of this population, which many believe faces increased challenges upon reintegration. While the Deployment Life Study does include Guard and Reserve families in its sample population, additional research to understand the unique needs of this population may be needed.

Although we've made progress in examining the short-term impacts of deployment on children, we do not yet understand the long-term effects of military life, including deployment and relocation, on military children over time and across developmental stages. It's also critical to employ comprehensive, multi-informant assessments of child outcomes. With few exceptions (e.g., Chandra et al., 2010; RAND Deployment Life Study Ref), the majority of surveys have only assessed children's well-being through parental reports.

Overall, it is important that representative and generalizable empirical data are gathered on military families across branches to guide policy and best practices to support their readiness and diverse needs in the future. For example, we need rigorously collected epidemiological data from representative samples of military families to understand sensitive, understudied issues affecting the population, including family violence (intimate partner violence, child neglect, etc.), suicide risk, etc. Currently, reports about these sensitive topics are limited to documented/reported cases, which likely underestimate the prevalence and extent of the problem and are thus ill equipped to inform policy solutions or prevention programs.

It's also essential that researchers across all sectors coordinate more closely as large-scale epidemiological and program evaluation studies are being designed. Beyond learning from one another, it will be important to coordinate and consider design and measurement issues to maximize collective learning and to address gaps in knowledge. For example, there is great variability in the literature in terms of the quality of measurement of key service member and spousal mental and behavioral health issues. While many have established collegial relationships and share to the extent allowable under their contract and grant mechanisms, it would be beneficial to create incentives (or at least reduce barriers) for more efficient coordination among the research community that need to be reconsidered.

18.4.4 Ensuring Lasting Impact of Military Family Research

The launching of several longitudinal surveys designed to assess the functioning of military families both before and after deployment is an invaluable and lasting accomplishment that will guide the field for years to come. The data that these studies produce may be used by the broader research community to analyze numerous outcomes and risk and resilience factors among military families. Over time results from these studies may reveal key priorities to guide allocation of resources and military family programming. We have learned that it can take years for these studies to "get to the field," and that ideally they should be conducted before conflicts begin so that we can detect changes associated with deployment, family reintegration, and other service-related changes.

The growing attention to military family issues in the past decade or so has led to increased cohesiveness among military family researchers, administrators, and advocates, facilitated in part by the work of organizations such as the Purdue Military Family Research Institute and the National Military Family Association. These organizations create and strengthen important linkages and enhance communication between various stakeholders, so that the research is informed by the most pressing needs "on the ground" and translated into action and policy reform.

18.5 Lessons Learned in Conducting Military Family Research

As we begin to look at the future of research priorities and strategies needed to support military families, it is first important to look back and take stock of the specific knowledge generated and disseminated over the past 15 years of conflict we discussed in the last section, but also of the lessons learned and challenged faced in the process of generating and disseminating it. In doing so, we hope to help our successors avoid similar challenges and benefit from our community's lessons learned. Perhaps, truly learning from these lessons and not repeating them can lead to greater clarity in future research studies and more impactful insights for supporting military families.

18.5.1   Poor Coordination and Little Strategic Portfolio Management

Over the course of the conflicts in Iraq and Afghanistan, multiple different entities across the services (those in the medical research arena, as well as those in the family support arena) initiated and supported research and analysis.[1] While this meant many studies were commissioned, it also meant there were multiple players moving in multiple directions, often going forward with little awareness of the other efforts underway and frequently with no coordination between efforts. This resulted in many "family research" portfolios and sometimes given the nature of the contracts, the inability to ensure that those working in the space could communicate with each other. This ultimately diminished the sectors' ability to create synergies and address gaps.

18.5.2   Scope and Design Issues Limited Generalizability of Findings

As noted earlier, research on military families over the past decade was often motivated to measure the scope of specific problems, to identify specific gaps in programs or initiatives, and to examine or assess the impact of some sort of intervention on outcomes. While important for understanding the impact of deployment and documenting need among the community, the results of this type of research focus also drove a narrative on military families as being broken or having problems, when in reality the rates of problems were often low overall (Cigrang et al., 2014; Karney & Crown, 2010; Trail, Meadows, Miles, & Karney, 2015).

At the same time, most research commissioned during the current war era focused on the use of cross-sectional data which really limited our ability to understand causal effects and impact. Where longitudinal data were employed by studies, they often relied only on administrative data sources (such as DEERS data or health care utilization records) that may be poor proxies for the outcomes of interest. In addition, many studies conducted over the past decade only looked at subpopulations

---

[1] Each of the services was conducting studies to understand how their families were faring, in addition to various defense agencies and different parts of the Office of the Secretary of Defense (e.g., Reserve Affairs, Military Community and Family Policy, Health Affairs).

(for example, Army wives or Marine Corps children) and lacked appropriate comparison groups as well. All of these design issues made it difficult to generalize from the studies to other populations or setting. For example, it is not appropriate to assume that a study focused on a group of Army wives living on a military installation generalizes to a population of Army wives living off-base, or Army wives of reservists, let alone spouses of other service members.

In the past several years, we also saw a proliferation in surveys conducted by nonprofit member based organizations (Blue Star Families, IAVA, American Legion, DAV) and other unofficial poles conducted by members of the media (Washington Post), all designed to identify challenges and issues facing their communities in an effort to shape dialog and decision-making for better support, benefits, etc. However, the convenience methods employed in these efforts may lack the rigor of some of those conducted by professional research organizations and this can have enormous impact with respect to the potential bias in the results.

18.5.3   Navigating Required Approval Processes Has Contributed to Significant Delays

Minimizing burden and risk associated with research is critically important in the conduct of studies on military families; ensuring appropriate privacy protections are in place is also critical to maintaining force readiness. And, in conducting studies that rely upon the participation of family members or access to data about them, research organizations are required to comply with all federal regulations (1991 revision to the U.S. Department of Health and Human Services Title 45 CFR 46 Subpart A: Common Rule; DoD Directive 3216.02). DoD and the VA each have their own sets of procedures and oversight bodies with responsibility to ensure this compliance; however, within DoD, there are multiple levels of oversight bodies that are often engaged in the review and approval of a single project (multiple IRBs, Privacy Offices, DMDC and WHS, the Chain of Command). For many studies, coordinating and navigating multiple different processes led to significant delays (which can be costly), conflicting guidance from different oversight entities, and exposed families to potential harm (Freed et al., 2015). The delays alone were quite severe and led to lags in our nation's ability to most effectively support families during an era of extended conflict.

18.5.4   Collecting and Sharing Data Was Challenging

As more research studies got underway, there became greater awareness of the need for consistent use of validated measures, as well as the development of new measures for evolving constructs. There were some attempts to identify and promulgate a common set of measures and metrics to be used in studies, particularly those in the health area (e.g., the NIH-funded PhenX Toolkit, www.phenxtoolkit.org; DCoE's efforts to standardize TBI measures, Wilde et al., 2010). Creating measure repositories also became popular as a means of facilitate research on military family issues. However, there still exists wide variability in how certain characteristics and outcomes are assessed, whether it be using different scales and scores for assessing PTSD or whether predictor variables are measured and included in analyses. In addition, comparing across data sets in the nation is difficult as the USA lacks a standard way for assessing military or veteran affiliation. These issues are essential for understanding what population any study findings reflect and how to compare findings across different studies.

The timing of data collection is also an important factor in interpreting data and study findings. The deployments to Iraq and Afghanistan were not static over the entire period of conflict, so it is inappropriate to believe that deployment experiences in 2003 were similar to those in 2012; not only was the makeup of the force different at these two time points, but the experience on the ground was vastly different for troops. This is another area where the reliance on cross-sectional data may contribute to blind spots in our understanding of how military families fared across this extended period of conflict.

The ability to access and share data is also often a hurdle. Not only can accessing DoD data be challenging due to various issues, but being able to share datasets and early findings across the research community can be difficult and counterintuitive in the competitive research environment. We mentioned earlier the multiple players conducting studies on military families, but in general there were very few opportunities for sharing and cross-fertilization of knowledge and findings (cite MFRI conferences and MSPAN summit). Many researchers relied upon their personal relationships to share informally and others had to wait until findings and data became publicly available to learn and build upon prior work. This inability to share may have minimized the field's ability to draw greater synergy and address gaps in the overall landscape in a timely manner.

18.5.5 Disseminating Findings to Inform Policy Requires Strategic Intention and Effort

Once knowledge is generated, in order for it to inform policy and program decision-making, it must be shared or disseminated with the appropriate audiences. In some cases for work conducted within the research and policy institute sector, the sponsoring agencies set specific restrictions or expectations around dissemination and publication. This often creates a set of mixed incentives with respect to what research gets publicly released or shared with appropriate stakeholders (even if not publicly available). While there has been a greater demand for transparency and program evaluation in the Obama Administration, many sponsoring agencies in the research and policy sector still would prefer to keep the knowledge or research results under wraps; sometimes even making it difficult for another part of the same agency to access the findings and recommendations. For those that do publish and disseminate the findings, making sense of what it means for policymakers is a challenge. In order to ensure that research can be translated into policy, intention is required to disseminate findings and recommendations through several mechanisms—beyond just publishing an article in a peer-reviewed journal. This often requires distilling complicated material into succinct materials and briefings, and disseminating them intentionally to appropriate stakeholders (versus letting them passively read about them in the literature). Toward this end, engaging the stakeholder community, and particularly the military and veteran support organizations, in the study process (and its dissemination) can be a critical amplifier and enabler of research-based policy decision-making.

18.6   Recommendations

In an effort to support military families effectively and efficiently now and in the future, we outline several recommendations for crafting and implementing research in a more strategic and informed manner.

18.6.1   Build Cross-Sector Support for Reliable Family Research Funding Stream

To create the conditions necessary to facilitate research studies that inform and support military families during periods of extended conflict, support will be needed across various sectors and organizations (governmental and nongovernmental). Building this support can help to galvanize the necessary resources and motivate policymakers and program officials to prioritize the importance of research, as well as ensure that resources are available in an ongoing, stable fashion. If this doesn't happen, the erratic nature of resources may force significant gaps in our knowledge base and support infrastructure.

18.6.2   Craft Strategic Research Agenda on Military Families

Understanding the gaps in the current knowledge base can help inform areas for new investment. At the same time, outlining different domains and areas of inquiry can be helpful for facilitating a more balanced portfolio approach. To this end, it will be important for the stakeholder community to come together to create a strategic plan for military family research. This work should involve not only the identification of research gaps that should be targeted in the future, but it should include the definition of key constructs, processes, and outcomes of interest.

18.6.3   Build and Maintain Representative Panel of Military Families, Cross-Service, Cross-Component

In order to ensure a consistent stream of data to inform policy and program officials on the issues affecting military families that may require additional attention, ongoing surveillance activities are necessary. While OSD has tried to add spouse panels to ongoing studies, like the Status of Forces Survey and the MilCo Study, the original sampling frame for those studies was based upon the overall military force. As such, it is not clear that the spouse participants in these studies reflect the overall population of military spouses. Therefore, there is high value in constructing and maintaining a representative cohort study of military families that includes periodic (although somewhat more frequent than once per year) data collection on topics relevant to the needs and issues affecting military families and force readiness.

18.6.4   Streamline and Modernize Regulatory Processes

As noted in the prior section, navigating the various approval processes caused significant delays for studies of military families. This included trying to coordinate among multiple Institutional Review Boards, gaining local and regional command/unit leadership buy-in, and getting through the information collection approval processes (DoD Directive 3216.02). While these regulatory processes are in place to protect/safeguard study participants and minimize burden, the fact that multiple layers are often required is redundant. To facilitate greater progress and more efficient knowledge generation, the DoD will need to streamline and modernize its procedures for ensuring compliance with appropriate federal regulations, to include creating and using rapid review procedures to ensure that the delays in conducting the research do not begin to inflict greater harm to the population that the burden of participating (Federal Register proposed rule 80 FR 53931: Federal Policy for the Protection of Human Subjects).

18.6.5   Facilitate Greater Access to Data and Findings

Informing good policy and program development or refinement requires having access to existing data or gathering new data. Several data sources already exist and can be helpful; however, accessing them for purposes of studies and analyses can often be quite challenging. At the same time, when new datasets are created, they often remain underutilized. Mechanisms and policies may be required to facilitate great access to and use of data on military families. We also need to work, as a field, more diligently to ensure that the findings generated from our research are shared with others in the research community, but also in the policy making community.

18.6.6 The Time Is Now

Research will continue to play an important role in supporting military families; however, to do so in a more efficient manner in the future, we will need an ongoing commitment to the creation and management of a strategic research agenda on military families across the federal government. We simply cannot afford to wait until the "next conflict" to design and initiate critical studies. Rather, we need to create environment of studying military family quality of life during eras of peacetime that can be used as a backbone and platform for studies during extended periods of deployment and conflict.

References

Allen, M. (2003, August 9). Bush cites 'progress' being made in Iraq; white house report on 'successes' in iraq counters criticism of postwar plan. *The Washington Post*. Retrieved from http://search.proquest.com/docview/409508382?accountid=25333.

Chandra, A., Lara-Cinisomo, S., Jaycox, L. H., Tanielian, T., Burns, R. M., Ruder, T., & Han, B. (2010). Children on the Homefront: The experience of children from military families. *Pediatrics, 125*, 16–25.

Chandra, A., Lara-Cinisomo, S., Jaycox, L. H., Tanielian, T., Han, B., Burns, R. M., & Ruder, T. (2011). *Views from the Homefront*. Santa Monica, CA: RAND Corporation.

Cigrang, J. A., Talcott, G. W., Tatum, J., Baker, M., Cassidy, D., Sonnek, S., et al. (2014). Intimate partner communication from the war zone: A prospective study of relationship functioning, communication frequency, and combat effectiveness. *Journal of Marital and Family Therapy, 40*, 332–343.

Crum-Cianflone, N. F., Fairbank, J. A., Marmar, C. R., & Schlenger, W. (2014). The Millennium Cohort Family Study: A prospective evaluation of the health and well-being of military service members and their families. *International Journal of Methods in Psychiatric Research, 23*, 320–330.

Davis, L. E., Polich, J. M., Hix, W. M., Greenberg, M. D., & Brady, S. (2005). *Stretched Thin: Army Forces for Sustained Operations*. Santa Monica, CA: RAND Corporation.

Defense Manpower Data Center (2012) Survey of Active Duty Spouses: Tabulations of Responses. Alexandria, VA Available at: http://oai.dtic.mil/oai/oai?verb=getRecord&metadataPrefix=html&identifier=ADA609606

DMDC (2015). Military Family Life Project: Active Duty Spouse Study Longitudinal Analysis 2010–2012 Project Report. Alexandria VA available at: http://download.militaryonesource.mil/12038/MOS/Reports/MFLPLongitudinal-Analyses-Report.pdf

Engel, C. C., Hyams, K. C., & Scott, K. (2006). Managing future Gulf War Syndromes: International lessons and new models of care. *Philosophical Transactions of the Royal Society of London B: Biological Sciences, 36*, 707–720.

Freed, M. C., Novak, L. A., Kilgore, W. D. S., Rauch, S. A. M., Koehlmoos, A. Ginsberg, J. P., et al. (2015, under review). IRB and Research Regulatory Delays within the Military Healthcare Setting: Do They Really Matter? And If so, Why and for Whom? *The American Journal of Bioethics*.

Glod, M. (2008, July 17). Coping with their parents' war; multiple deployments compound strain for children of service members. *The Washington Post*. Retrieved from http://search.proquest.com/docview/410234597?accountid=25333.

IOM. (2013). *Returning home from Iraq and Afghanistan: Assessment of readjustment needs of veterans, service members, and their families.* Washington, DC: The National Academies Press.

Karney, B. R., & Crown, J. S. (2010). Does deployment keep military marriages together or break them apart? Evidence from Afghanistan and Iraq. In S. M. Wadsworth & D. Riggs (Eds.), *Risk and resilience in U.S. Military Families.* New York: Springer.

Loeb, V. (2003, December 28). Pace of casualties in Iraq has risen; counterinsurgency costlier than combat. *The Washington Post.* Retrieved from http://search.proquest.com/docview/409528206?accountid=25333.

McCarroll, J. E., Ursano, R. J., Liu, X., Thayer, L. E., Newby, J. H., Norwood, A. E., & Fullerton, C. S. (2010). Deployment and the probability of spousal aggression by U.S. Army Soldiers. *Military Medicine, 175,* 352–356.

McIntyre, J. (2005, June 8). War takes toll on military marriages. *CNN.* Retrieved from http://www.cnn.com/2005/US/06/08/military.marriages/.

Ross, S. M. (2010). Fighting two protracted wars. In S. Carlton-Ford & M. G. Ender (Eds.), *The Routledge handbook of war and society: Iraq and Afghanistan* (pp. 9–19). New York: Routledge.

SteelFisher, G. K., Zaslavsky, A. M., & Blendon, R. J. (2008). Health-related impact of deployment extensions on spouses of active duty army personnel. *Military Medicine, 173,* 221–229.

Tanielian, T., Karney, B. R., Chandra, A., Meadows, S. O., & Deployment Life Study Team. (2014). *The deployment life study: Methodological overview and baseline sample description.* Santa Monica, CA: RAND Corporation (RR-209). Retrieved from http://www.rand.org/pubs/research_reports/RR209.html.

Trail, T. E., Meadows, S. O., Miles, J. N., & Karney, B. R. (2015). Patterns of vulnerabilities and resources in U.S. military families. *Journal of Family Issues.*

Weinick, R. M., Beckjord, E. B., Farmer, C. M., Martin, L. T., Gillen, E. M., Acosta, J. D., et al. (2011). *Programs addressing psychological health and traumatic brain injury among U.S. military servicemembers and their families.* Santa Monica, CA: RAND.

Wilde, E. A., Whiteneck, G. G., Bogner, J., Bushnik, T., Cifu, D. X., Dikmen, S., et al. (2010). Recommendations for the use of common outcome measures in traumatic brain injury research. *Archives of Physical Medicine and Rehabilitation, 91,* 1650–1660. e1617.

Chapter 19
Military Families Research: Department of Defense Funding and the Elements of a Fundable Proposal

Carl A. Castro and Kathrine S. Sullivan

Today's US Military consists of more than two million service members and almost three million family members (Department of Defense [DOD], 2015). It has long been understood that the health of the military family is critical to the well-being of our service members and to overall mission readiness (Park, 2011). Since 2001, however, military families have been exposed to an unprecedented host of stressors, including repeated overseas deployment of loved ones, combat-related physical and mental health injuries, and frequent relocations (Burrell, Adams, Durand, & Castro, 2006; Cozza & Lerner, 2013). Concerns about how military families would respond to these stressors sparked a surge of research into the functioning of these family systems. Despite this surge, empirical efforts to understand the functioning of military families still lag behind in comparison to research efforts focused on service men and women (Park, 2011). In order to address gaps in our knowledge, new, larger and more robust empirical studies of military families must be undertaken.

This chapter will focus on describing the basics of DOD's research funding process, including a review of the Psychological Health Research Continuum (Castro, 2014), as it pertains to military families research. Further, we will discuss important elements of a fundable research proposal from the perspective of the DOD, including a review of relevant family theories with the goal of providing a useful framework for future proposals aimed at addressing gaps in the military families knowledge base. Lastly, we will discuss challenges in military families research including ethical issues and the time and costs associated with conducting research with military families.

C.A. Castro, Ph.D. (✉) • K.S. Sullivan, M.S.W.
University of Southern California, Suzanne Dworak-Peck School of Social Work,
Los Angeles, CA, USA
e-mail: cacastro@usc.edu; kate.sullivan@usc.edu

© Springer International Publishing AG 2018   323
L. Hughes-Kirchubel et al. (eds.), *A Battle Plan for Supporting Military Families*, Risk and Resilience in Military and Veteran Families,
https://doi.org/10.1007/978-3-319-68984-5_19

19.1   The Basics of DOD Funding

In the broadest sense, the Department of Defense (DoD) funds research and development that is relevant and often unique to its mission. This research falls predominantly into the hard sciences, involving weapons systems development. However, the DOD also funds medical and social science research. For the purposes of military families research, it may be most useful to understand the Military Psychological Health Research Continuum (Castro, 2014) as this framework provides a common language, has been adopted by the White House to shape interagency research strategy, and is being used to guide research priorities. This continuum was initially developed in response to concerns regarding the mental health of service members in the contexts of the wars in Iraq and Afghanistan, but is equally applicable to future research aimed at addressing aspects of military families' social and psychological well-being.

The continuum, presented in Fig. 19.1, consists of seven domains that build on one another, including foundational science, epidemiology, etiology, prevention and screening, treatment, follow-up care, and services research (Castro, 2014). Each of these domains will be discussed briefly. *Foundational science* involves discovery of mechanisms and biological processes that cause disease. As families research is largely focused on social processes, proposals are unlikely to be classified as foundational science. Yet, family researchers should not shy away from applying for such research funding. *Epidemiology* studies are concerned with the incidence, patterns, and causes of health conditions at the population level. These studies tend to be descriptive, large-scale, and prospective, like the Millennium Cohort Family Study, whose goal is to follow over 10,000 service members and their spouses for 21+ years in order to evaluate the impact of military-related stressors on family life (Crum-Cianflone, Fairbank, Marmar, & Schlenger, 2014). *Etiology* studies are focused on the biological, social, or environmental causes of disease. Research in this category might focus on biomarkers or the origins of mental health diagnoses in adverse childhood experiences. *Prevention and screening* efforts are focused on reducing and preventing risk of adverse outcomes,

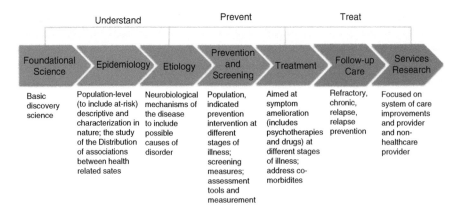

Fig. 19.1 Military psychological health research continuum (Castro 2014). Used with permission

improving resilience capacity, and reducing stigma. Screening, specifically, may be focused on evaluating measures and assessment tools. *Treatment*-focused efforts are largely concerned with ameliorating symptoms or other adverse outcomes, including evaluating interventions and medication. Efforts to evaluate family-based treatment modalities would fall into this category of research. *Follow-up care* research involves evaluating long-term outcomes from treatment and relapse prevention. Lastly, *services research* is focused on large-scale changes to systems of care, including access, utilization, and delivery of services (Castro, 2014).

At DOD, gaps are identified within these seven domains of research and are prioritized based on a number of factors, including the number of service members or their dependents who are affected, the severity of the identified problem, and the existing state of the science in that particular area (Castro, 2014). Given the competition for DOD funding, particularly in medical and social science research, before developing a full proposal, it is critical to understand where a particular research question or problem fits into the continuum described above and to assess the potential for funding through the DoD. Only research questions or problems that address a critical research gap in one of these research domains should be pursued.

It is important to appreciate that military family program development, sustainment, evaluation, and assessments are not considered research. All too often military family advocates believe that simply collecting data to show that their current family program is useful constitutes "research." While conducting such studies is important, these studies do not constitute research, and thus will never be funded by DOD research programs.

19.2 Elements of a Fundable Proposal

Once the decision has been made that a particular military families-focused research question meets the criteria described above and is worthy of the effort involved in developing a research proposal, potential DOD funding applicants should ensure that their proposal includes the following critical elements: (1) a clear definition of what constitutes a military family for the purposes of the proposal; (2) a solid definition of the problem that the proposal intends to address; and (3) a robust theoretical orientation or framework that provides a justification for the proposed hypotheses. Each of these elements of a fundable proposal will be discussed in detail below.

19.2.1 Defining the Military Family

Conceptual murkiness around who is and is not considered part of a military family could be a fatal flaw in a research proposal. Depending on the source and purpose, how the military family is defined varies widely. Political definitions tend to be broad. For example, the President and the Joint Chiefs of Staff have defined military families to include: "active-duty service members, members of the National Guard and Reserve, and veterans, plus the members of their immediate and extended families, as well as the families of those who lost their lives in service to their country" (Cozza & Lerner, 2013, p. 4). While this certainly has political value, from a research perspective, very inclusive definitions like this one are not helpful in the development of research proposals. For the purposes of DOD policy decisions and program eligibility, military families are defined more narrowly as those dependents (spouses and children) who are registered in the Defense Enrollment Eligibility Reporting System (DEERS). Eligible spouses include married (and divorced in a few special cases) partners of active duty, guard/reserve and retired service members, including same sex spouses. Eligible children include biological, adopted, and stepchildren (as long as the sponsor is married to their biological parent) until their 23rd birthday (Tricare, n.d.). Researchers engaged in military families research have tended to use a definition that closely resembles this policy definition. For the purposes of military families research, a clear definition of the military family includes spouses and dependent children (until their 23rd birthday) of service members on active duty or in the National Guard and Reserve (Cozza & Lerner, 2013). Many researchers also broaden this definition to include the families of military veterans in acknowledgement of the ongoing stressors that military experience can have on the family system following separation from service. However, though veteran families are certainly a population worthy of study, a narrow definition focused on active duty, Guard and Reserve families is likely more amenable to DOD funding.

19.2.2 Defining the Problem

While clear problem definition is the hallmark of any good study, research proposals aimed at the DoD should clearly articulate a capability that the military currently lacks which the proposed research will develop. Thus a research question or a research problem, even one that is clearly defined, is not sufficient for a fundable proposal from the perspective of the DOD. Rather, a successful DOD proposal should articulate how the capability the proposal will develop serves the mission of the DoD.

19.2.3 A Strong Theoretical Orientation

Previous scholars have noted the lack of explicit theory that characterizes much existing military families research (Park, 2011; Riggs & Riggs, 2011). Indeed, military family theory is underdeveloped. Nevertheless, theory serves an important purpose in a fundable proposal. In addition to previous empirical evidence, a robust theoretical framework justifies the proposed hypotheses and provides a rationale to funders as to why the proposed work is likely to be successful. In order to support the use of theory in future military families proposals, the next section will review a number of theories that could be applicable to military families research.

19.3   Military Family Theories

In this section we will describe a number of theories, which may be of use in developing military families research proposals. Some of the reviewed theories have more explanatory utility than others, but all of them at a minimum could be used to inform an explanatory conceptual framework and guide variable selection. Further, this is not intended to be an exhaustive list of useful theories but rather an illustration that useful theoretical perspectives exist. First we will review several general family theories that have been used to understand military family functioning in previous research. Second, we will review a number of theories designed explicitly to understand the dynamics of military families.

19.3.1   General Family Theories

Family Systems Theory

Military families researchers invoke family systems theory as a useful framework through which to view the impact of military-related stressors on families (DeVoe & Ross, 2012; Paley, Lester & Mogil, 2013). This theoretical orientation suggests that the causes of behavior are not a function of the individual alone, but are determined, at least in part, through interactions with the family (Cox & Paley, 1997; Minuchin, 1974). Family systems theory assumes that members of the same family system will have an ongoing and reciprocal impact on each other through the active stabilization processes that maintain family homeostasis (Cox & Paley, 1997; Minuchin, 1974).

Circumplex Model

The circumplex model (Olson, 2000) assumes that balanced families will function more successfully than unbalanced families. Family balance is determined by where families fall on three dimensions: cohesion, flexibility, and communication. *Cohesion* is essentially the family's sense of togetherness or emotional bonding and ranges through four levels (disengaged, separated, connected, and enmeshed) with the middle two levels considered more balanced than the extremes. *Flexibility* concerns the amount of change the family can tolerate and also ranges through four levels (chaotic, flexible, structured, and rigid). Again, the middle two levels are considered more balanced. Finally, communication facilitates a family's movement across the preceding two dimensions. The circumplex model is the foundation for the FACES self-report instruments that assess family functioning.

Family Stress Theory

Family stress theory is actually a group of theories that all derive from Reuben Hill's ABC-X model, developed through work with veterans of World War II and their families (Hill, 1958). This group includes the double ABC-X model (Patterson & Mccubbin, 1983), the family adjustment and adaptation response model (FAAR; Patterson, 1988), and the contextual model of family stress and coping (Boss, 2002). As a group, these theories attempt to explain why some families adapt and thrive despite exposure to stress while other families may experience crisis. Generally, these theories suggest that a family's resources, both internal and external, and their capacity to make meaning out of stressor events determine their ability to successfully cope with a single stressor or, more likely, the pileup of both large and small stressors that most families face.

19.3.2 Military Family Theories

Military Family Fitness Model

The military family fitness model (Bowles et al., 2015) applies concepts from both the circumplex model and family stress theories to military families specifically. This framework distinguishes resilient families, who have overcome stressors, from fit families, who are ready to meet demands but have yet to experience significant stressors. The military family fitness model posits that family demands (e.g., deployments) require the mobilization of internal and external resources at multiple levels (individual, family, external) to promote adaptive outcomes (e.g., well-being). Maladaptive outcomes result when demands exceed resources.

Conceptual Model of Military Career and Family Life Course Events

This theory builds on life course theory, the stress process model, and Segal's greedy institutions hypothesis, which posits a potential conflict between the military and the family, both "greedy institutions" that place large demands on service members (Segal, Lane, & Fisher, 2015). This model assumes that events within or intersections among four dimensions of the life course (military, family, child, and major life events) will determine well-being. The impact of events or intersections on well-being outcomes may be mediated or moderated by several factors, including demographics, military contextual variables, and resources.

The Emotional Cycle of Deployment

This is a stage model that describes the social and psychological aspects of military deployments as experienced by service members and their families (Pincus, House, Christenson, & Adler, 2001). The model hypothesizes five stages to the deployment cycle and specifies a time frame and particular social/emotional tasks, which must be mastered at each stage. The stages include pre-deployment, deployment, sustainment, redeployment, and post-deployment. As this model was proposed prior to the start of combat operations in Afghanistan in 2001, there are aspects of this model, particularly the time frames proposed for each stage, that are out of date with the current experiences of many military families. However, the deployment cycle concept and the emotional tasks at each stage are still relevant to many families experiencing one or multiple deployments.

Family Attachment Network Model

This is a complex model that builds on family systems theory, attachment theory, and diathesis stress models to describe the adaptation of military families during the deployment and reintegration process (Riggs & Riggs, 2011). In this model, the attachment style of the military spouse determines his or her coping strategies during the service member's deployment and ultimately shapes parenting, family processes, and child outcomes, including well-being, internalizing and externalizing behavior. This perspective also describes three different archetypal family systems: (1) the fit for duty family, which adapts well to deployment stressors, (2) the closed-ranks family, in which maladjustment to deployment is characterized by rigidity and disengagement; and (3) the open-ranks family, in which maladjustment is characterized by diffuse boundaries and inappropriate communication.

Resiliency Model of Role Performance

This model distinguishes between resilience, a process which reflects one's ability to perform roles despite adversity or to recover following challenging experiences that overwhelm role performance, and resiliency, which reflects the outcome of that process and can be observed at the individual or family level (Bowen & Martin, 2011). A successful outcome of this process is defined as role performance, referring to one's overall performance of responsibilities as a service member, spouse, parent, etc. In this model, social connections and individual assets have both a direct impact on resiliency (operationalized as role performance) and an indirect effect through self-orientations and behavioral health. These variables may also moderate the impact of stressors and risks.

While the reviewed theories offer a foundation on which to build, future research that advances military family theory development is desperately needed. It would be extremely valuable, for instance, to develop a program of research that pits one of these theories against another so that poorly performing theories may be discarded or modified. Ultimately, it would be useful to unite the military family research community around a guiding theoretical framework.

19.4 Ethical Issues in the Conduct of Research with Military Families

Among many reasons that could explain the paucity of empirical research with military families are the ethical issues inherent in conducting research with this population. According to Department of Defense Instruction Number 3126.02 (DOD, 2011), both DOD personnel and children are protected research participants. With regard to service members, this instruction prohibits superiors from influencing their subordinates' decision with regard to research participation. With regard to children, this instruction directs potential investigators to the Code of Federal Regulations, Part 46, Sub-Part D. This regulation provides that, in most cases, research with children involving greater than minimal risk must present the prospect of direct benefit to the actual research participants (Protection of Human Subjects, 2009). This regulation, while justified and certainly well intentioned, nevertheless makes it very difficult to involve children in original research and particularly in randomized controlled trials (RCTs).

While these ethical challenges may deter many potential investigators from undertaking empirical research with military families, there is a counter-balancing ethical obligation that we encourage researchers to consider. The ethical requirements inherent in conducting research with this population, and particularly with military-connected children, has the unintended consequence that many programs designed to meet the needs of military families have not been adequately evaluated (Park, 2011). Thus, many families may already be participating in programs that may or may be suitable to actually meeting their needs. Thus, as researchers, our ethical obligation to protect research participants from harm must be balanced against our obligation to save lives and alleviate suffering, which includes our obligation to provide service members, families, and children with evidence-based care.

19.5 Time and Costs Required to Conduct Military Family Research

Another important consideration in conducting military family research is the time and costs it takes to conduct research. The funding cycle within DOD is 2 years from the initial identification of the idea to receipt of funding by the investigator. This timeline does not include the time it might take to receive human subjects approval and the time to collect, analyze, and report the research findings, which could easily take an additional 3–5 years. Realistically, a military families research study will take a minimum of 5–7 years to complete.

Additionally, the cost to conduct a rigorous military families research study may vary considerably. A small pilot study may cost as little as $200,000, while a large treatment or services research study could easily cost $10 million. It is rare that a single study can solve a critical research problem or provide a needed capability. Indeed, several studies are typically required. Thus, the investment in time and money required to solve a single, critical military families issue could take 15–21 years, costing $20–30 million. While many readers may view such costs and time estimates as ridiculous or absurd, DOD has well over a decade of data supporting such cost and time estimates. This finding argues for the continuation of military families research well after the wars in Iraq and Afghanistan end, as well as the identification and prioritization of the most pressing military family issues that research can address.

19.6 Way Ahead

Science is hard. There are no shortcuts or easy approaches. In this chapter, we have outlined some of the enduring elements that make family research proposals successful in obtaining DoD funding. As funding opportunities decline, it will become even more challenging to secure research funding focused on the military family. However, we mustn't despair. The DoD has always allotted funding to military family research. Our task will be to incorporate these basic elements into our military family research to ensure that are allotted are well spent.

References

Boss, P. (2002). *Family stress management*. Thousand Oaks CA: Sage.

Bowen, G. L., & Martin, J. A. (2011). The resiliency model of role performance for service members, veterans, and their families: A focus on social connections and individual assets. *Journal of Human Behavior in the Social Environment, 21*(2), 162–178.

Bowles, S. V., Pollock, L. D., Moore, M., Wadsworth, S. M., Cato, C., Dekle, J. W., et al. (2015). Total force fitness: The military family fitness model. *Military Medicine, 180*(3), 246–258.

Burrell, L. M., Adams, G. A., Durand, D. B., & Castro, C. A. (2006). The impact of military lifestyle demands on well-being, Army, and family outcomes. *Armed Forces & Society, 33*(1), 43–58.

Castro, C. A. (2014). The US framework for understanding, preventing, and caring for the mental health needs of service members who served in Combat in Afghanistan and Iraq: A brief review of the issues and the research. *European Journal of Psychotraumatology, 5*, 1–12.

Cozza, C. S. J., & Lerner, R. M. (2013). Military children and families: Introducing the issue. *The Future of Children, 23*(2), 3–11.

Crum-Cianflone, N. F., Fairbank, J. A., Marmar, C. R., & Schlenger, W. (2014). The Millennium Cohort Family Study: A prospective evaluation of the health and well-being of military service members and their families. *International Journal of Methods in Psychiatric Research, 23*(3), 320–330.

Department of Defense. (2011). *Department of Defense Instruction: Protection of Human Subjects and Adherence to Ethical Standards in DoD-Supported Research*. Retrieved from http://www.dtic.mil/whs/directives/corres/pdf/321602p.pdf.

Department of Defense. (2015). *2014 Demographics Profile of the Military Community.* Retrieved from: http://download.militaryonesource.mil/12038/MOS/Reports/2014-Demographics-Report.pdf.

DeVoe, E. R., & Ross, A. (2012). The parenting cycle of deployment. *Military Medicine, 177*(2), 184–190.

Hill, R. (1958). Generic features of families under stress. *Social Casework, 49*, 139–150.

Minuchin, S. (1974). Families and Family Therapy. Boston, MA: Harvard Press, and London: Tavistock.

Olson, D. H. (2000). Circumplex model of marital and family systems. *Journal of Family Therapy, 22*(2), 144–167.

Paley, B., Lester, P., & Mogil, C. (2013). Family systems and ecological perspectives on the impact of deployment on military families. *Clinical Child and Family Psychology Review, 16*(3), 245–265.

Park, N. (2011). Military children and families: Strengths and challenges during peace and war. *American Psychologist, 66*(1), 65–72.

Patterson, J. M., & Mccubbin, H. I. (1983). The impact of family life events and changes on the health of a chronically III child. *Family Relations, 32*(2), 255–264.

Patterson, J. (1988). Families experiencing stress: The family adjustment and adaptation response model. *Family Systems Medicine, 6*(2), 202–237.

Protection of Human Subjects. (2009). *Code of Federal Regulations, 45 C.F.R. Part 46, Sub-part D.* Retrieved from http://www.hhs.gov/ohrp/regulations-and-policy/regulations/45-cfr-46/.

Riggs, S. A., & Riggs, D. S. (2011). Risk and resilience in military families experiencing deployment: The role of the family attachment network. *Journal of Family Psychology, 25*(5), 675–687.

Segal, M. W., Lane, M. D., & Fisher, A. G. (2015). Conceptual model of military career and family life course events, intersections, and effects on well-being. *Military Behavioral Health, 3*(2), 95–107.

Tricare (n.d.). Tricare eligibility. Retrieved from: https://www.tricare.mil/Plans/Eligibility.

Chapter 20
Rules of Engagement: Media Coverage of Military Families During War

Karen G. Jowers and Patricia N. Kime

20.1 The Dynamic Role of News Organizations

In the early days of the Iraq war, a Military Times photographer took a picture of a mortally wounded soldier as he was being rushed to treatment. The photo was a compelling, moving portrayal of the agony of war (Neill, 2015). Alex Neill, who was until 2016 executive editor of Military Times, remembers spending hours on the phone with Army officials and the soldier's grief-stricken family, who asked him not to run the photo. It was late in the editorial process and the decision already had been made to run the picture—small, on the inside of the papers, and not on the front cover, as the Army and family feared. During the conversations with military officials and family members, Neill said he learned much about cultural sensitivity regarding military families and the military community.

Neill is no stranger to this military world; he is a Navy veteran who has worked at the Military Times media organization for nearly two decades. His years of covering the military have only strengthened his belief that cultural sensitivity and awareness is integral to the coverage. Every day, he and other journalists who write about the military must question and analyze the words, photos, and videos used to tell the public about war.

The authors thank the countless military families we have known in our personal lives and professional lives who have contributed greatly to our understanding of and respect for this unique community. Any opinions, findings, conclusions, or recommendations expressed in this chapter are those of the authors and do not necessarily reflect the views of Military Times.

K.G. Jowers, B.A. (✉)
Sightline Media Group, Vienna, VA, USA
e-mail: kjowers@militarytimes.com

P.N. Kime, B.A.
Arlington, VA, USA
e-mail: patriciankime@gmail.com

© Springer International Publishing AG 2018
L. Hughes-Kirchubel et al. (eds.), *A Battle Plan for Supporting Military Families*, Risk and Resilience in Military and Veteran Families,
https://doi.org/10.1007/978-3-319-68984-5_20

Every news organization makes decisions about coverage. Just as Military Times editors chose to run that photograph, they, like editors at the Washington Post and New York Times, have held or delayed release of information at the request of military leaders—or decided to run stories regardless of the Pentagon's wishes—but only after great discussion and thought.

With the prolonged conflicts in Iraq and Afghanistan, news outlets have covered not just the early and continued fighting, but some lasting effects on service members and families, which are addressed in other chapters in this book. The purpose of this chapter is not to provide blanket advice to news outlets on covering military personnel and family members, but to raise some issues and questions to consider. News organizations differ widely in their approaches to writing, filming, and photographing the military community. Different circumstances including war, training, budget climates, and operational tempo often dictate how a media organization will handle coverage day to day, weekly, monthly, and yearly. This chapter does not propose to be last word on how to cover the military community. Instead, it pulls together some of the lessons learned from the previous 15 years of war that may help future media outlets as they make assignment decisions, cover military personnel and families in their communities, and report on this community, both in peace and in wartime. In wartime deployments, military families face heavy burdens with fears about the risk of injury or death of their service member. But that's not the whole story of the military family lifestyle, which is often filled with disruptions. On orders from the military, service members frequently relocate their families to a new duty station, causing major changes and adjustments in families' lives, such as uprooting children from schools and disrupting the careers of non-military spouses. Deployments even in peace time cause logistical challenges for the spouse left behind who in effect becomes a single parent while managing the stress. In some cases with dual-military couples, both parents are deployed, and they've had to make arrangements for other family members or friends to care for the children. It is also important to remember that the military family is not just spouses and children, but parents, grandparents, siblings, and other relatives. Military personnel have left communities across the country to serve in the armed forces, and the relatives they leave behind in these communities also feel the effects. Other relatives of military members may not have the kinds of support from the military establishment that spouses and children have. There are many different situations, and it helps journalists to talk to families to begin to understand how stressful and difficult these wartime deployments are.

For civilians and non-journalists, including organizations that work with and support military personnel, veterans, and their families, this chapter may provide a glimpse of some of the issues the ever-evolving media face, including doing more with fewer resources. Some news outlets cover the military community around the world day in and day out, during war and peace and in the aftermath of war. In communities where a large military installation exists, some journalists may primarily cover the military community regularly. Some media organizations, however, may not have enough manpower to assign someone regularly to the military beat. But even if covering the military is a smaller portion of someone's beat, it is important that the person assigned the task has some level of understanding and expertise with the military, regardless of the size of the newsroom, according to Kirsti Marohn, a reporter who worked for the St. Cloud (Minnesota) Times from 1998 until 2017. Her advice? "Having someone with sources, even in peacetime. …Following Facebook [or other current social media platform], knowing which units have people in your community, so you're not starting from ground zero on deadline" (Marohn, 2015).

More than 2.4 million people have served in the Iraq and Afghanistan wars. As of mid-2016, 4425 had died and 32,380 were wounded. Military personnel live and work in bases around the world, yet they make up less than 1% of the US population. A surprising number of US citizens know no one who has served in the US armed forces; news organizations face the issue of educating the public on the warriors and families in their midst. Media outlets need to report about the military and their families as part of their role in society—not just reflecting the views of those in the majority, but those without a voice. The task is anything but easy. Journalists new to the beat will find that cracking the code on the military is a challenge and may prove elusive until trust is earned. For example, many service members are required by their commands to contact their public affairs officers if they are approached by a member of the media. It is the job of the services' and Department of Defense's (DoD) public affairs professionals to interface with the media and provide the official response to media questions. Often, public affairs officers help reporters gain access to information and people, but often they pose an impediment to speaking with the troops, acting as the gateway for access and information. It is the job of public affairs officers to provide strategic communications, and this often means ensuring that the information disseminated supports whatever official message is decided on. Even if a journalist breaks through this barrier, the top-down military culture often means active duty troops are reluctant to speak with journalists. But some military personnel are comfortable talking to reporters, a characteristic that varies by rank, military position, branch of service, and individual. Reporters might find they will be chastised by public affairs officers for going directly to a source within the military, but this is a military policy, not a journalism policy, and journalists should provide these service members the opportunity to speak. It is the job of the media to get at the truth. Bringing issues to light from the military community, and going to military leadership for their response, could be an important step in addressing the issues. This is where having multiple sources inside and outside the military official channels is essential.

Journalists must remember that family members are not under the same obligation to public affairs officials. While they can request assistance from their sponsor's public affairs officer if they are uncomfortable with an interview, they are never required to do so. This is a key point in covering the military: the spouse and parent network can serve as an invaluable source for understanding what may be happening to a unit, on a military base or in the military community. During the Iraq and Afghanistan wars, the spouses were among the first to recognize the long-term impacts of traumatic brain injury, the failure of the Veterans Affairs Department to care for personnel with head injuries, or the lifelong struggles their service members have with post-traumatic stress or combat-related depression.

Early in the Iraq conflict, when the brunt of the fighting was being waged by US soldiers and Marines, many U.S. Army wives contacted Military Times seeking advice on how they could help their soldiers when they returned. Their service members were relaying stories from the desert of the carnage they witnessed and their combat experiences. The wives could sense the effect it was having but weren't sure where to turn. As with every war, an ongoing issue for spouses has been figuring out how to help their returning service members. Each generation has handled the aftermath of war differently. World War II members returned home to family and friends, and although they experienced a high rate of post-traumatic stress disorder—28 per 1000 to 100 per 1000, depending on assignment, according to the 2008 Rand Corp. report, "The Invisible Wounds of War," they recovered largely with the benefit of family, friends, and spiritual counselors (Tanielian, California Community Foundation, & Rand Corporation, 2008). Many Vietnam veterans were able to successfully transition to civilian life while others struggled with mental health issues and received no support for their combat-related mental health trauma (Tanielian et al., 2008). Some Persian Gulf War veterans came home with vague symptoms that have affected their long-term health. Iraq and Afghanistan veterans have come home with traumatic brain injuries that present challenges for families to address, since many have gone undetected. No one can predict what the next war's "signature wound" will be. But the early calls to news outlets from concerned family members often serve as the canary in the coal mine. Listening to these voices often can spur needed changes.

During the recent conflicts, military spouses whose soldiers came home with severe injuries and were not getting proper treatment at Department of Veterans Affairs (VA) were among the first to alert USA Today reporter Gregg Zoroya about the extensive problem of traumatic brain injury (Zoroya, 2005, 2007). Reports from families on problems with the casualty notification process led to improvements in the system. Reports on impediments to the public's ability to make donations to injured troops and their families helped change policies that restricted these offerings. Reports on service members and veterans dying after returning home from multidrug toxicity prompted DoD and VA to improve prescription monitoring and change guidelines regarding medications. These stories came to light through issues raised by military family members. A few years into the wars, families also raised concerns about the long-term effects on children of prolonged, continuing war-time deployments, and asked for help to mitigate these effects. Little information was available then, but researchers have since been looking at the issues. News outlets covering the next conflict would best serve their audience by cultivating these valuable sources, building relationships, and being a voice for them in the community.

20.2   Report, then Verify?

One of the continuing issues for the media is the warp-speed spread of information through social media and real-time posting of events to both reputable and unsavory websites. The competition to break news is as fierce as ever in the 24-h news cycle. Retired Marine Col. Dave Lapan, a public affairs officer whose last position in the military was director of the Pentagon press office, recalled an incident when a US news outlet picked up a report from Abu Dhabi TV about an incident involving an American service member. The report cited its source as Abu Dhabi TV, "drawing that little distance, saying this isn't theirs," Lapan said, but the original report was not true, and several additional news outlets had reported it after the first US report. "News organizations are saying we can't wait because our competitors are reporting it, and we can't not report it, so you have this echo chamber where everybody is saying this stuff," Lapan said. "It's that kind of discussion across the breadth of military operations, whether it's casualties, whether it's incidents, whatever it is. Because of the way information flows and the speed of information, do you have time to verify and validate things before you report them? Or do you pass along information based on what others are reporting, or that you see on Twitter?" (Lapan, 2015).

In some cases, major outlets have agreed to delay publication of a story if it puts a military operation or personnel at risk. The Washington Post, in 2009, agreed to hold a report on Afghanistan at the request of the DoD (The Washington Post, 2009). Any reports on military service members have a profound effect on family members concerned that their loved one was involved, hurt, or worse, especially since initial reports do not contain the names of service members. It is not unusual for news stories to appear in some outlets but not others, because many media outlets prefer to use their own sources rather than rewriting a story from another news outlet. Each media outlet should consider clarifying its own policies on using other news sources as the basis for stories, especially when it comes to reporting on casualties that affect the local community. "Our paper was not comfortable with reporting what other media said, or social media" said about casualties, Marohn said. "Maybe if AP reported it, yes. But if it was local TV, we wanted to do more reporting. What if the family didn't know, or the report was wrong? We didn't have a lot of casualties, but we would try to get confirmation from the family and from the funeral home. We would tell the funeral home to ask the family if they wanted to talk to us."

Casualties are the most sensitive reports to verify but any incident where service members may be hurt should be treated with the same respect. Journalists should be prepared when making a cold call to a family, because, despite the best intentions from the military commands that they notify the family first, a reporter may be the one informing the family, said Bonnie Carroll, president and founder of Tragedy Assistance Program for Survivors (TAPS). That organization has guidelines on its website for journalists. "Be sensitive, and be aware that's a possibility." The DoD issues releases identifying those killed in combat, but only after notifying next of kin, a process that can take hours, days, weeks, or longer.

Families may also find out about their loved one's death by watching the news. Carroll recalled the local crash of an Airborne Warning and Control plane that happened at 7:47 a.m., and it was the lead story on television media by 8:00 a.m. "That's how a lot of families found out. One wife was at her kitchen sink when her mother-in-law called and asked if her son was flying. The wife replied, 'Oh, yeah, he'll be back tonight.' Then she looked out [her] window and saw black smoke. There's really no good way to find out. Everybody in the military tries to do it the best way they can, but we're in a whole new information age," Carroll said. (Carroll, 2015)

Early identification of casualties in battle or accidents often is a relief for families whose loved ones were not killed. The DoD standard is to publish a release with the name and personal information no sooner than 24 h after the next of kin are notified. "But if the family talks to the press at the 10-h mark, we don't say we're going to go with it," Lapan said. "We kept it [the 24-h policy] the same, and said that's up to them. If the family wants to talk, they don't have the same constraints that we do."

The speed of information flow and the prevalence of social media platforms have made it much more difficult to keep casualty information "non-public" until the military service can make a personal notification—in person for deaths, and over the phone in many cases for wounds, Lapan said. Yet, "I think there is still an obligation to the families to inform them as soon as possible, in person, regardless of the changes in the media/information environment," he said (more about casualties and military families later.) Lapan said he has learned that families of those killed want to talk about their loved ones, often early, before DoD makes the official announcement through a press release.

In trying to tell the human story of the service member, journalists often contact and quote friends, neighbors, or others familiar with the person. This may provide some relief for grieving family members, who in some cases even assign their own spokesperson or point of contact. In some of those cases, though, families may feel that the stories are written "around" the family, providing an inaccurate picture. Carroll urged journalists to give family members the opportunity to talk about their service member, and said a call to the family, while tough, should be an imperative, because "families want to tell the story of their loved one and they want it written well."

The flag-draped coffin is an iconic image that stirs Americans' hearts. On Feb. 26, 2009, the Obama Administration repealed a policy dating to the 1991 Persian Gulf War that prohibited media coverage of US war casualties arriving home to Dover Air Force Base, in Delaware. The policy came under fire as the number of fallen troops returning to US soil rose, and the media fought to have the policy reversed. Some critics had accused the Bush administration of trying to obscure the true cost of war; but one reason given by the administration was to protect the privacy of families of the fallen. Families were mixed in their opinions about the policy. Some felt the nation should be allowed to grieve their fallen, too. Others felt families should be able to grieve privately in this moment when they saw their loved one's coffin for the first time. In the end, the administration struck a balance: The new policy left it to individual families to decide whether they will allow media coverage of the return of their loved ones' remains.

The issue was something many families weren't even aware of, said Carroll, president of TAPS, who was among those who worked with defense officials to come up with a solution. "In most cases, families wanted to have press there, we found. Families wanted their loved ones to be shared, wanted to tell the story. They were in favor of it being open to the press being there," she said. "Some wanted their hometown press there.... But families want to tell the story of their loved one and honor their life."

This particular episode is somewhat symbolic of the relationship between Americans and the military, Carroll said. She noted that even in cities where there isn't a large military presence, newspapers run pictures of the flag-draped casket in full color on the front page. "It shows how America grieves, even if it's momentarily, with the family. ... What is it about military sacrifice that so captures the national consciousness? That's why what (journalists) do telling that story, then telling the story beyond the flag-draped casket, of the family that's mourning a loss and will forever miss that person, is so important. Telling that story about who that person was in life, why they joined the military, what they were like growing up. That really speaks to so much of what we do at TAPS as an organization. ...It's amazing how that is such an iconic image in America" (Carroll, 2017).

20.3   Veterans, Spouses Can Be an Asset in the Newsroom

Not long after the invasion of Afghanistan, former Military Times editor Chuck Vinch, an Army veteran and also a former reporter for Stars and Stripes newspaper, spearheaded the launch of a casualty database, including information and photos of every fallen service member. He went to great lengths to track down a photo of each troop. When the casualty flow became heavier from 2005 to 2008, Vinch couldn't single-handedly keep up with the photos but he made every effort to track them down. "I am as proud of that database as I am of any other initiative I ever worked on during my 16 years at Military Times. As a veteran myself, I simply thought the Americans who volunteer to serve their country and end up making the ultimate sacrifice deserve to be honored by Military Times—and by every other American," he said. At St. Cloud Times, when the newspaper began covering the reintegration of service members into the community, they included an employee who was a National Guard spouse in their planning discussions. The spouse is a graphic artist who worked with them on their Scars of Service veterans' project. That military family member was "a really good sounding board," Marohn said. "We were much more comfortable going to press knowing she'd seen what we did. She read everything we wrote and said we captured the issues well. We're also worried about finding the right tone, not stereotyping. The best praise we got was from her husband in an email afterwards. That meant a lot to us."

20.4   The Fact Is, Many Military Families Are Strong and Resilient

The percentage of Americans who have served in the military or know someone who has served declines each year. Phillip Carter, an Iraq veteran who directs the Military, Veterans, and Society Program at the Center for a New American Security, a nonpartisan think tank in Washington, D.C., has called military bases the country's "most exclusive gated communities." With this divide, the potential for misunderstanding the military community is high. During times of war, especially, there may be a tendency in the civilian community to feel sorry for military personnel and family members and even see them as victims of a government that has sent them to war or helpless individuals who had no other choice but join the military. While some military families—especially those whose service member has been physically or mentally injured as a result of service—need extra support, many are resilient, balanced, patriotic citizens who embrace their military lifestyle. Media outlets must be conscientious to avoid portraying military families and veterans as victims, unless, of course, they are actually the victims of crime or malfeasance.

Journalists should educate themselves about the numerous programs available to support military families, not just in the government, but in the civilian community. (Some of those resources are discussed elsewhere in this book.) This will improve their reporting and increase their credibility in the military community; no journalist should be that reporter who fails to research available resources. During deployments and increased operations, the DoD and military services often bolster their family support programs, as they did during the Iraq and Afghanistan wars. Among the most helpful, according to military families, was the Military and Family Life Counseling Program, which provides free short-term, nonmedical counseling to service members and families. Other programs abound for military family members, from free mental health treatment provided through nonprofit organizations like Give an Hour, to those focused on child care, employment, and education. The Military Spouse Employment Partnership program links spouses to vetted employers who are seeking military spouses to fill vacancies. Military family support groups, military relief societies, Military OneSource, and nonprofits like Fisher House Foundation, Operation Homefront, Blue Star Families, National Military Family Association, Wounded Warrior Project—these are just a fraction of the resources and organizations set up to assist military families.

"Don't assume they're the victims and not getting the support," said Professor Ellen Shearer, co-director of the Medill National Security Journalism Initiative for Northwestern University's Medill School of Journalism. "Are they really as badly damaged as the anecdotes depict? Don't take it at face value. Maybe the real problem is the family hasn't checked it out. A lot of it comes back to reporters who are not full time on the military beat. They get thrown in, and it's hard to figure out."

Overall, military families don't want to be perceived as victims. If there's a bias in that regard, the stakes could be high. Families are concerned that if the media portrays them that way, this could persuade the public that these service members, spouses, and children are "damaged goods." Could that perception affect veterans' abilities to get a job after leaving the service? Could it affect spouses' abilities to find employment? What effect could that have on children? These are questions journalists should consider when considering how to portray a service member or family member.

20.5 Military Families May Be Skeptical of the Media

Another concern among some military families is that they are being exploited by the media, according to the study, "Greedy Media: Army Families, Embedded Reporting, and War in Iraq" (Ender et al., 2007). Researchers noted that local, national, and international media outlets posted reporters and cameras at a popular café just outside one Army post. "I feel like they exploit the wives that are left behind—'oh, well what does your husband do? What does your husband say?'" one Army wife told researchers. "I am like, 'Look, can I just do an interview and tell my husband that I love him? I don't really want to answer any questions or nothing, I just want to tell him that I love him.' I think that they exploit the situation to the point that it is almost sickening."

The researchers who conducted the "Greedy Media" study found an "overwhelming negative impact of mass media on military families" using their study design. They noted that they were careful about overstating their findings, and that the sample size was small, and wives of career soldiers were overrepresented in the sample, conducted early in the unit's deployment. The study authors also noted that they suspect there are more positive impacts worth exploring (Ender et al.). Nevertheless, journalists should be aware that troops and families are often very skeptical of the media and may believe the media is "anti-military" if they write something different from their point of view. When interviewing a family member, a journalist may seem sympathetic, but it doesn't mean the journalist is a friend or that the story will be written from the family member's viewpoint alone, Shearer said. This doesn't mean a story should have been handled differently, but the issue may come up after the story is published or aired. In some cases, military public affairs officers provide advice to educate military members and families about the process used to create an article, but family members may not know such information is available or seek it.

20.6 "Please Help Military Families"

After the post-9/11 wartime deployments began charitable organizations moved to assist the families left behind and provide goods and services for deploying troops. New charities seemingly popped up each week. Some of these groups have proven invaluable to military families and will be around to serve them for years to come. But not all these organizations are legitimate. And some that might have had laudable motives lack the infrastructure to carry through on promises. As a reporter, it's often difficult and time-consuming to vet these organizations but it is necessary. If the organizations are in the local area, a reporter can try to visit, interview executives and see their operations. Reporters can check with local authorities for complaints made against the organization. The charity will make financial information available if it is transparent. Also, with legitimate charities, organizations such as

Charity Navigator, Guidestar, and Charity Watch can be used to vet these groups, but it takes time for new ones to be reviewed by these bodies.

The questions become: How can a journalist vet a charity before writing about one to make sure that these groups are legitimate and aren't just playing to the public's sympathies to line their own pockets? Would a story about this charity direct a military family to an organization that does not have the ability to help them or may even cause harm? Is the charity in question touting a service that already is being provided by DoD? Companies often contact media outlets, Military Times included, expecting that stories be written about them because they plan to donate a portion of the proceeds from sales to a military charity. Should a reporter pursue a story on such a company, it is imperative that the charity named be contacted to verify their involvement, that the companies actually define what "a portion of the proceeds" means and whether it is a percentage of sale of an item, percentage of profit, of gross, etc. In one instance, for example, a company admitted that it was donating less than one cent for each of the compact discs sold. Reporters should do due diligence whenever they are writing on companies that have attached military families to their marketing materials.

20.7   Embed Program: Unexpected Benefits

From the beginning of the Iraq war, journalists were embedded with military units. More than 700 US and international journalists were placed with US military and coalition units during initial combat operations phase. Planning for this program began in late 2002, when defense officials started meeting with media bureau chiefs to get their input. In these meetings, officials made it clear that no decision had been made to go to war but the planning was prudent for any future decision. The process began partially because media organizations were unhappy with the access they had to troops in Afghanistan, according to Lapan, who was a key player in development and implementation of the media embed program.

As part of the discussions, the idea arose to develop "boot camps" for journalists, training sessions to prepare civilian reporters who did not have much experience reporting on military operations for combat situations. Media outlets were told up front that attendance at the boot camps weren't "access cards" that would be required for journalists to embed with the troops but neither did they guarantee access. According to Lapan, journalists' copy was not censored or read by military officials before publication. "But as part of the ground rules, we made clear there were things you can't report," Lapan said. "For example, there were times when journalists were brought into a tent for a briefing about an operation with the understanding they couldn't report this. You can't tell the enemy we're coming."

The embed program came under much fire, with some critics saying that placing journalists in close quarters with troops could erode objectivity in the media's coverage of the war and deflect attention from the larger question of whether the USA should be going into war in Iraq. Military Times' Alex Neill said to some extent this was how it played out as well before troops deployed, as much of the focus among media outlets was jockeying with the Pentagon over inclusion and positioning in the embed program. But Neill said concerns about objectivity were unfounded. "They reported and photographed everything they saw, good and bad, to the point that it sometimes created tensions with military leadership in the war zone and in the Pentagon, when media reported on stories they viewed as negative. That full scope of coverage in fact served to lend credibility to the war-zone reporting. Being in the action with the troops also deepened journalists' understanding of everything from combat operations to the culture and concerns of those wearing the uniform. It built two-way respect between the troops and the media." And war coverage isn't limited to coverage in theater—it also involves the President, Congress, the Pentagon, critics, military facilities such as installations and hospitals.

Pentagon officials and media outlets alike found that the program had a positive effect on the morale of the home front. Families were thirsty for any news from the war zone; often, journalists living alongside service members would sometimes write about them from the human interest perspective. "I think one of the unexpected benefits of the program was that reaction you got from families," Lapan said. "I don't think we really thought through that this is going to help our families understand what their sons and daughters, husbands and wives were doing. So that's sort of a byproduct, that access of the media will help on the home front by keeping families informed about what's going on."

Many troops also expressed appreciation to journalists who joined them in the war zone to tell their stories. Marohn, with the St. Cloud Times, said her newspaper got a lot of positive feedback from families when reporters were embedded with their local units and writing stories about them. "Going overseas, embedding even for a few weeks, helps build trust and credibility and a great list of sources," Marohn said. "People in our community still talk about that."

According to Lapan, the program also gave DoD firsthand accounts of what was going on across the country, because reporters were in places reporting on events they normally wouldn't have had access to. Since DoD knew Iraq ruler Saddam Hussein would rely on using propaganda to try to manipulate the news coming out of the country, the Pentagon felt the best way to counter this was having objective third parties in place to describe events. The plan proved successful when Iraqi Information Minister Mohammed Saeed al-Sahhaf proclaimed, on camera, that the US military was not in Iraq. One broadcast news organization aired a split screen with the declaration, alongside a journalist who had been embedded with an Army unit inside the Baghdad city limits, saying, "We're right here."

One of the toughest challenges facing embedded journalists and journalists covering war in general is reporting on casualties. The way the media reports deaths can have a profound effect on military families. The DoD set ground rules in the embedding program for a range of activities, including reporting on casualties. Lapan said internet cafes were shut down and there were communication blackouts so troops couldn't communicate back home that people had been killed. Likewise, embedded journalists had strict rules for reporting casualties, often facing blackouts as well until families had been notified. "We don't want families to find out through a news media report," Lapan said, adding that many military officials were upset when media coverage identified a unit too closely. "The philosophical wrestling we did was, is it better for everyone in the unit to think something's up, or to narrow it down so that only a few people are freaked out? Which is better?"

Social media created its own set of issues. Often, families posted information before a formal press release went out. Or immediately following a death, the media and others would access the person's various social media pages—Facebook, primarily, during the Iraq and Afghanistan wars—to get information, said Carroll, president of TAPS. People sometimes posted statements on the service members' pages before family members were notified. "Some families found out when reading, 'Rest in peace,'" Carroll said.

Embedded journalists were required to adhere to guidelines, with some questioning their stringency and others discovering some rules were inviolable. One national TV journalist was ejected from a unit and sent home after drawing a map in the sand while on air, showing troop locations and planned movements. Marohn's embedded reporters were more careful, Marohn said. "Our policy would have been not to do anything to put anyone in danger."

20.8 Other lasting effects of war adjustment

Casualties are not the only effect of war that has a profound, lasting impact on families. Wartime injuries may be devastating and reporting on them can present challenges for the media with their complexity and long-term effects. Depending on the length of the conflict and the impact on the community, media outlets should consider having their consumer health or health care reporter, if they have one, take on the task of at least following military and veterans' health care, since it may have a huge impact on their readership and community. Marohn learned the VA medical facility in their community was a draw for Minnesota veterans as well as those throughout the upper Midwest. It took the wars in Afghanistan and Iraq for her to understand the scope of veterans influence on the community. "There may be more veterans in your community than you think. They're coming back from Afghanistan and Iraq and not all are going back to where they started from," she said. According to Marohn, the St. Cloud Times invested resources to study the issues facing these veterans, and staff members spoke with numerous sources within the VA, student veteran organizations, veteran centers, law enforcement, as well as veterans, to understand veterans and their families.

20.9 Reporters also Spent a Lot of Time with the Veterans and Their Families

"You can't swoop in for a day or two and tell a story about how war changed lives. We were there multiple times in the home—how they interacted with families and kids, at appointments at the VA. Don't underestimate the importance of spouses. The spouse is the glue that held the family together. They helped convince the vet talk to us," Marohn said.

Family members not only may be able to provide access to a veteran, they also can offer perspective and insight into the pulse of the veterans' community. Largely through spouses, parents and family members seeking help for their veteran service member did media organizations find out about health concerns facing veterans, including traumatic brain injury and post-traumatic stress and cognitive disabilities.

Newsrooms should consider a broader range of stories that may be of interest to the military, veteran, and civilian communities regarding injuries. For example, news of medical advancements are of interest to veterans and family members and reporting on those can provide a valuable service to readers—including the local medical community.

20.10 Wartime Journalism Is Dangerous

It goes without saying that journalists who cover a conflict are at risk themselves, for both physical and mental wounds. Newsrooms must take tremendous care and precautions when considering sending one of their staff members to a combat zone, spending untold thousands on training and protective gear, as well as insurance policies. In "A Mighty Heart," Marianne Pearl wrote that her husband, Wall Street Journal reporter Daniel Pearl, was pressing senior editors at the publication to craft policies regarding dangerous assignments overseas. Pearl was killed by Al-Qaeda on Feb. 1, 2002, while investigating the link between the organization and Richard Reid, the "shoe bomber."

"You don't know who's on what side … journalists are more targeted," said Professor Ellen Shearer, co-director of the Medill National Security Journalism Initiative for Northwestern University's Medill School of Journalism, whose students included freelance reporter James Foley. Foley graduated from the master's program at Medill and embedded with the Indiana National Guard to go to Iraq. Later, while working in Libya as a freelancer, he was captured and held for 44 days. After a brief stay in the United States, he returned to Libya. He eventually made his way to northern Syria, where he was captured on Nov. 22, 2012 and held for 2 years before being executed in 2014 in a grisly beheading broadcast on the internet. "When he was taken, it was not clear how much journalists were targeted," Shearer said, adding that this lack of understanding may have led to his capture. "I think of Jim a lot in terms of what and how I teach students," Shearer said. "We have strengthened our national security reporting track and we have changed our hostile environment training to reflect the new realities and dangers of reporting in conflict areas. Reporters are now deliberately targeted as part of terrorists' or enemies' strategy. That requires different thinking about how to react if kidnapped."(Shearer, 2015).

In many ways, the stories of journalists and military families intersect with ABC journalist Bob Woodruff. He also was an embedded journalist in Iraq in January 2006, when he was severely injured by an improvised explosive device. He received medical care through the military for more than a month after the injury, from his evacuation to Landstuhl, Germany, back to Bethesda National Medical Center. Woodruff's is a unique perspective of a journalist in a situation similar to those of troops severely injured, and being covered by other journalists. Together, he and his wife Lee wrote "In an Instant," in which they described the events surrounding the attack and their subsequent recovery, individually and as a family. One section describes the decision of two Boston Globe reporters, Kevin Cullen and Michele McDonald, not to take pictures of him when he was being transported to Bethesda. "Michele told Kevin that she had ethical concerns about taking photos of us. She worried that my family might see a photo of me before they could see me in person," Bob Woodruff wrote. "I will always be grateful that she and Kevin put Lee and the children above getting a picture of me for her story. That's a tough balance to achieve, especially with bosses back at headquarters demanding the story. She put herself in my shoes that night as a parent." (Woodruff, Lee and Bob, 2008)

But other media outlets did carry pictures, including wire photos when he arrived in Germany, with a "NO BONE FLAP" sign posted above his head to alert his trans-porters of precautions they needed to take because part of his skull was missing. "My twelve-year-old daughter Cathryn, would see this in People magazine that week and burst into tears when she learned the specifics of my head injury," Woodruff wrote. "As one accustomed to covering an unfolding story, I had suddenly become the subject of one."

Lee Woodruff wrote that she and Bob "became the temporary faces for what so many others had been through before us. The support and backing we had from ABC and from friends and family made us luckier than most. Yet we would also be uncomfortable with the attention Bob's injuries received."

"To us, what we were going through was no different from all the military fami-lies who had walked in our shoes. I thought of those families every single day, and I still do."

Their experience led the Woodruffs to establish the Bob Woodruff Foundation, dedicated to helping members of the military who have sustained injuries during service to their country, and their families.

Journalists', unseen wounds

When journalists return safely from conflicts, like service members, they may have lingering effects from war. The impact may not initially be evident and will differ between people. Military Times' Neill said in some cases, staff members need time off to adjust and in other cases, the effects last longer, with some journalists not being as focused as they were before they went on assignment. "It was a learning process for everyone," said Neill, who spent 6 weeks in Iraq in 2005. Some report having a surreal experience returning to a newsroom cubicle after serving alongside troops in combat. It's important to understand that an adjustment period is war-ranted for staff members who go to the war zone and they should be encouraged to seek counseling if behavioral or emotional problems persist. It is the responsibility of editors to ensure that their journalists are aware of the potential effects of war on mental health and encourage them to seek help if needed.

20.11 Recommendations of Questions for Newsrooms to Consider

The following is a list of recommended questions to consider for newsrooms in communities affected by combat deployments:

- Discuss the newsroom's policy for reporting on events that could be painful to families, including deaths and injuries. What verification will the publication require if the Defense Department hasn't made an official announcement? Will these events be reported based on other media outlets? On social media? As rapidly as technology advanced in past 15 years, it is guaranteed to be even faster and more pervasive in the future. Newsrooms must anticipate this.
- What is the newsroom's policy for identifying family members? Is a name necessary? With increasing concerns about the security of military families, and a growing feeling within the Defense Department to protect the names of military service members, newsrooms must set their own ground rules for identifying sources in stories on active duty military personnel and their families. If a family member asks that his or her name be withheld because they are concerned about reprisals that could hurt that service member's career, what will be your response?
- What policies and processes does the newsroom have for dealing with questions of whether a story should be withheld, or details of a story, because of operational security or sensitivity to families? Having an established relationship with military public affairs officials and an open dialogue with military commanders before these issues crop up is essential.
- What is the newsroom's policies for reporting on local deaths, including murders or accidents? Will the policies for military operations be different? How and why?
- What questions will editors ask in determining whether to publish explicit photos or pictures of wounded troops? Are the subjects easily identifiable? Does the photo tell a story and what purpose does it serve? What are the ethics of deciding to use a photo to draw in readers?
- If the media outlet decides to send journalists into a war zone, has the organization considered adopting the international protection standards for journalists published by A Culture for Safety Alliance? These standards are aimed at ensuring that journalists, especially freelancers, do not go into dangerous reporting situations and take unnecessary risks because they believe editors and news directors expect exclusive stories, according to Professor Ellen Shearer, a member of the ACOS committee and co-director of the Medill National Security Journalism Initiative.
- Will the outlet send journalists to training to prepare them for hostile environments? Although the Defense Department held media "boot camps" for journalists, and had a structured embed program in these wars, there's no guarantee DoD will have a similar program in the next conflict. Private companies often fill in the gap, however, offering paid courses.

- Does the newsroom have the resources to support journalists while they are over-seas and after they return home, possibly with physical or mental injuries?
- Does someone in your newsroom have a working knowledge of the resources and benefits that troops and families have? Beyond their basic pay, troops get a host of other pays, such as housing allowances. Some extra pays and benefits are offered to deployed troops as well. There are countless other benefits afforded to troops and families, yet they often don't know what is available to them, espe-cially young families. And the military is constantly changing, with a constant influx of new members.
- If you report on charitable efforts to help troops and families, will you vet these organizations before writing about them? How?
- Have you checked within your organization to see if there are veterans and/or military spouses who could provide input on issues?
- Do you have mechanisms in place for hearing the voices of the military com-munity—including active duty, Guard, Reserve, veterans, and spouses?

A journalist's experience in covering the military and military families will vary from base to base and from branch to branch. Access and openness often depends on the individual, the unit, or the command. Covering the community takes tenacity, skepticism, and a willingness to learn. For more on the subject, Navy veteran Ed Offley, who covered the military for the Seattle Post-Intelligencer and served as edi-tor of Stars and Stripes, published an invaluable primer for those hoping to land the beat, *Pen & Sword: A Journalist's Guide to Covering the Military,* in 2002.

References

Carroll, B. (2015, November). Interview with founder and president, Tragedy Assistance Program for Survivors regarding media coverage of military families during wartime. (K. Jowers, Interviewer).

Carroll, B. (2017, June). Interview with founder and president, Tragedy Assistance Program for Survivors regarding media coverage of military families during wartime. (K. Jowers, Interviewer).

Lapan, D. (2015, October). Interview with retired Marine Corps colonel who formerly served as director of the Pentagon press office regarding media coverage of military families during wartime. (K. Jowers, P. Kime, Interviewers).

Marohn, K. (2015, November). Interview regarding St. Cloud Times coverage of military and veteran families during wartime. (K. Jowers, Interviewer).

Ender, M.G., Campbell, K. M., Davis, T. J., & Michaelis, P. R. (2007). Greedy media: Army fami-lies, embedded reporting, and war in Iraq. *Sociological Focus, 40*(1), 48–71. https://doi.org/10.1080/00380237.2007.10571298.

Neill, A. (2015, October). Interview regarding Military Times coverage of military and veteran families during wartime. (K. Jowers, Interviewer).

Shearer, E. (2015, November). Interview with co-director of Northwestern University's Medill School of Journalism's Medill National Security Journalism Initiative regarding journalists' coverage of military and veteran families during wartime. (K. Jowers, Interviewer).

Tanielian, T., California Community Foundation, & Rand Corporation. (2008). *Invisible wounds of war: Summary and recommendations for addressing psychological and cognitive injuries.* Santa Monica, CA: RAND, Center for Military Health Policy Research.

The Washington Post. (2009, September 23). *At Pentagon's request, Washington Post delayed story on.* The Washington Post: Afghanistan.

Woodruff, Lee and Bob. (2008). *In an Instant.* New York: Random House.

Zoroya, G. (2005, March 6). Brain injuries range from loss of coordination to loss of self. *USA Today.*

Zoroya, G. (2007, September 25). Brain injuries from war worse than thought. *USA Today.*

Index

© Springer International Publishing AG 2018
L. Hughes-Kirchubel et al. (eds.), *A Battle Plan for Supporting Military
Families*, Risk and Resilience in Military and Veteran Families,
https://doi.org/10.1007/978-3-319-68984-5

PGMO 09/26/2018